*The
Arts
of
Costume
and
Personal
Appearance*

Grace Margaret Morton

The Arts of Costume
and Personal Appearance

by Grace Margaret Morton

Third Edition, revised by

Mary E. Guthrie / Viletta Leite / June Ericson

Department of Textiles, Clothing and Design
School of Home Economics
University of Nebraska

New York · London · Sydney   John Wiley & Sons, Inc.

COPYRIGHT, 1943 BY GRACE MARGARET MORTON

COPYRIGHT, 1955 © 1964 BY UNIVERSITY OF NEBRASKA FOUNDATION

All Rights Reserved
This book or any part thereof
must not be reproduced in any form
without the written permission of the publisher.

6 7 8 9 10

All of the author's rights of Grace Margaret Morton (deceased) in the book *The Arts of Costume and Personal Appearance* have been granted by her heirs to the University of Nebraska Foundation, to be owned and used by it for the benefit of the "Grace Margaret Morton Scholarship Fund" of the University of Nebraska.

Library of Congress Catalog Card Number: 64-20077
Printed in The United States of America
ISBN 0 471 61845 4

"There is no intellect that does not desire to create continually, and the pleasure in the perception of a new or unaccustomed form of unity is comparable to that of original achievement."

HERBERT LANGFELD, THE AESTHETIC ATTITUDE

GRACE MARGARET MORTON was head of the textiles and clothing division at the University of Nebraska for over twenty years. During that time, she was appreciated by her students and fellow faculty members as a person of unusual talents. A scholar of wide interests, she had a vision that placed her ahead of her time in sensing the psychological and economic implications possible in a study of clothing.

Her expressed goal in her teaching of both undergraduates and graduates was to help students to recognize and value beauty, to strive to bring it into their surroundings, and to achieve real creative satisfaction in their use of color, line, and texture in their study of clothing.

Grace Morton was born in Washington, Pennsylvania, and received her bachelor's and master's degrees from Columbia University. In addition she did further graduate study in many places, such as Pratt Institute in Brooklyn and the International School of Art in Vienna.

A tall and striking figure, Grace Morton evidenced her creative abilities in her own manner of dress and in her beautiful home. Both showed the distinction and elegance which were a part of her unique personality. Her untimely death came a few months after the publication of *The Arts of Costume and Personal Appearance* in 1943. Through the generosity of her family, the rights to the book were given, ten years later, to the University of Nebraska as a memorial to her. The accumulated royalties have provided a substantial addition to the Grace Margaret Morton Scholarship Fund.

The University Foundation is indebted to three of Miss Morton's friends and colleagues for their gratuitous "labor of love" in the revision of the book for the Second Edition. These were Bess Steele (now deceased), head of the Design Division, Carolyn Ruby, head of the Textiles and Clothing Division, and Mary Guthrie, all of the Home Economics Department at the University of Nebraska.

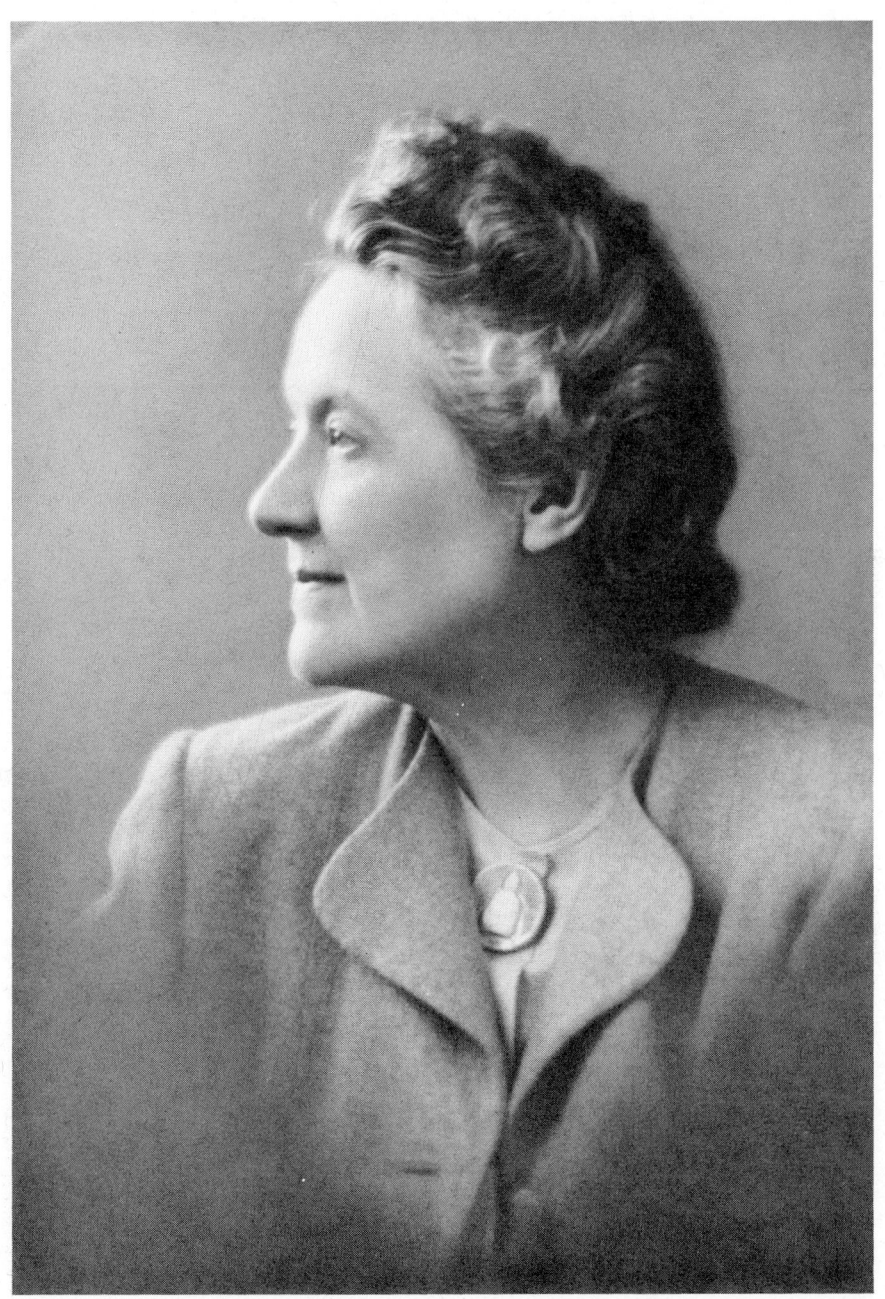

Grace Margaret Morton

Preface

TEXTBOOKS, and especially textbooks devoted to costume and fashion, need revision from time to time. The farsighted vision of the author, Grace Margaret Morton, has made it possible to incorporate an appreciable amount of the original material. Especially notable was her application of basic principles and discriminating aesthetic sensitivity in selecting timeless illustrations. An attempt has been made to retain Grace Morton's philosophy as well as the scholarly way in which the first edition was written.

We again wish to mention the kindness of the Morton family in their gift of the rights to the manuscript to the University of Nebraska Foundation. Royalties from the book have made possible the establishment of a substantial scholarship fund in the name of Grace Margaret Morton. The fund is available for both undergraduate and graduate students in Textiles, Clothing and Design, School of Home Economics.

Many people have given of their time and assistance in the preparation of this revision, and we wish to acknowledge our indebtedness to them. The present book is submitted in the hope that it will fill a need in the same way as have the two previous editions.

MARY E. GUTHRIE
VILETTA B. LEITE
R. JUNE ERICSON

Lincoln, Nebraska
May, 1964

Contents

One	Personal Appearance Values	1
Two	The Meaning of Style	10
Three	Self-Made Beauty	19
Four	Expressing Personality Through Costume	46
Five	Design Essentials for Good Costume	67
Six	Principles of Composition	94
Seven	Texture and Texture Combination	117
Eight	Dark and Light	145
Nine	Fundamentals of Color	174
Ten	The Art of Combining Colors	194
Eleven	Enhancing Personal Coloring	205
Twelve	Creating Illusions	221
Thirteen	Hats and Hairdressing	247
Fourteen	The Wardrobe	277
	Appendix A	293
	Appendix B	295
	Appendix C	298
	Index	315

One

Personal Appearance Values

THE *Arts of Costume and Personal Appearance* is devoted to one of the important and absorbing pursuits of modern society. This book deals with the techniques of improving natural beauty or of achieving its illusion; it is written for those whose interest is personal and for those who look forward to careers of helping others make the most of their personal appearance. When women have cultivated the inner graces and have made themselves outwardly as pleasing as possible, their minds are freed for more productive pursuits.

Ever since primitive people began to adorn their naked bodies with colored clays, men and women have been occupying themselves more or less with the attaining, enhancing, and preserving of external beauty in themselves. In the tombs of ancient Egyptians are found toilet sets which are marvels of workmanship: rouge pots and perfume bottles, countless ointment jars of alabaster and gold, and mirrors of burnished metal with richly carved handles. We are informed that the ladies of Egypt rouged their cheeks and lips, penciled their eyebrows, shaded their eyelids, and applied to their bodies creams and oils to prevent perspiration.

This tendency of men and women to try to make themselves beautiful in each other's eyes is seen also in ancient Crete. Here three to four thousand years ago a rich and luxurious civilization was already old in arts and wiles. In those days men were distinguished by wasp waists and handsome headdresses, turbanlike, with one tall waving plume. As though to rival the men, women resorted to "stiff corsets which gathered their skirts snugly around their hips, and lifted their bare breasts to the sun. It is a pretty custom among the Cretans," writes Will Durant, "that the female bosom should be uncovered, or revealed by a diaphanous chemise; no one seems to take offense. The bodice is laced below the bust, opens in a careless circle, and then, in a gesture of charming reserve, may close in a Medici collar at the neck. . . . The skirt, adorned with flounces and gay tints, widens out spaciously from the hips, stiffened presumably with metal ribs or horizontal hoops." [1]

A marvel to modern eyes is the delicacy of taste and mastery of the needle arts revealed in Cretan murals and figurines. The jewelry, too, of these prehistoric Cretan men and women is very elegant. From figurines and portraits of the time we find that Cretan women used hairpins of copper and gold and stickpins decorated with gold flowers and crystal beads. Fillets of precious metals bound their hair; pendants fell from their ears and chains from their breasts. The men flaunted "great rings with scenes of battle or the chase. . . . Everywhere in Cretan life man expresses his vainest and noblest passion—the zeal for beauty." [2]

Quite as interested in making themselves beautiful were Greek women of the early days. We are informed they wore soles of cork, padded out their deficiencies, compressed themselves by lacing, and supported the breasts with cloth brassières to create the illusion of more perfect proportions, which they so greatly admired.

Coming down to later times, there is further evidence of preoccupation with adornment. The desire for the beautiful silks and jewels and other rich things brought by European traders from the East played a large part through the centuries in making western Europe the seat of progress and culture in modern times. And it is generally conceded that a very potent factor in the exploration and final settlement of our North American continent was the demand of the European bourgeoisie for the beaver and sables of the New World.

These instances are cited to show how great was the interest in adornment before our time, and how intimately dress and the arts of personal appearance have been associated with social and economic life. The persistence of this interest in adornment at different stages of culture has brought anthropologists and sociologists to recognize it as an impulse common to us all.

---

[1] Will Durant, *Life of Greece,* Simon and Schuster, New York, 1939, p. 9.
[2] *Ibid.,* p. 10.

In our time the possibilities of self-improvement through the arts of personal appearance are within the reach of almost every level of society. In the United States modern scientific invention and business enterprise have put fashion and cosmetics among our foremost industries. If there seems to be a certain madness in modern women's pursuit of beauty, it is because of greater leisure and the means to indulge the natural urge to fulfill their role in the evolution of the race and to make the most of their lives and attributes. Changes in our society have come rapidly in the twentieth century; since the Second World War, the pace of those changes has been enormously stepped up. The increased mobility of population, the increased leisure, the increased numbers of women working, and the spectacularly increased individual buying power, all contribute to the rapidity of change in opinions and outlooks. It becomes more imperative that people find the values that are important to them in assuming their place in society.

When life moves at double-quick speed, we have little time to form opinions of people leisurely. We must evaluate others with nothing to influence us but how they look and speak, so that first impressions make a tremendous difference. A woman's appearance is very revealing of her skill, taste, and imagination. If she fails to comprehend the importance of personal appearance, she is missing a great opportunity to create the kind of impression she wants to make.

CLOTHING AND SOCIAL VALUES

The study of clothing as an important part of man's environment has claimed the attention of many sociologists, psychologists, and economists, especially in recent times. Many casual writers on the subject give the following reasons for wearing clothes: first, for protection; second, for modesty; and third, for decoration. Lawrence Langner, in his entertaining book *The Importance of Wearing Clothes,* calls attention to many primitive societies where the decorative feature has long preceded the need for protection. He dismisses modesty by quoting an anonymous writer who said, "modesty is a feeling merely of acute self-consciousness due to appearing unusual, and is the result of wearing clothing rather than the cause."[3] Langner ascribes to clothing an exceedingly important place in the development of civilized so-

---

[3] Lawrence Langner, *The Importance of Wearing Clothes,* Hastings House, New York, 1959, p. 72.

cieties. "Man from the earliest times has worn clothes to overcome his feeling of inferiority and to achieve a conviction of his superiority to the rest of creation . . . and to win admiration and assure himself that he 'belongs'." [4]

A well-known psychologist with the Menninger Clinic calls clothing "a means of making real the role that is to be played in life. . . . This utilization of clothing in the enactment of roles that begin in later infancy remains a life-long preoccupation. . . . Primarily, people are still classified largely by their occupational status; one must dress up to his status role." [5]

Russell Lynes asserts that the "mood and morals and mores of a people are portrayed by their clothes even more readily than by their arts, because clothes are essentially ephemeral and respond easily and quickly to changes in the public temper." [6] "A man's problems of dressing, now that the standard uniform of earlier days has been discarded, are not unlike a woman's problems when decorating her house. Both have to decide who they are, what public effect they want to create, what kind of society they live in, and with whom they are going to compete." [7]

George Dearborn, one of the early theorists on the psychology of clothes, writes, "One's habits in life as far as social communications are concerned are more determined by clothing than many have ever stopped to think or to realize. Clothes determine how much one 'goes out' both into the street and into society . . . the company one invites to his home. . . . Clothes help people to get jobs and to hold them; but they help others to miss positions and to lose them. . . . The way we clothe ourselves is one of the surest indices of substantial intelligence.[8]

DEVELOPMENT OF ONE'S CLOTHING BEHAVIOR

The urge in young people to conform to their group in clothes and manners is observed as one of the strongest forces in the development of one's pattern of choices in clothing. In a study of adolescent boys and girls, Vener and Hoffer concluded that clothing is of crucial importance as one of the "signs" which serve to distinguish the social positions of individuals in a

---

[4] *Ibid.*, p. 12.
[5] Gardner Murphy, *Personality*, Harper & Brothers, New York, 1947, pp. 495, 518.
[6] Russell Lynes, *The Tastemakers*, Harper & Brothers, New York, 1949, p. 305.
[7] Russell Lynes, *A Surfeit of Honey*, Harper & Brothers, New York, 1953, p. 77.
[8] George Dearborn, "Psychology of Clothes," *Psychological Monographs*, Vol. 26, No. 1, Whole No. 112 (1918), pp. 29, 70.

community. They found that movies, television, and sports celebrities have some impact on young peoples' dress behavior; but the people whom they know personally and intimately influence them far more directly. It was observed that twelfth graders as a group tended to refer less frequently to specific other persons in their responses to the clothing referral items than did the individuals in the lower grades. It was therefore suggested that by the time the youth reaches the twelfth grade, approved rules related to dress behavior have become habitual.[9]

Some young women of real ability fail to realize the value of a good appearance. Sometimes they are absorbed in intellectual pursuits and regard themselves as superior to so-called feminine frivolities. But frequently this kind of young woman misses a great opportunity to make herself socially effective. Think what added attractiveness she could have if she were to provide her fine mind with a beautiful setting! Many women in society and the arts are noted for their feminine charm and beautiful appearance quite as much as for their intellectual attainments. Chapter Four will give you several examples of women in public life who have learned this secret of charm.

It might be a stimulating experience for a strong-minded, intellectually self-contained person who feigns indifference to clothes to learn how average people are affected by clothes and personal appearance. It will be well for her to realize that impulses older than civilization impel people to varying degrees of preoccupation with adornment, and that the insights she can gain through an understanding of human nature are the very basis of any real service to family or society. Many writers on anthropology and sociology see fundamental reasons why the beautifying of the person is important to society. They have observed that competition among women for status and for men has existed through the ages. It was not only recognized but sanctioned in medieval Europe. A certain German bishop who was also a duke once stated in a sumptuary edict regarding the luxurious dress of certain notorious women of Wurzburg that "Respectable women have a right to dress luxuriously, not only that girls may find husbands, but that married women may become more pleasing to their husbands' eyes and may make sure that their husbands do not roam and find other lovers."[10]

---

[9] Arthur M. Vener and Charles R. Hoffer, *Adolescent Orientations to Clothing,* Technical Bulletin 270, March 1959, Michigan State University Agricultural Experiment Station.

[10] German Document, "Prohibition of Bishop Rudolph Von Scherenberg," Wurzburg, 1449.

APPEARANCE AFFECTS ONE'S STATE OF MIND

Besides the influence of our personal appearance upon others there is also its subjective aspect, or what it does to the inner person—at least to those who are sensitive. Dearborn found that clothes help to protect us from fears; fear of ridicule, of the estimation of inefficiency, of lack of taste, or lack of charm. He believes "fear is one of the very worst enemies of our race's civilization, as well as of our personal comfort, and moreover of our efficiency. . . . Protection and relief from such fears . . . I take to be *la raison d'être,* the real reason and purpose of the wearing of clothes. And that is of importance." [11]

Pertaining to this same thought, Dearborn adds in another connection that self-respect and self-confidence "are intimately part and parcel of the essential initiative of every individual. . . . If a man has not self-confidence he will not have initiative. He will not 'start' things, or keep them going. . . . In my deliberate opinion, self-confidence for the great masses of men and women is to some extent obviously dependent on being well dressed." [12]

Another keen observer of human nature writes in her book on personality, "There is undoubtedly a confused, half-apologetic state of mind, an uncertainty of bearing, a preoccupation of manner—a general reduction of the personality to something negative and vague which comes from not realizing completely and to one's own satisfaction one's picture of one's outward self." [13]

Social workers and physicians often see a therapeutic value in an improvement of personal appearance in their patients or clients. No one can claim that new clothes can effect a "cure" of a mentally or emotionally disturbed person; but the improvement may be a contributing factor along with other more fundamental treatment. John Robert Powers described an early experiment of his organization in relating beauty to mental health. Members of the staff worked with semidisturbed female patients in a large New York mental hospital. "The slovenly, suspicious and disinterested women who filed into the hospital's gymnasium for the beauty clinic left that room with their heads held higher, some smiling for the first time in months. Since

---

[11] Dearborn, *op. cit.,* pp. 51–52.
[12] *Ibid.,* p. 66.
[13] Marjorie Barstow Greenbie, *Personality,* The Macmillan Company, New York, 1932, p. 88.

then, beauty routines have become an accepted form of therapy in progressive mental institutions. Doctors agree that when a woman will take an interest in her appearance, it is proof that she has not completely forsaken interest in herself." [14]

An experiment in a "Glamour Treatment for the Mentally Ill" was carried out by the Fashion Group at a state hospital near San Francisco. Patients were treated by professional stylists, were given beauty treatments, and were encouraged to attend style shows of the latest creations by professional designers. Dr. Miller, Director of the hospital, found that many of the patients started to improve. "Some way or other," he admitted, "the fashion thing works. . . . There is no evidence," he continued, "that this fashion therapy by itself will cure any of our patients. But combined with all our other treatments . . . it can contribute tremendously." An unexpected side effect was noted also: "When these patients start looking better, their sons and daughters and relatives start visiting them more often and we see the re-establishment of old family ties." [15]

Social workers also note a connection between personal appearance and social behavior. Teachers from the Powers School have donated their time to the teaching of the principles of good grooming, hair styling, and the use of make-up to teen-agers in the settlement houses and youth centers. "These girls, often the product of broken homes and poor environment, are without a home source of guidance on good taste, manners, and comportment. This kind of inspiration often gives a girl the chance to rise above her background, prepare for a decent job, and plan a better life for herself." [16]

Dr. Richard C. Guilford says, "People who are brought to the attention of the social worker often come with very little idea of their own worth. . . . People with no hope, no self-respect, almost seem to court censure. An improvement which the social worker may help to bring about in financial outlook and future life plans is nearly always reflected in an improvement in personal care and personal appearance, greater pride in home surroundings, and increased interest in other people. All these serve as signposts to the social worker of the beginning of a general 'cure'." [17] On the other hand,

---

[14] John Robert Powers, *How to Have Model Beauty, Poise and Personality,* Prentice-Hall, New York, 1960, p. 20 ff.
[15] Milton and Margaret Silverman, "Glamour Treatment for the Mentally Ill," *Saturday Evening Post,* August 26, 1961, p. 80. © 1961, The Curtis Publishing Co.
[16] Powers, *op. cit.,* p. 23.
[17] Dr. Richard G. Guilford, Director, University of Nebraska Graduate School of Social Work. Personal interview.

he suspects that efforts to rehabilitate a person by cleansing him and "dressing him up" will not have a lasting effect unless the person has begun to change inwardly, because of his own change of heart and outlook on the world.

Helen Meiklejohn states most aptly the part she thinks the right clothes can play in allaying intangible fears and establishing a feeling of confidence: "Clothes are so intimate, obvious, and omnipresent a part of our personality that no other expenditure of equal amount can contribute so much to the satisfaction of our deep desire for personal recognition and to the sense of personal security always under threat in this uncertain world. Like players on a stage who know their parts badly, we feel that we might improvise a little if only we knew that we looked all right." [18]

A good personal appearance, then, achieved by taking advantage of the abundant means our civilization offers for the improvement of grooming, posture, and quality of voice, and for learning the secrets of becoming dress, is within the reach of all. Discovery of the techniques for making herself a more interesting-looking individual has started many a girl on the road to broader and richer experiences. The woman who is intelligent, clever, and aware of the times in which she lives will see the values which come from a continuing interest in her appearance—from youth to age—and will apply her imagination to presenting an appearance as smart and attractive as her ability and finances will permit.

One who plans a profession in the field of clothing or textiles will realize the values of a good personal appearance in the lives of average people, will understand the impulses which impel many people to search for satisfactions through appearance, and will use her influence to guide others into sane and desirable attitudes.

Below are some interesting references you will enjoy because of their bearing on this subject.

Quentin Bell, *On Human Finery,* Hogarth Press, London, 1947.
John Carl Flügel, *Psychology of Clothes,* Third Impression, Hogarth Press, London, 1950.
Elizabeth B. Hurlock, *The Psychology of Dress,* Ronald Press, New York, 1929.

[18] Helen Meiklejohn, "Dresses," in Walton Hamilton et al., *Price and Price Policies,* McGraw-Hill Book Co., New York, 1938, p. 304.

Lawrence Langner, *The Importance of Wearing Clothes,* Hastings House, New York, 1959.
Russell Lynes, *A Surfeit of Honey,* Harper & Brothers, New York, 1953.
Russell Lynes, *The Tastemakers,* Harper & Brothers, New York, 1949.
Vance Packard, *The Status Seekers,* David McKay Co., New York, 1959.
Kimball Young, *Social Psychology,* Third Edition, Appleton-Century-Croft, New York, 1956.

Two

The Meaning of Style

Today concern with style or fashion has expanded beyond the limits of wearing apparel until it has become an integral part of every product and service marketed. The interest in personal appearance alone is substantiated by a fashion industry in the United States which ranks third in dollar value of product. Fashion often goes unrecognized as a major industrial force, as the individual firms contributing to the enormous total output are relatively small. The textile and ready-to-wear industries developed out of craft traditions long before other enterprises emerged in the gigantic patterns we associate with modern business. Historic structure consequently has influenced the size of fashion firms. The fashion industries have of necessity remained relatively small to permit the flexibility necessary to cope with constantly changing fashions and to supply the diversity of products found in the fashion market. Currently there is a trend in the fashion industries, made imperative by economic considerations and changes in styling, to integrate; thereby the number of smaller units has been decreased. The magnitude of the fashion industry becomes apparent, however, only when we realize the quantity of products manufactured, the vast number of persons employed in the industry, and the sums of money spent by consumers on products. Fashion is in reality a "big business."

Rare is the instance in our contemporary society when a woman disdains interest in her personal appearance; but ask women to express frankly what they most desire in personal appearance, and the vague answers received might be typical responses such as, "I should like to have style," "to have individuality," or "to be considered smart." What is this mysterious, elusive quality which is such a desirable ingredient in today's conception of good appearance? Perhaps the discovery of some of its secrets may enable us to achieve it for ourselves.

Try to find out what style is by considering what it is not. Style is not applying make-up in public, indulging in a passion for ornament, or rushing out to purchase the latest design in a fashion product. Nor is style the ignoring of social conventions, such as going without a hat or gloves on city streets or other places good taste indicates they should be worn. Style is not wearing slacks or shorts, or head scarves, or going without hose on these same city streets. Style is not wearing our evening finery during working hours. Style is not wearing hair curlers and unattractive garments among family members so that one can be a ravishing beauty for strangers.

Nor is style attained by lavishing a great deal of money on clothes, hair dressing, and beauty products. One cannot deny that money is important when it is spent with discretion. With it one more easily purchases quality fabric, excellent construction, and creative design, all of which contribute to style. Lack of money does not exclude personal style, but it means that on a budget it takes more thoughtful planning and purchasing to avoid costly mistakes. Anne Fogarty states that, "Good taste and the amount of money spent are interrelated but not necessarily dependent on each other. Expense does not assure good taste, nor is 'good' taste necessarily expensive to acquire."[1]

After examining some of the practices of dress which do not constitute style, consider some of the accepted definitions of fashion terminology as a beginning for the study of making the most of personal appearance. Currently there is a tendency to use terms loosely and interchangeably, but there has evolved among professional people working in the fashion industry a precise vocabulary.

> *Style* is generally understood to be a particular form of art expression recognizable by distinguishing traits or characteristics.
> *Fashion* is the current style or accepted mode in favor at the moment. The word "accepted" carries the connotation that the style is used or worn by an appreciable segment of the population.

[1] Anne Fogarty, *Wife Dressing*, Julian Messener, Inc., New York, 1959, p. 81.

Mode is a synonym for fashion.

Fads are short-lived fashions in unimportant elements of dress such as accessories or minor details.

Taste is the ability to discern and appreciate what is beautiful and appropriate.

Good taste in dress indicates the ability to adapt the elements of fashion most becoming and suitable to an individual's personal characteristics, way of living, and circumstances.

STYLE VERSUS FASHION

Every art period has a characteristic style by which it is recognized. Greek sculpture, fifteenth century Italian brocades, eighteenth century musical forms are all known by distinguishing characteristics. Directoire ornament, late Victorian furniture, and the 1920 feminine figure are so distinct and characteristic in their modes of expression as to be known as styles. Sometimes past styles reappear in the fashion picture. The easy, flowing movement of the princess lines of the Directoire period and the sumptuous elegance and rich ornamentation of the Elizabethan era recur from time to time. By this we do not mean that the style is revived in toto, as any art form is an expression of the philosophy of the period in which it prevails. The distinguishing and recognizable traits are maintained in the revival, but the style is modified in conformity with the cultural ideals of the time at which it returns to fashion.

Fashion is the living version or current chapter of a style. As any past style is the reflection of the ways people thought and lived, so fashions of today are molded by the social forces of our time. They are the reflection of our mode of living and thinking, of our manners and morals, of the changing kaleidoscope of events in our time. And as life today moves with increasing rapidity, so do our fashions evolve and bring changes in taste more frequently than ever before in history. Fashion change is directly related to industrial development; therefore, it is not surprising to find that America produces the greatest quantity of fashion goods and that our fashions change more rapidly than those in any other country.

Much has been written and said about changing fashion during the centuries society has recognized the existence of this element. Change has been condemned as being immoral and wasteful of time and money, but words have never stayed the force of innovation. Lawrence Langner comes to the defense of fashion; he feels that in countries where fashion plays a part, women have become more accomplished, more useful, and more capable. By contrast, in the less developed areas where fashion remained static, the women have not taken their places in the professions and in politics; nor have they learned about sanitation or the education of children. He credits fashion with enabling men and women to achieve and maintain the goal of superiority which is one of the chief reasons we wear clothes.[2]

Fashion can be followed by nearly everyone in our affluent economy, but it is not a blind devotion to fashion that develops the qualities of "style," "individuality," or "smartness" indicated as desirable characteristics of dress. Recently there has been a spate of writing concerning the force of mass advertising directed toward selling mass-produced fashions to a mass-behavioral public who little need the products they are encouraged to purchase. Who is to deny the excitement of a new fashion purchase or the boredom of the old? This is a normal human reaction. Fashion is fun, but use it intelligently. Don't be swayed by fashion advertising.

Individuality of style requires the expression of personality. Stanley Marcus once wrote, "Fashion leaders . . . are the anonymous women of taste in all classes. If one follows the whims of fashion in silhouette, color, and coiffure, one may attain what is known as chic; but true elegance and distinction result when judgment and skill are used in adapting the best in fashion to one's particular needs. This is one of the secrets of personal style."[3]

STYLE AND A SENSE OF VALUES

The woman of style and a limited income plans before she buys, so that her costume is the result of thought and not of impulse. Careful planning becomes increasingly important as we are ever faced with greater quantities of fashion merchandise and a barrage of advertising campaigns psychologically motivating us to buy the latest fashion. Mme. Elsa Schiaparelli, on a recent trip to New York, is quoted by a news reporter as saying, "For a

[2] Lawrence Langner, *The Importance of Wearing Clothes,* Hastings House, New York, 1959, p. 285.
[3] Stanley Marcus, "Fashion Is My Business," *Atlantic Monthly,* December 1948, p. 43.

woman to be smart, she must buy very little, and only what suits her, what goes with what she has. I don't mean a hat that matches shoes—that is not smartness, but boredom."[4] In another interview several years ago, Mme. Schiaparelli was quoted, ". . . If your budget is slim, have a couple of good things rather than many cheap ones." Quality clothing will retain its appearance with frequent wearing long after the cheap garment has become shabby.

Young people feel the need for frequent change far more than older women, and their purchases of clothing are important to the garment industry. Designing, merchandising, and advertising cater to their whims. The thought of wearing the same fine suit, coat, or dress for four years may not disturb the older woman, whereas the college girl could hardly be expected to be happy in the same garments with which she started her freshman year. In this span of years she has matured immeasurably, and stepping into young adulthood requires different clothing.

All too many women cling to the teen-age habit of preferring a closet full of inexpensive clothes to a few good costumes. Statistics prove that today we spend less on individual items of clothing but buy a greater number; this is due partly to our greater leisure and diversified activities. Nor do people today buy garments chiefly because they will give good service, since long before they wear out they will have gone out of style. Here surely is one place the average American woman misses her chance to achieve style. It takes ability to recognize enduring quality, ageless fashion, and truly functional apparel that will not become obsolete overnight despite the fact that we are constantly pressured by advertising to succumb to industry's built-in obsolescence.

STYLE AND SOCIAL CONVENTION

Although standards of good taste in dress tend to change, good taste will have regard for the conventions which have been established by the accumulated experience of cultivated people. If you are unaware of these established conventions, refer to Chapter Fourteen, as well as to other authoritative references available on the accepted etiquette of dress.

People with taste realize the importance of wearing the right clothes for the right occasions, and provide themselves with those items that are suited

---

[4] Courtesy Mme. Schiaparelli, Paris, France, letter dated July 30, 1963.

to their way of life. Convention has progressed far beyond the state of everyday clothes and clothes for "best." Today there are rather sharp distinctions among costumes suited to different occasions; this has been brought about in part by our greater leisure activities, our greater mobility in traveling from place to place, and our enjoyment of a wider sphere of activities. Increased use of transportation has tended to internationalize fashion and erase local idiosyncrasies of dress. And because of our mobility there has been a trend toward designing multipurpose costumes and all-weather apparel. Nevertheless, there are limits to the many faceted garments, and the standards of good dress in modern life require that our clothes be suited to the occasion, the time of day, and the vicissitudes of weather. The woman on a budget will do well to consider purchasing clothing which will serve more than one occasion, but she still must plan for all the activities in her way of life.

STYLE AND PLANNING

Previously the necessity for planning purchases of a few items of quality was brought out as a means of achieving style. Consider again the women of adolescent tendencies with closets full of clothes. These too are the women with a wide assortment of shoes, hats, and accessories purchased willy-nilly without plan. In the midst of this seeming plenty they are often heard to lament that they "have nothing to wear." And in a sense, their complaint is valid. What was the isolated, "cute" little dress, purchased on impulse, becomes the closet "ghost," because it isn't suitable. Likewise the treasure trove of accessories will harmonize with nothing else. The selection and purchase of a total ensemble takes time and thought in planning, and time in shopping with discriminating judgment for just the right articles to present a beautifully costumed look. This, too, expresses style.

STYLE AND QUALITY

The importance of good fabrics cannot be overemphasized, as good lines cannot be achieved in cheap or shoddy materials. Quality fabric is frequently so distinctive in character, color, or texture that it becomes the inspiration for the final garment or design.

As fabrics play an important role in style, so do fit and workmanship;

cheap workmanship and poor fit can never be concealed. Through a study of fitting and a thorough analysis of one's own figure and proportions, a consciousness for well-fitted clothing is developed. A garment may have been expertly designed, carefully cut, and meticulously constructed; but it has been designed for an average figure. If it is not right in grain, balance, and ease for your figure, it will lose all its smartness. An ill-fitting garment may be uncomfortable and certainly never appears well.

Good workmanship is recognized through studying clothing construction methods or by observing the manner in which quality ready-to-wear is constructed. Too often lovely fabrics and designs are spoiled by telltale evidences of inexperienced home dressmaking or by cheap construction of ready-made garments, which are produced to sell at a low price. It does take study to learn to recognize quality construction, but the effort pays off, since such construction is one of the tangible evidences of style.

STYLE AND YOU

In the arts of personal appearance, clothes should be chosen for self-expression and for identification of the wearer with beauty. Clothing should not be used for display, evidence of wealth or power, or, as is so often currently discussed, identification with the social stratum to which one belongs or with which one wishes to identify himself. Individuality of costume style certainly transcends herd instinct.

The costume which supports self-expression of the modern woman eliminates all nonessential and extraneous trimming applied without regard for structural lines. The costume presents a clear-cut, streamlined simplicity, fusing with the wearer and enabling her to stand out vital and alive. Well-designed contemporary costume, like well-designed contemporary furniture, architecture, and decorative articles, is dependent upon judicious use of line, interesting shapes, honest use of materials, and subtly blended colors that make extra decoration absurd. Our clothes and our homes become vehicles of self-expression and a well-bred background for us. Contemporary costume must be carefully assembled: the right hat with the right dress, harmonizing gloves and shoes, and some tellingly effective ornament not at once noticed, but when noticed, not easily forgotten. These meticulously ordered clothes are never more important than the individual; they reiterate the individuality that is you.

All too few people today seem to have a flair for achieving results which embody style. There are those who are impeccably correct but have no spirit in their carriage; or who are neatness personified but have a kind of old-maidish taste; or who have no eye for color; or who with good color sense, lack a feeling for line and silhouette.

But here and there is one who embodies all the elements of style. She is seldom pretty. In the eyes of many people she is plain; but she is intelligent, interesting to know, and cosmopolitan. She has a clothes sense too, either acquired or innate, which enables her to discover and appropriate the thing which has significance and meaning. It may be a memorable note of color, an exquisite ornament, a skill in combining garments. Some people would say that style results more from the way one's clothes are worn than from the clothes themselves. There must be something personal in one's manner of wearing them—some kind of flair—the hat's jaunty angle, a dash of nonchalance, an enviable air of pride or authority or elegance which expresses the spirit and vitality within.

Stanley Marcus, in a statement formulated especially for this book, says of individuality of style, "The main trend since the war has been the complete internationalization of fashion. Today it is difficult to identify the country in which you may be visiting by the dress of its women for they are all wearing versions of the contemporary successful silhouette from Paris.

"One of the problems of today and of the years to come is the trend towards conformity in dress brought about by mass production of fabrics and clothes. A woman can maintain individuality in her appearance, but it is no longer as easy to accomplish as it was in mother's day."

The following references are suggested:

Pauline Arnold and Percival White, *Clothes and Cloth,* Holiday House, New York, 1961, Chaps. XI–XII.

Lincoln Clark (editor), *Consumer Behavior,* Vol. 3, Part I, Harper & Brothers, New York, 1958.

James F. Dewhurst and Associates, *America's Needs and Resources,* The Twentieth Century Fund, New York, 1955, Part II, Chap. VI.

Anne Fogarty, *Wife Dressing,* Julian Messner, Inc., New York, 1959.

Elizabeth Hawes, *It's Still Spinach,* Little, Brown and Co., Boston, 1954.

Edith Head, *The Dress Doctor,* Little, Brown and Co., Boston, 1959.

Lawrence Langner, *The Importance of Wearing Clothes,* Hastings House, New York, 1959.

Claire McCardell, *What Shall I Wear?*, Simon and Schuster, New York, 1956.

Eve Merriman, *Figleaf; the Business of Being in Fashion*, J. B. Lippincott, Philadelphia, 1960.

Vance Packard, *The Hidden Persuaders*, David McKay Co., Inc., New York, 1957. (Also Pocket Books, Inc., New York.)

Vance Packard, *The Status Seekers*, David McKay Co., Inc., New York, 1959. (Also Pocket Books, Inc., New York.)

Exercises

1. Study the women in some public place, noting those who may be considered to have style, and try to decide in each case what it is that gives them this quality.
2. Make a list of examples of fashions of the past which are now known to us as styles.
3. What styles of the past can you think of which have been revived?
4. Would you subscribe to the theory that there are no unbeautiful women—only those who do not know how to look beautiful? Expand this idea.
5. Analyze yourself to see if you can determine wherein you do or do not possess qualities of style. Think through a program for yourself whereby you may acquire, in the years just ahead, a greater measure of the intrinsic qualities of style.

Three

Self-Made Beauty

Today few want to be merely pretty. Like the creative artist, intelligent people see beauty in what may have been considered homeliness in former days. We appreciate plain features if they are possessed of humor and vitality, imagination, and mobility of character. We know that real beauty comes from within. Surface prettiness is largely a transitory attribute of the young; beauty is an ageless quality. Plain women of intelligence study to make themselves intellectually interesting as well as physically attractive. Contemporary beauty may be just as much a job of skillful attention to the person as a gift of nature.

John Robert Powers, creator of the famous "Powers Models," gives the following "seven golden rules of glamour."[1]

1. Make the most of your face and hair.
2. Strive for good posture and physical condition.
3. Walk smoothly with grace and rhythm.
4. Sit and stand gracefully.
5. Dress to suit your face and figure.
6. Speak in a well-modulated and unaffected voice.
7. Develop your mind as a vehicle of self-expression.

[1] John Robert Powers. Quoted by permission.

Self-made beauty is attainable to an appreciable extent by all who are intelligent and willing to undergo the physical and mental discipline necessary to its achievement.

PERFECTION IN GROOMING

The first requisite of being a truly attractive person is thorough cleanliness. What the fashion magazines call the American Look is one of health, vitality, efficiency, and freshness. This well-scrubbed, well-polished look begins with a fastidiously clean body. A daily bath is imperative, as are regular use of a deodorant and removal of superfluous hair. Shampoo the hair as frequently as it needs it, rather than trying to get by just another day or waiting until the end of the week. Woman's crowning glory appears so only when sparklingly clean, not when it is oily and straggly. Nails, too, must be manicured or pedicured when the need arises. Women on the go frequently engage in activities destructive to a manicure. There is nothing attractive about chipped nail polish. The teeth and mouth are not to be overlooked in this cleanliness regimen. Following the dentist's advice and brushing the teeth after eating is excellent for beauty and for health.

Perfection in grooming is evidenced in hair which always appears to have just been brushed and combed and in make-up that is as fresh as though it had just been applied. Correctly applied make-up stays intact over a longer period of time. The face should be thoroughly cleaned and freshly made up when it needs repair. The application of make-up and grooming of the hair are matters to be taken care of in private rather than in public.

Perfection in grooming extends beyond the body to clothing. Outer garments should be kept spotlessly clean through frequent dry cleaning or laundering. It is also important that they be kept faultlessly pressed, brushed, and repaired. It is emphatically important that absolute cleanliness extend to all articles of underclothing and hosiery. Don't believe that just because they don't show, they aren't important to perfection in grooming. Shoes need always to be shined and in good repair. Gloves must never appear soiled; purses need cleaning inside and out; scarves need frequent laundering; and dingy costume jewelry can mar an ensemble.

Some people have a freshness in every detail with a clean-cut look. This appearance is not accidental, but results from setting aside time for grooming. It means getting out of bed in sufficient time in the morning to begin the day faultlessly groomed before leaving for work or school, and it will contribute to a more enjoyable day. It means managing time during the day to cleanse the face, teeth, and hands. It means time before bed for a bath and care of the face, hair, and nails. In a busy life faultless grooming means efficient use of time. Begin now by making a list of all required weekly activities including the details of personal care and care of clothing. From this list formulate a realistic time schedule to accomplish your goals; the plan at the same time should be flexible enough to take care of emergency shampoos and manicures. Once the plan has been made, hold religiously to it. Surprisingly much more can be accomplished in an ordered existence. Each one has experienced the lift she felt when at her shining best; make this feeling yours throughout each day of the year.

Poise and assurance result when one is well groomed. A run in a stocking, a broken shoulder strap, a conspicuous stain, and chipped nail polish do not contribute to self-assurance or permit the mind to function on a level above petty annoyances. If one's appearance is neat and orderly, one's thinking is more often organized. If one's appearance is slovenly, it is safe to assume that the mind behind it is unorganized or ill disciplined. Smartness through perfection in every detail of grooming is an expression of an alert and tidy mind, one that can be relied on for constructive contributions on the job. Immaculate grooming can be of value in getting and holding positions and is essential in social relationships.

A PLEASANT FACIAL EXPRESSION

Many times the remark has been made that a charming woman is the most fascinating thing in the world. In analyzing charm, a common attribute that all charming women possess is an expressive, responsive countenance.

This demand of self-made beauty is worth pondering. What does your face reveal to the world? Are warmth and animation in it? In the theatrical world faces which are not responsive, which never change, never reflect thoughts or emotions, are called "dead pans." Do you have a sensitive, mobile countenance which expresses warmth and generosity?

A very wise saying from the past is that after forty a woman is responsible for her face. Youth and beauty are qualities of mind and soul. When they remain on the face it is an indication of kindness, nobility of character, and patience with life's discipline. Youth is not a time of life; it is state of mind. It is a quality of imagination, of vigor, of freshness of outlook. People grow old by deserting their ideals, by worry, doubt, fear, and despair. Caroline Duer in her charming essay, "Our Enemy the Wrinkle," tells us that there are two kinds of wrinkles: "those of the skin" when the "sun and wind have had too much their way," and "wrinkles of the soul." Wrinkles of the soul she thinks come from holding grudges and being envious and uncharitable, and getting overtired. She thinks that a great many "line-making habits" are under our control. There is a "buoyancy of spirit which comes from taking most things amusedly and all others as philosophically as possible." [2]

Many a handsome face has been enhanced or marred by the philosophy behind it. A study of one's own face without make-up in a good light may reveal many things. Ask yourself, "What does my face reveal?" Understanding, spontaneity, generosity, and patience are traits of feminine charm which have made some women notable. Are you studying to discover and cultivate them within yourself?

A PLEASING VOICE

A beautiful, well-modulated speaking voice is one of the important aspects of charm. To the listener it can seem a reflection of warmth, sincerity, and humor. Speech to a remarkable extent draws or repels, influences or dissuades people. Meanings are conveyed as much by the inflections of the voice as by words themselves. A voice too high or too loud suggests tenseness, excitement, anger; a low, muffled voice gives the impression of fatigue, weakness, boredom. Faults of speech largely result from poor habits and can be improved. Every young woman should learn to "place" or pitch her speaking voice agreeably. A middle ground, in both pitch and volume, gives more opportunity for expressiveness; for it permits the raising or lowering of pitch to express thought or emotion. In varying the pitch care must be taken to avoid a singsong effect.

As today good speech is an asset in social situations and in so many occupations, it is more important than ever for young people to learn to speak in a clear, pleasant voice, free from affectations, free from provincialism, and

---

[2] Caroline Duer, *How to Tell the Fashions from the Follies,* Charles Scribner's Sons, New York, 1925, pp. 54–57.

with a discriminating choice of words. As one scholar who was also a fine speaker remarked, errors of pronunciation or of grammar assault the ears as unpleasantly as evil odors the nose. The subject matter of speech and conversation is of equal importance; it can reveal as much as the face. Those who talk of themselves, of others, of petty frustrations, and of trivia show little depth of character. Reading and a sincere interest in the world about one contribute much to intellectual speech.

The first recording or taping of one's voice is a startling experience, and seldom does the owner recognize it when it is played back. An analysis of the recording aided by a trained voice teacher is a start on the way to needed improvements. Most schools and colleges have departments of speech with classes and clinics available to all students.

It must be remembered that general health, posture, and mental attitude are reflected in one's speech; and improvement of all these contributes to a more interesting personality. In the final analysis, nothing will take the place of genuine interest, enthusiasm, and sympathy for others in making one's voice a pleasure to the listener.

A SOUND HEALTHY BODY

The modern idea of good looks demands a sound and supple body, healthy and with abounding vitality. Good health imparts radiance and enthusiasm which are contagious. It is recognized in clear eyes, smooth transparent skin with overtones of color, and lustrous hair.

A good skin ranks next to personal cleanliness as a mark of beauty. It may be lightly tanned, olive, or fair, but it must be clean with a gloss that comes from radiant health. It goes without saying that it should be fine grained, soft to the touch, and unblemished by immoderate eating. A dermatologist should be consulted for guidance in the care of troubled skin, which is frequently experienced by young people.

Diet plays a large part in appearance. It is reflected in all the manifestations of a healthy body which in itself is beautiful; and it is reflected in weight. Unquestionably, no girl or woman can be as attractive as it is possible for her to be unless her weight is somewhere near what is considered "normal" for her height and build. Refer to Table 1. It is a rather sad commentary on American discipline to note the frequent incidence of over-

TABLE 1 HEIGHT-WEIGHT TABLE *

HEIGHT (inches)	WEIGHT (pounds)		
	LOW	MEDIAN	HIGH
60	100	109	118
61	104	112	121
62	107	115	125
63	110	118	128
64	113	122	132
65	116	125	135
66	120	129	139
67	123	132	142
68	126	136	146
69	130	140	151
70	133	144	156
71	(137)	(148)	(161)
72	(141)	(152)	(166)

Weights were based on those of college women 20 to 24 years old. Measurements were made without shoes and other clothing. The range from "low" to "high" at a given height included the middle 50 percent of the cases. Half the weights were below the median and half above. Body build will determine where, within the ranges given, normal weight should be. Weight at any age probably should not exceed these values by more than 5 pounds for the shorter adults and 10 pounds for the taller ones.

* The United States Department of Agriculture, *FOOD The Yearbook of Agriculture,* The United States Government Printing Office, Washington, D. C., 1959, p. 182.

weight. Obesity can place added strains on the body and shorten the life span.

As diet influences our bodily appearance, so can exercise. In the words of a leader in the field of women's physical education, "The medical profession tells us that maintenance of vital capacities (the heart-lung complex) is based upon nerve-muscular reactions. Maintenance of body condition is, therefore, definitely a phase of preventive medicine. After a physical examination, every woman should construct for herself, under expert direction, a set of simple body exercises that will help her keep muscle tonus. Retention of adequate physical condition is a personal responsibility so that she will have enough energy to pursue each day and to enjoy any leisure after working hours."[3]

[3] Dr. Dudley Ashton, Head, University of Nebraska Department of Women's Physical Education.

Very important to self-made good looks is the habit of relaxing periodically. All rushing and no resting help to make one look old before one's time, for beauty is lost when there are signs of strain. A relaxing period, no matter how short, helps to take wrinkles from the face, ache from tired muscles, the edge from the voice. The mind responds too; what seemed like a mountain before becomes a mere hurdle. Some suggestions for a ten-minute freshener that can work wonders in giving a new outlook are given below:

Forget all frustrations and pressures.
Stand up at an open window and give yourself a mighty stretch—stretch the body from right hand to left foot, then from left hand to right foot.
Bend your waist and rotate your trunk to the right and then to the left.
Bend at the hips and let your arms and head dangle limply down to the floor until fresh blood surges to your face.
Remove old make-up and put on fresh.
Touch up your hair with a comb.

The availability of a longer period of time will permit removal of clothing and ten minutes in a supine position. Elevating the feet and legs to a position higher than the head will stimulate circulation. Other forms of relaxation should be planned for in well-rounded living. Active sports, creative pursuits, community service, and ever continuing education through a reading plan or adult classes help keep a healthy perspective and balance, which are reflected in face, voice, and bearing.

In the plan of a busy life, adequate time for sleep must be allowed. Not all people require the same amount to awaken refreshed. After sufficient sleep it is possible to meet the day with enthusiasm, a clearly functioning mind, and a tolerance of others and all the problems which may arise.

GOOD POSTURE

How rarely do we see a perfect figure, perfectly poised! Many men and women with intelligent faces, who are well dressed and prosperous looking, have poor carriage. Both physicians and physical educators recognize that good posture can be both cause and effect in relation to good health. One of the positive indications of health is seen in good posture and carriage; reciprocally, posture affects the suspension and function of the organs. Aside from the health standpoint, good posture has three other values: economic

26 *The Arts of Costume and Personal Appearance*

(the mental alertness of the job applicant is evaluated by the mannerisms of standing and walking); social (a fine body and beautiful carriage are always attractive); and spiritual ("The glory of the rising sun is never seen by one walking with protruding head and abdomen."[4]).

There is no single good posture; there are many good postures, in the sense that each person is a distinct individual mechanism and that the body is constantly in motion in the performance of many feats. Good posture, however, means a perfect balance of the various units of the human framework and a perfectly articulated body mechanism. There are basic principles in the efficient movement of the body which contribute to health and at the same time produce a more aesthetic, graceful appearance. *The Victory of Samothrace,* in the Louvre, is a classic example of youthful, exuberant motion. Humanity is not cast in one mold; yet each individual can work toward an optimum posture. In their departments of physical education, college girls have the advantage of professional help in posture analysis and in well-planned exercises for correction of posture and for the improvement of body mechanics. Many posture problems result from unconsciously copying family members and from incorrect use of the body. An erect posture is always in good taste, regardless of the fashion of the moment.

Standing Posture

Good figure alignment requires that the body always be relaxed and that its various parts be in the proper relationship to one another. A line drawn through the profile of the human figure should pass through the center of the ear lobe, the shoulder, the hip, the knee, and the ankle (Figure 1). If one of these points of articulation is out of line, it will throw other parts of the body out of position and will place extra strain on the muscles.

A simple device for checking posture is that of standing against a wall. The back of the head, the flat surface of the shoulders, the small of the back, the hips, and the heels should all lie flat against the surface. If your body is not in this position, begin the correction by placing one hand on the abdomen, at the same time pulling it in; place the other hand on the back of the hips and tuck them under while slightly flexing the knees. This is a surprisingly simple beginning to good alignment: the chest assumes its proper elevated position. The shoulders are another point for special attention. The posture

---

[4] Jesse Feiring Williams, M. D., and Gloyd Gage Wetherill, *Personal and Community Hygiene Applied,* W. B. Saunders Co., Philadelphia, 1950, p. 169.

of youngsters who are told to "throw their shoulders back" results in high, tense shoulders, pinched muscles between the shoulder blades, head thrust forward, and hips flaring out in back. Once the shoulders have been placed flat against the wall, pull them toward the floor in a relaxed position. Reach for the ceiling with the top of the head. Check points during practice include head tall, shoulders back and down, chest up, abdomen in, hips under, and knees slightly flexed. The arms will hang a bit in front of the hip bones and not awkwardly on top of them.

Good standing posture requires that the alignment of the body be maintained and that the feet be kept close together to give a slender tapering look. When standing at rest for a period of time, the weight may be carried over the ball of one foot, the other dropped back a little and resting lightly for balance. The heel of the forward foot carries little of the weight; the heel of the other is clear of, or barely touches, the ground. In this position the weight of the body may be shifted gracefully from the ball of one foot to that of the other in readiness to move, as in dancing. For greater stability, stand with the feet close together and parallel and distribute the weight between the balls of both feet. When it is necessary to stand for a long period of time, a frequent shift in position will be found restful.

Walking Posture

The rhythm of walking is such an individual matter that most people can be recognized by their gaits or even the sound of their footsteps. The long, flowing stride of the tall, athletic woman will contrast with the staccato steps of a short, active person. The quick, energetic walk of the soldier seems purposeful, efficient. A hesitant waddle can suggest shiftlessness and apathy; a shuffling gait, age and fatigue.

A good carriage in walking is light, rhythmic, and graceful, never heavy and swaying. It demands that the

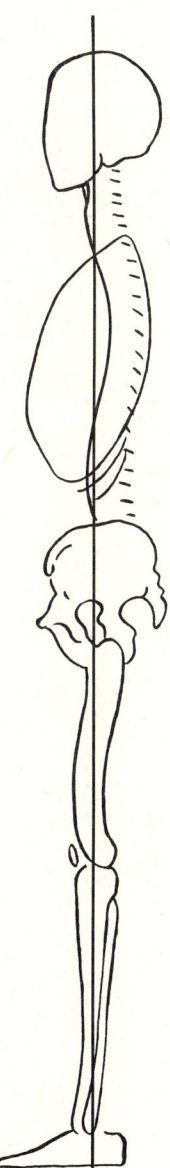

Figure 1. Human framework in correct balance.

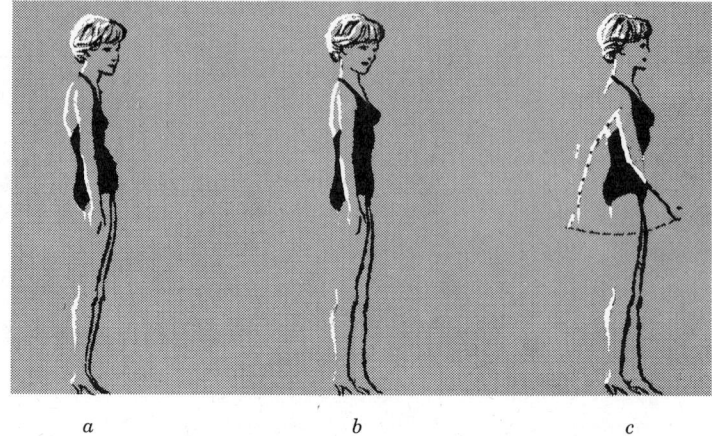

Figure 2. Posture as you stand and walk.

feet be pointed straight ahead, and not at an angle like those of the opera singer who wrote in her memoirs of being trained to stand with her toes "at a quarter to two." The legs should swing from the hip joints in propelling the body, while the knees are kept flexed. The feet are placed one ahead of the other in a single line, and the weight is rolled rapidly from the heels through the balls and toes of the feet.

Frequently women walk with their knees snapped back, throwing the entire body out of alignment; walk on their heels, so that it seems as if each step jars the entire body; place their feet in two separate lines of locomotion, so that the body bobs sideways in a most unattractive duck waddle; or thrust their head forward, as though it could arrive before their feet. Length of stride is dependent upon height; learn to take steps neither too long nor too short for your stature. A graceful walk includes maintenance of the body in perfect alignment while it is propelled smoothly forward, seeming to function as one unit, with no sideward motion or up and down bounce. Let the arms hang free so that they can swing slightly, but rhythmically, in opposition to the swing of the legs (Figure 2c). If burdens such as school books must be carried, divide the weight or shift it from the right to the left arm.

Climbing or descending stairs correctly is nothing more than the continuation of good walking posture. In ascending stairs keep the back in perfect alignment and at a right angle to the surface of the steps; let the legs do the work. Do not make yourself appear years older by stooping or bending forward. The same principles apply in descending. Keep the body in perfect alignment; and with the head held high, look forward and not down at your feet. Pause a moment to get your bearing if necessary, and float down as though making an entrance at a grand ball.

Sitting Posture

The sitting posture which is hygienic also presents an attractive appearance and indicates good breeding. Slide all the way back in the chair so that the hips are close to the back. The torso rests upright above the pelvis and is never permitted to double up or collapse. Tuck the buttocks under to act as a cushion. The weight is born by the pelvic bones and not the spine. The feet are invariably kept close together. Both feet may be on the floor, one slightly in advance of the other; or they may be crossed at the ankles (Figures 3a and 4c). When the legs are crossed, cross them above both knees so that the flesh of the calf is not pushed out increasing its apparent size. The top leg drops down in the same general direction as the under leg. In leaning forward when seated, the torso should swing forward from the thigh joints so that the spine is not bent at the waist (Figure 3c). The fatigue of desk work can be minimized when this basic principle is observed.

To be seated, turn the back to the chair, and place one foot slightly ahead of the other; the back leg is close to the chair. Keep the torso in an erect position, and gradually lower the body into the chair. In rising, the back leg takes the weight and the thighs do the work. Do not thrust the hips

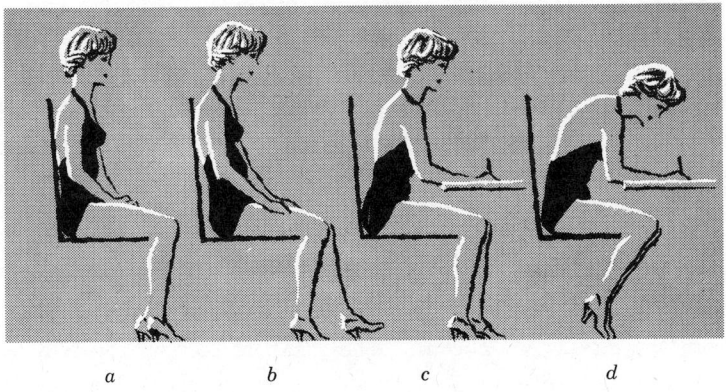

Figure 3. Posture as you sit and write.

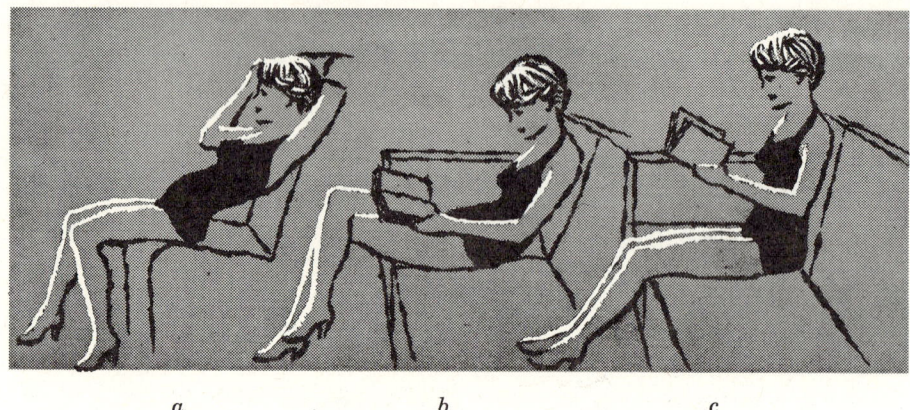

a   *b*   *c*

Figure 4. Posture as you read.

upward in an ungraceful position in being seated or in rising. This mannerism, along with seeming to heave the body from a chair with the arms, can add years to one's appearance.

The same basic mechanics apply in stooping to lift a weight; bend the knees and maintain good back posture (Figure 5a). There is nothing particularly lovely about a woman's derrière rising in the air as she retrieves some dropped article.

FIGURES AND FACES

There probably never was a time when women were more conscious of their figures or more eager to improve them. Before any comprehensive study of figure problems can be made or any constructive guides can be given for improving the effect through choice of apparel, one must first consider the characteristics of the ideal feminine figure.

All great civilizations have had their ideals of feminine beauty, which seem to have expressed their time. There was the Greek figure, slightly more rounded than ours, still a criterion of beautiful proportions, as seen in the lovely *Venus de Milo* or the *Venus Cyrene* (Figure 6). Differing considerably from the classic was the medieval ideal, as seen in the tall, elongated figures of sculptured madonnas (Figure 1 Chapter Five) or in the Fra Angelico angels (Figure 7). In northern Europe in the fifteenth century, strange as it may seem, the ideal was the pregnant figure pictured by Albrecht Dürer and the Flemish masters (Figure 8). During the Renaissance the standards of beauty of those wealthy and luxury-loving aristocrats are revealed through Rubens' corpulent women. Coming nearer to our own time, there was the Second Empire ideal of Empress Eugénie with sloping shoulders and eighteen-inch waist (Figure 9). During the Gay Nineties appeared the sway-back stance and the sleek, poured-in, molded line. Differing from all the others was the slender, boyish figure of the 1920's with its flat chest, debutante slouch, and air of disillusionment.

Women throughout the centuries have molded their figures into many strange and different shapes. Each seemed beautiful in its day; like our predecessors, we are inclined to think none quite so lovely as today's.

Contemporary Figure Ideals

Our contemporary ideal calls for a figure less buxom and taller than the *Venus Cyrene* (Figure 6). The most enviable height is five feet five or six. Other characteristics of the contemporary ideal figure include an oval head and face; slender arms, tapering from wrist to elbow and very little, if any, larger above the elbow; shoulders and hips the same width; waistline well curved; thighs the same width as the hips, tapering to gracefully proportioned calves; slender ankles and slender feet. Other characteristics in our conception of ideal proportions are a neck one-third the length of the face and not wider than the jaw; shoulders approximately three times the

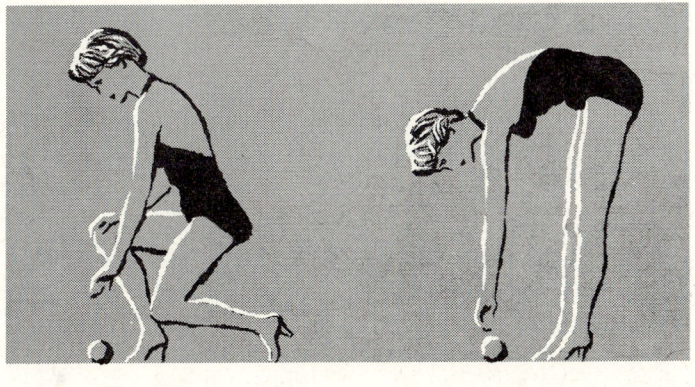

Figure 5. Posture as you kneel.

32　*The Arts of Costume and Personal Appearance*

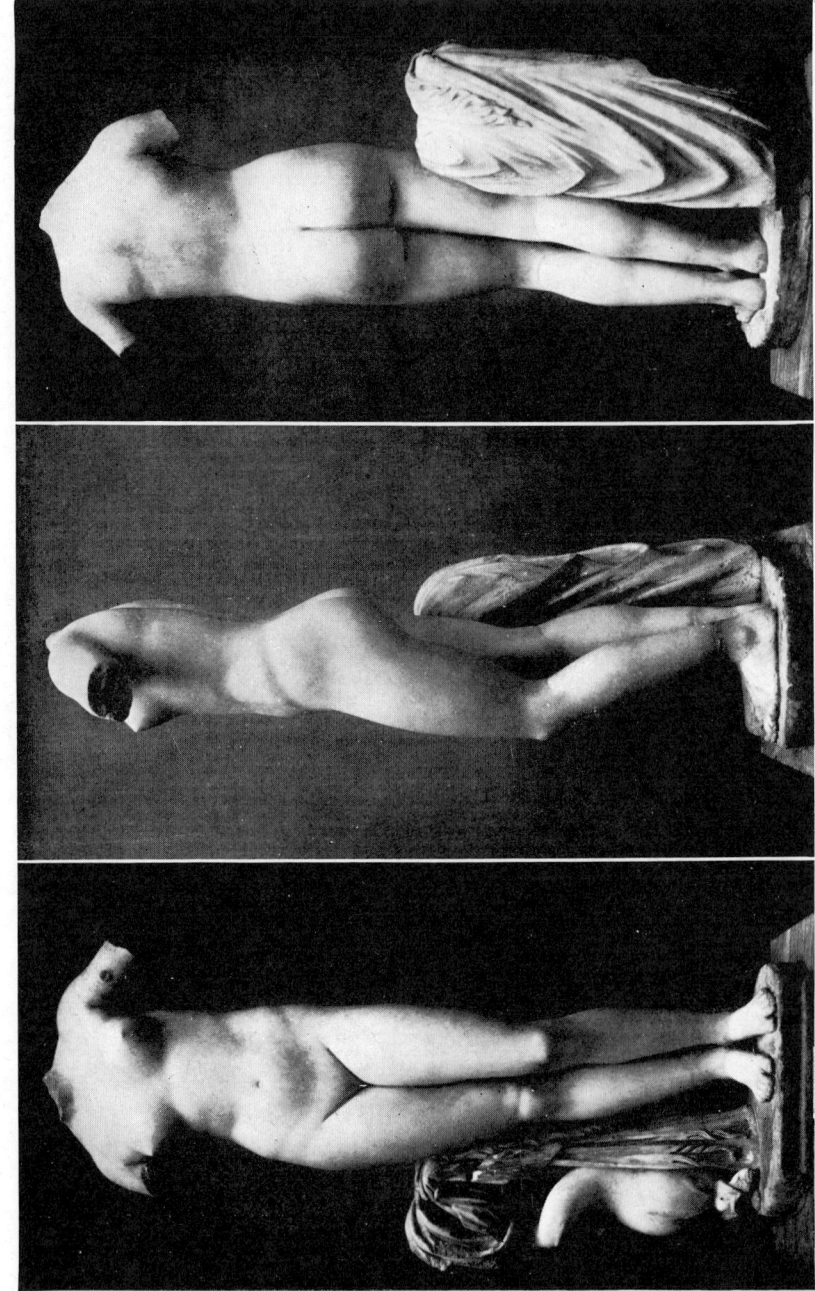

Figure 6. Three views of the Venus Cyrene. Found in Crete during the Italian wars in Tripoli, this Venus is a symbol of beautiful feminine contours. Museum Delle Terme, Rome.

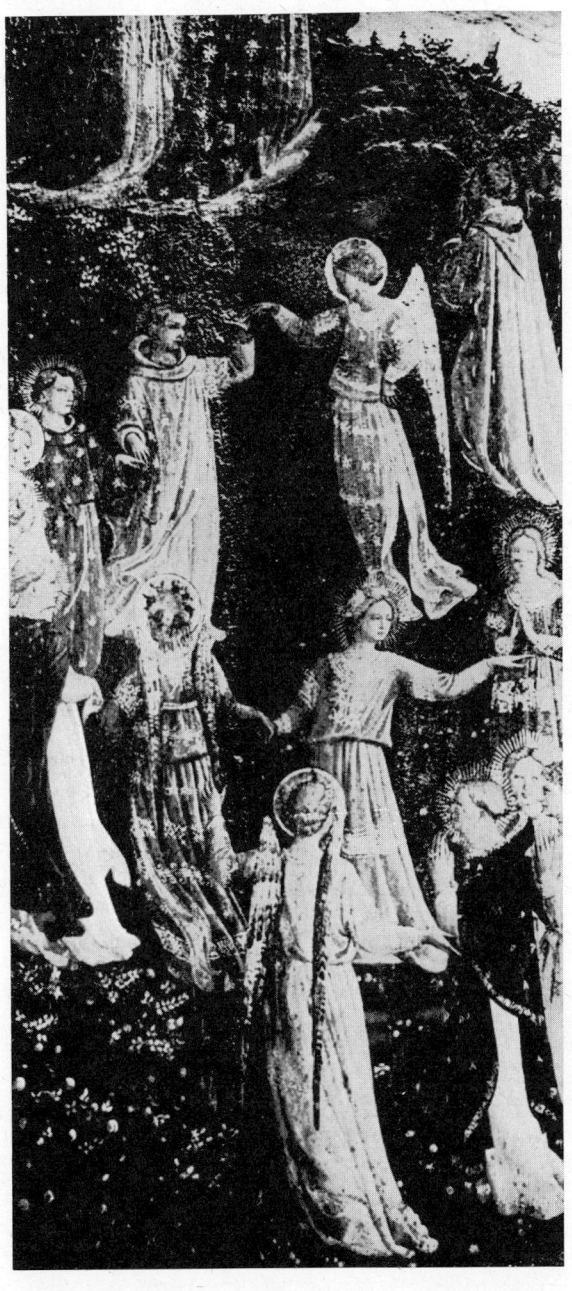

Figure 7. Fra Angelica *angels,* The Last Judgment, *left panel.* Berlin Museum. *The tall, attenuated figures of these heavenly beings are typical of the medieval ideal.*

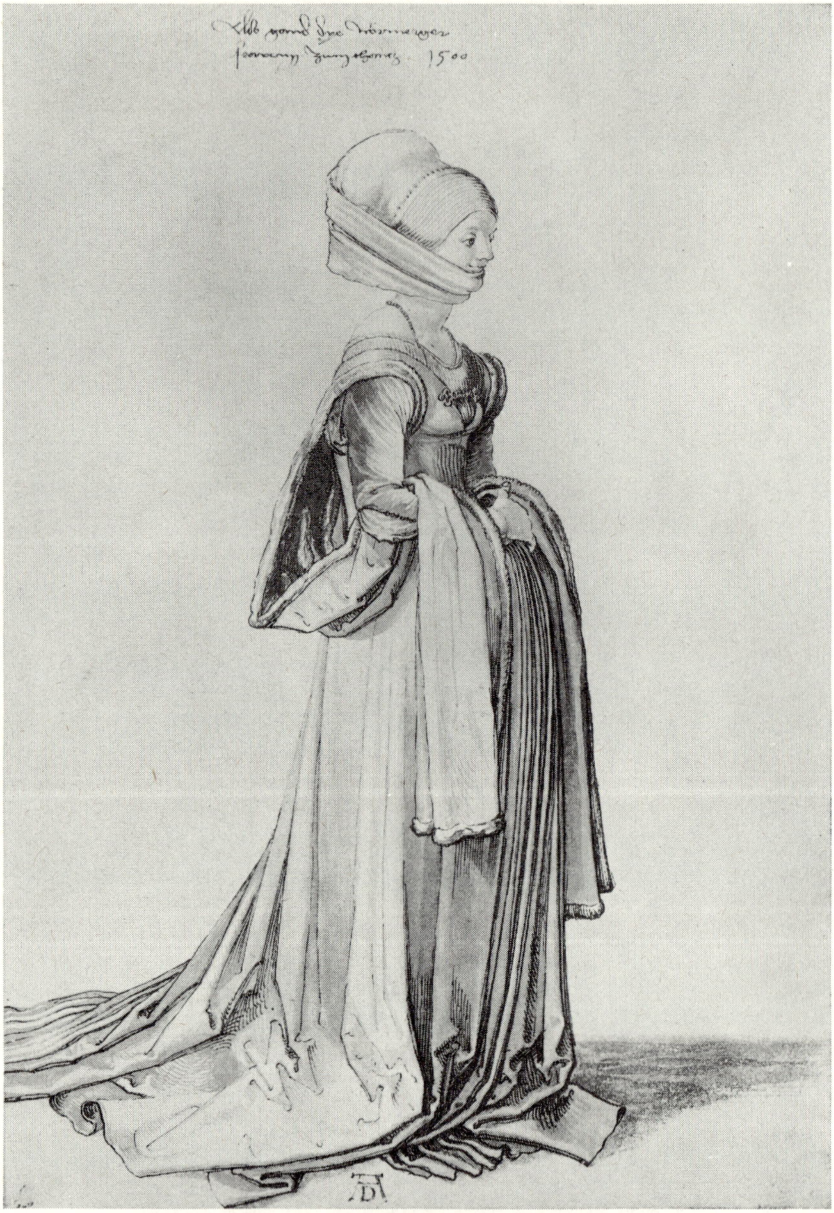

Figure 8. A hausfrau of 1500 arrayed for a ball. A graceful version of the elaborate costume of the bourgeois class of that material age.   Albrecht Dürer.

SELF-MADE BEAUTY 35

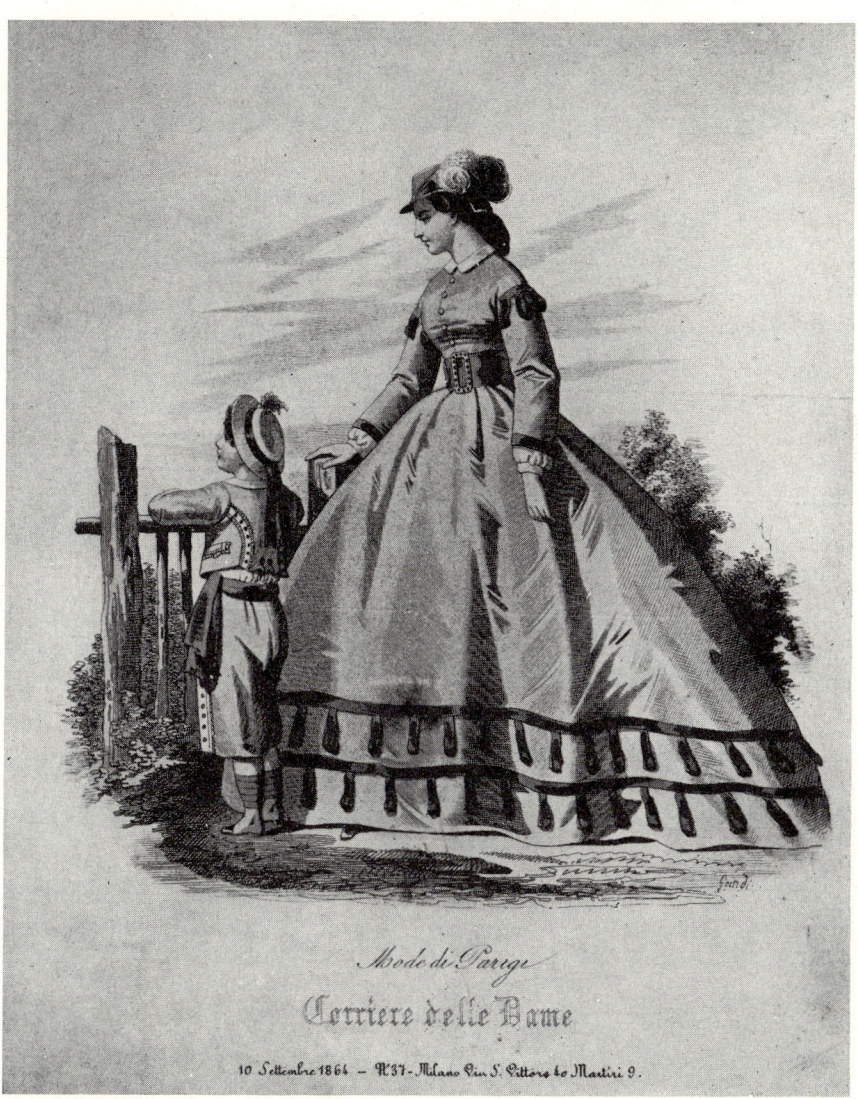

Figure 9. Fashion plate from Milan, September 10, 1864 (the era of wasp waists, sloping shoulders, and extravagantly wide and concealing skirts).

width of the head; elbows coming to the waistline; wrists coming to one-half the height of the figure; hands the length of the face; and the width of the hands, when placed flat with fingers straight, equivalent to the widest part of the foot.

The concept of a beautiful figure includes several aspects of the human body. The influence of good posture in creating a more pleasing, graceful appearance has been discussed.

Articulation is concerned with the juncture of parts of the body. There is charm in the perfect joining of a well-shaped hand to a slender wrist, or a rounded shoulder to a curving breast, or a slender ankle to a well-shaped foot.

Bone structure is a part of our inheritance. Fundamentally it cannot be altered, but it may be enhanced. The accumulated length of bones determines stature, which may range from short to tall. The time has passed when optimum weight was determined by height alone. Differences are now recognized in body framework in determining height-weight relationships. Bone structure is classified as small, medium, or large; and a small-boned person is no longer expected to weigh as much as one with a much heavier structure.

The covering of the skeletal structure is muscle and flesh—sometimes adequate, sometimes excessive. This covering may enhance or destroy the charm of a fine bone structure. An inadequate covering may reach thinness, even angularity, where body lines tend to approach straight lines. On the other hand, a covering too excessive suggests the full, round curves of the rococo. Ideal body contours will approach restrained curves; they will be neither angles nor circles, but ovals.

The question of weight is a popular topic both of conversation and of innumerable writings. Unfortunately, much that is printed in relation to diets is without scientific basis; beware the fad diet that ignores essential body needs. The principles of good nutrition should be studied and practiced by all. Good nutrition is the foundation of a healthy body. There is no magic formula to weight reduction; sensible weight loss is a slow and gradual process. It demands that the individual exercise discipline until the objective has been accomplished. If an appreciable amount is to be lost, place yourself in the hands of a physician. It might be said with little reservation that obesity is a matter of inadequate exercise and overeating. There are very few instances of metabolic causes, and these instances can be controlled under a doctor's guidance and sensible diet. Do not blame heredity for overweight merely because you have family members who are also overweight. Eating habits, like many posture habits, are learned through imitation. Aside from copying a bad family habit, overeating may indicate a psychological involvement. Some overeat to reward themselves; others, because they are unhappy for a host of reasons. Overeating because you are fat and left out of things can be disastrous to your beauty.

Dr. Leverton, a nutrition authority, in writing about weight says, "Excess weight is inconvenient; it can spoil your looks, threaten your vanity, and put you on the defensive about life in general. Also, it can be a health hazard. Compared with people of normal weight, those who are overweight are more likely to have gall bladder trouble, diabetes, gout, and arthritis; they are poor surgical risks and less resistant to infections. They are more likely to have hardening of the arteries and high blood pressure than lean people. Overweight also places an extra burden on the heart. . . . Being underweight can mean lowered resistance, no reserve to use in emergencies, undue fatigue, and poor physical and emotional stamina." [5]

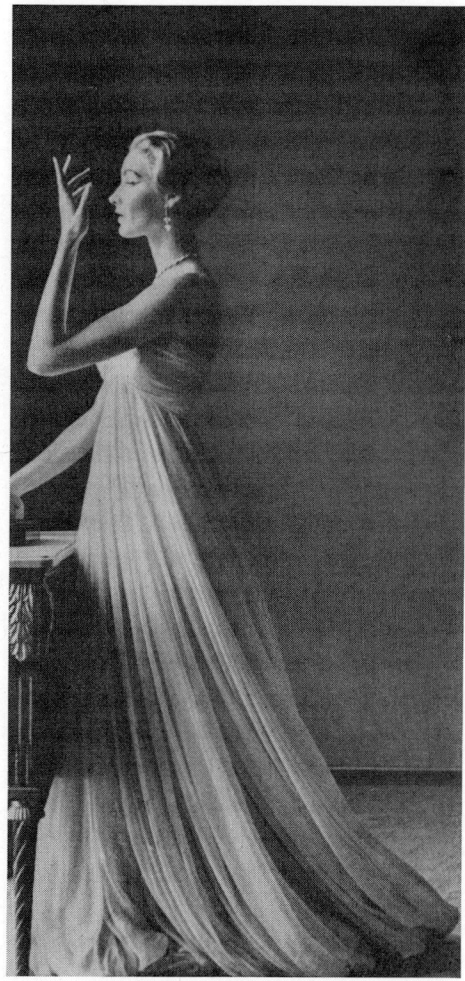

Figure 10. Rose colored chiffon by Jacques Griffe. Courtesy of Harper's Bazaar. *Photograph by Karen Radkai. A contemporary gown derived from the silhouette ideal of the Directoire period.*

The appearance of the seriously underweight person is affected through the habit of not eating enough to meet the demands of the body and add

[5] Ruth M. Leverton, *Food Becomes You,* Iowa State University Press, Ames, Iowa, 1960, pp. 48–49, 71.

TABLE 2 MODEL WEIGHT CHART*

HEIGHT	SMALL FRAME	AVERAGE FRAME	LARGE FRAME
5′	95	100	105
5′1″	100	105	110
5′2″	105	110	115
5′3″	110	115	120
5′4″	115	120	125
5′5″	120	125	130
5′6″	125	130	135
5′7″	130	135	140
5′8″	135	140	145
5′9″	140	145	150
5′10″	145	150	155
5′11″	150	155	160

* John Robert Powers, *How to Have Model Beauty, Poise and Personality,* Prentice-Hall, Inc., Englewood Cliffs, N. J., 1960, p. 93.

weight. In a few instances it is as difficult for this person to put on pounds as for another to take them off. This problem, however, is not frequently encountered.

TABLE 3 COMPARISON OF THE VENUS DE MILO WITH THE AMERICAN WOMAN

	VENUS DE MILO *	AMERICAN WOMAN †
Weight		133.48 lb.
Stature	64 in.	63.16 in.
Neck girth	12.5	15.27
Chest girth	33	34.77
Bust girth	37	35.62
Waist girth	26	29.15
Hip girth	38	38.82
Thigh girth	22.5	22.24
Calf girth	13.2	13.45
Knee girth	15	13.96
Upper arm girth	12.5	11.37
Forearm girth	9.5	9.75
Wrist girth	5.9	6.01
Ankle girth	7.4	9.31

* Ida Jean Kain, ℞ *for Slimming,* David McKay Co., Philadelphia, 1940, p. 16.
† "Women's Measurements for Garment and Pattern Construction," Miscellaneous Publication 454, U. S. Department of Agriculture, 1941, p. 27.

The truly remarkable results of correct diet in transforming figures have been seen by everyone.

The normal or desirable weight for each person depends on age, height, and body build. If the weight is within the normal range at age 25, it should not change appreciably after that. Height-weight tables are helpful in assessing your relationship to the average person of the same height and bone structure. The statistics in Table 1 were obtained through a study of average young women who in general tend to be somewhat overweight. For that reason the weights in this table are higher than those in Table 2 for models who display garments to the best advantage on their ideal figures. In using Table 1, those weights under the column "Low" may be used by those of small bone structure; those labelled "High," by those of large bone structure.

Proportion of the various parts of the body structure to each other and to the total physique play an important part in perfection of figure. "Large hips," "short legs," and comparable complaints are frequently expressed. Some figures differ in being comparatively wide from side to side but more thin than ordinary from front to back. Other figures are thick from front to back, and appear more rounded than ideal. Actual measurement studies of women throughout the United States reveal that the mean of women's measurements is far from ideal. She is both shorter and heavier than most

TABLE 4 MODEL MEASUREMENT CHART *

	HEIGHT			
	SHORT (under 5'4")	AVERAGE (5'4" to 5'6½")	TALL (5'7" to 5'9")	VERY TALL (over 5'9")
Bust	32–33	34–35	35–37	38–39
Waist	22–23	24–25	25–27	28–29
Hip	32–33	34–35	35–37	38–39
Upper thigh	18½	19	19½	20
Calf	12½	13	13½	14
Ankle	7½	8	8½	9
Upper arm	8½	9	9½	10

Note: for accuracy, measure over a bra but without a girdle. The hip is measured 7" to 8" below the waistline. The upper thigh is measured just below the groin. The calf is measured at the widest part, the ankle at the ankle bone, the upper arm is measured about midway between the elbow and the shoulder joint.

* John Robert Powers, *How to Have Model Beauty, Poise and Personality,* Prentice-Hall, Inc., Englewood Cliffs, N. J., 1960, p. 104.

women would like to be and is apt to have a poorly proportioned figure in many ways. Table 3 makes a comparison of the average figure with that of *Venus de Milo,* who is also more rotund than our contemporary figure ideal; Table 4 gives the ideal proportions sought in fashion models.

Louis Hippee of Warner Brothers uses the wrist as a unit of measurement. He says that "the wrist varies in size with one's bones, and on the weight and size of these depends the correct measurement for each person." [6]

The wrist is measured at the point where it joins the hand. This figure may be used in establishing the desirable measurements of various parts of the body; consult Table 5 for this ideal proportional relationship. Table 6 may be used to determine bone size on the basis of wrist circumference and height.

Although American women are conceded to have the best figures in the world, few women are fortunate enough to have a face and body of perfect proportions. Table 7 lists some characteristic physical traits that indicate

TABLE 5 RULE OF THE WRIST

Chest measures 5½ times the wrist
Waist measures 4 times the wrist
Hip measures 6 times the wrist
Thigh measures 3½ times the wrist
Calf measures 2½ times the wrist
Ankle measures 1¼ times the wrist

TABLE 6 BONE SIZE BASED ON WRIST MEASUREMENT

HEIGHT	SMALL-BONED WRIST	LARGE-BONED WRIST
Under 5′3″	Less than 5½″	Over 5¾″
5′3″ to 5′4″	Less than 6″	Over 6¼″
Over 5′4″	Less than 6¼″	Over 6½″

TABLE 7 SOME TYPICAL FIGURE IRREGULARITIES

STATURE AND BUILD	HEADS
Very tall, thin, and angular	Large in relation to body size
Tall and heavy-boned	Small in relation to body size
Short and slight	Round
Short and plump, small-boned	Square
Stout and heavy-boned	Long, narrow

[6] Statement in a letter, Warner Brothers, Hollywood, July 1, 1952.

TABLE 7 (*Continued*)

FACES
- Long, narrow
- Square or round with heavy jaws
- Heavy features
- Small features for body size
- Receding chin
- Prominent chin
- Prominent ears

NECKS
- Long and thin in proportion to head and shoulders
- Short and thick in proportion to head and shoulders
- Dowager's hump and neck forward

WAIST
- Flat and wide from side to side
- Thick through from front to back
- Long-waisted in proportion to height
- Short-waisted in proportion to height
- Abdomen prominent

HIPS
- Large in comparison with torso above waist
- Wide from side to side
- Low slung
- High slung
- Sway-back with prominent posterior
- One hip higher

ARMS AND HANDS
- Square hands and fingers
- Long, bony hands
- Short, thick hands
- Fleshy upper arms

NOSES
- Large, prominent
- Bulbous
- Roman
- Short and broad
- Short and thin
- Retroussé

MOUTHS
- Small, thin lips
- Straight and determined
- Weak
- Full lips

SHOULDERS
- Square and high
- Sloping
- Narrow
- Very wide in relation to head
- Prominent collar bones
- One shoulder lower than other

BUST
- Large, full
- Small
- Flat or no bust
- Low and flabby
- High in relation to waistline

LEGS, ANKLES, AND FEET
- Long in proportion to body
- Short in proportion to body
- Bowlegged
- Thick ankles
- Heavy thighs, calves, and ankles compared with above-waist proportions
- Legs set far apart, knees not together
- Square, wide, and peasant-like feet
- Short feet in relation to body proportions
- Knock-knees

POSTURE
- Flat chest
- Head held forward
- Round shoulders
- Knees snapped back tensely
- Body out of balance
- Prominent abdomen
- Lordosis curve

a lack of what is considered ideal. Means of minimizing figure problems will be discussed in Chapter Twelve.

Facial Contours

In silhouette the ideally shaped face is an ovoid, slightly flattened at the sides. The widest part of the face should come between the cheekbones, and the width should be approximately three-fourths the length of the face. In the accompanying illustration seven types of facial silhouettes are depicted together with descriptions (Figure 11). In determining face type it is important to observe that the face has four planes: the frontal plane, in which are the eyes, cheekbones, nose, and mouth; the forehead; and the other two areas, on either side of the face from the cheekbones to the hairline.

The profile of the ideal face is one that is nearly a straight line from forehead to chin, with the chin parallel to the floor. Deviations from this straight line are not unusual. A prominent nose may give the appearance of a line slanting backward from the tip of the nose to the hairline; a protruding jaw, a slanting line from chin to forehead. The combination of a receding forehead and chin and prominent nose produces a profile in which lines slant backwards from the tip of the nose. In evaluating the profile, especially in relation to hair style, there are some important balance lines to be considered. The distance from the crown of the head to chin should appear to equal that from the forehead to the nape of the neck; another point of balance is that from chin to ear and ear to the nape of the neck.

Proportion is another aspect of face structure. Features such as nose, eyes, and mouth vary considerably in size in relation to each other and to the total facial area. The placement of the brows and nose in the ideal face divides the area from hairline to chin into three parts. When this does not occur, there are such deviations as the high forehead. The placement of eyes may vary; they may be set farther apart or closer together than the ideal. It is, however, these individual differences that give faces their charm and distinction. Use of make-up and becoming necklines for various face shapes will be discussed in Chapter Twelve; and hair styles and hats, in Chapter Thirteen. Table 7 includes some of the common differences noted in faces.

The relationship of the head to the body should be considered as well as the contour of the face. The proportion of the head to the body is sometimes expressed in units of head lengths. A head length is the measurement from the chin to the crown of the head. The average person is seven and one-half head lengths in height; in other words, the total height may be

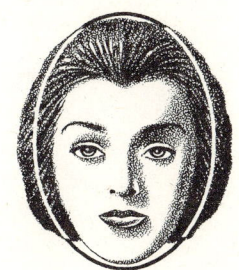

OVAL
The oval contour is the ideal shape.

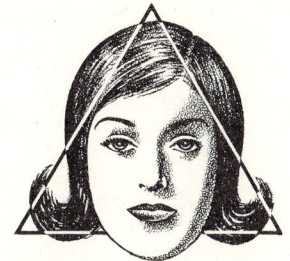

TRIANGLE
The forehead appears very narrow and tapering, and the jaws are very broad and wide.

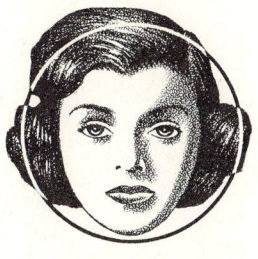

ROUND
This type appears quite full and has a rounded jawline and forehead.

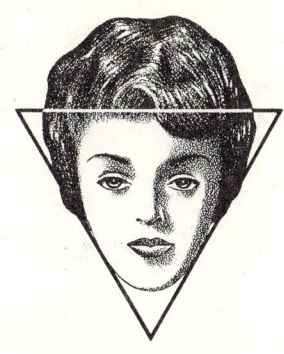

SQUARE
The horizontal line of the broad jaws and square chin is repeated in the square line across the forehead hairline and at the temples.

INVERTED TRIANGLE
The forehead is very broad, and the face tapers from the cheekbones to the jaws and chin line quite abruptly. The chin is usually pointed.

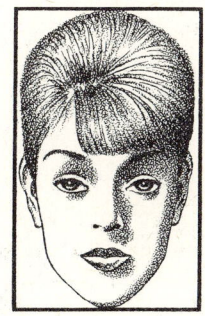

OBLONG
This is a long, thin face; the forehead is only slightly wider than the chin.

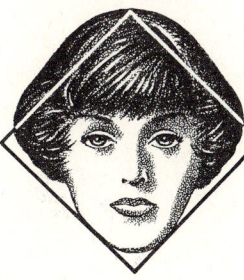

DIAMOND
Extreme width through the cheekbones, a very narrow forehead, and a pointed chin characterize this type.

Figure 11. Seven basic types of faces.

divided seven and one-half times by the length of the head. Fashion drawings may be done on figures of eight heads, but few women have faces this small in relation to total body length. The attenuated fashion figure does, however, display garments to the best advantage. Very high fashion drawings may be done on figures which are eight and one-half, nine, and ten heads.

CULTIVATING BEAUTY

Poise is a result of being at ease because one knows the accepted behavior and dress in social situations. Dress conventions will be dealt with in Chapter Fourteen. If in doubt about the social graces, consult books on etiquette to feel more confident.

As Rome was not built in a day, so you cannot become a more attractive person in all aspects overnight nor with one application of a cosmetic. The pathway to a more charming personality begins with the sincere desire to improve and requires planning and discipline. Faultless grooming takes constant attention over a lifetime. Correction of posture, weight, and voice problems results from practice; and once the objective has been reached, allow no slackening of standards. And as good grooming is a lifetime pursuit, so is the development of personality and the nourishing of the mind.

These, then, are the fundamental secrets of charm: scrupulous cleanliness, fine posture and carriage, an attractive voice and manner of speaking, and a pleasant facial expression reflecting inner graces. It is a comforting thought for the many who were born without a large measure of physical beauty that this kind of good looks is within reach of all, and that it is something which the world today recognizes and deeply admires. Without charm, all the lovely clothes money can buy will have little meaning or value.

The following list of books is suggested for further reading to help you in your quest for self-made beauty.

Marion R. Broer, *Efficiency of Human Movement*, W. B. Saunders Co., Philadelphia, 1960.
Anne R. Free, *Social Usage*, Appleton-Century-Croft, New York, 1960.
Ruth M. Leverton, *Food Becomes You*, The Iowa State University Press, Ames, Iowa, 1960. (Also Dolphin Books, Doubleday & Company, Inc., Garden City, N. Y., 1961.)
E. W. McHenry, *Foods Without Fads; A Common Sense Guide to Nutrition*, J. B. Lippincott, Philadelphia, 1960.

Ethel Austin Martin, *Nutrition in Action,* Holt, Rinehart and Winston, New York, 1963.

John Robert Powers, *How to Have Model Beauty, Poise and Personality,* Prentice-Hall, Inc., Englewood Cliffs, N. J., 1960.

Carolyn Hagner Shaw, *Modern Manners: Etiquette for All Occasions,* E. P. Dutton & Company, Inc., New York, 1958.

C. Raymond van Dusen, *Training the Voice for Speech,* McGraw-Hill, Inc., New York, 1953.

Katharine F. Wells, *Kinesiology,* Third Edition, W. B. Saunders Co., Philadelphia, 1960.

Eva D. Wilson, Katherine H. Fisher, and Mary E. Fuqua, *Principles of Nutrition,* John Wiley & Sons, Inc., New York, 1959.

Exercises

1. Honestly keep a list of all activities for a week and the time spent in each. Study this record, and from it formulate a workable plan for the more efficient use of your time.
2. With a friend or with several friends listen to each other speak. Is your voice pleasantly pitched, expressive? Do you enunciate distinctly? Is your speech free of provincialisms, slang, and grammatical errors?
3. Study your face in a mirror. What does it say about you? Are you a happy, considerate person or are you cross and selfish?
4. Before a full-length mirror, or preferably a triple mirror, examine your posture. Stand, walk, sit down, and arise. Are all your motions graceful and rhythmic?
5. Compare your height and weight with those of Tables 1 and 2. Evaluate your bone structure by the principle of Table 6.
6. Determine your body measurements and compare them with those given in Tables 3, 4, and 5.
7. Study your face to determine its characteristics of silhouette, profile, and individual features.
8. Divide your height by head-height. Crossed L-squares or an L-square and ruler will help in obtaining the head-height measurement.

Four

Expressing Personality Through Costume

Having been introduced to the values of personal appearance and the distinguishing qualities of style, we have yet to examine that culminating aspect of taste which may be reflected through dress as a means of personal expression. In order to achieve this goal, we must have not only an understanding of personal characteristics but also a working knowledge of the parts design, color, and texture play in harmonizing apparel with appearance and expression. To accomplish this harmony, we must first recognize that no two women are alike, even though their height, weight, general body structure, and coloring may be almost identical and their grooming equally meticulous. What is this personal quality which makes one individual different from another? The psychologist calls it personality, and defines it as "the study of the individual as a whole and of the interplay between him and other individuals in the normal course of living."[1] A new theory that draws heavily on sociological concepts tells us that personality differences are expressed in social roles. Cultural background and participation in a particular social structure determine the knowledge one has of a particular social

[1] Clifford T. Morgan, *Introduction to Psychology,* Second Edition, McGraw-Hill Book Company, Inc., New York, 1961, p. 467 (used by permission).

role, one's ability to perform, and one's motivation concerning it. Applied more specifically to one's appearance and choice of costume, this theory may be interpreted as the total impression or picture the individual presents to others.

America's dramatic fashion personality and acute observer of life, Valentina, believes that the designer must know and understand the people, because fashion reflects their whole life. A woman is far more interesting and distinctive if her clothes are made to express her own individuality than if they merely express a type or reflect the prevailing fashion. Selecting and designing costume becomes a problem of recognizing individual differences as well as searching for the line, the silhouette, the color, and the texture which best reflect or accent these physical and emotional traits. In this way she will attain a personal style by which she may be recognized. When costume reflects the whole personality, becomes unique, then and only then can it be considered a work of art.

PERSONAL EXPRESSION—ITS RELATION TO COSTUME SELECTION

How often have we heard the comment, "That dress looks exactly like Sally Smith." There may be certain suggested qualities of likeness; but you do not mean that the dress is five feet six inches tall and weighs 125 pounds, or that it has the beautiful rich warm coloring that makes Sally Smith so strikingly distinctive. You do, however, mean that the dress suggests the sophisticated youthful dignity, charm, and richness in coloring that Sally Smith means to you. Such a comment indicates that there are certain personal traits and modes of expression which are significant in the selection of costume.

Just as the person schooled in the art of flower arrangement presents a planned relationship between all component parts—the various flowers and the foliage, the particular form, texture, and color of the container, the completed arrangement and its background—so should the costume artist endeavor to key the component parts of the costume to the personality of the wearer. At all times it must be appropriate to the individual and the spirit of the occasion.

EVIDENCE OF OPPOSING CHARACTERISTICS

To those who enjoy watching streams of passers-by on city streets or groups of men and women in social gatherings, the study of visible evidences of masculinity and femininity in men and women is very interesting. Some women give the impression of delicacy of form and texture and gentleness of breeding: others are vital, forceful, compelling. Some men appear aesthetic and almost feminine in bearing, and others are extremely masculine in their physical vigor and reactions. Whether in man or woman, the impression may come from gesture, voice, or the positions taken by head, arms, or legs. It may be the facial expression which helps us to glimpse something of the individual's inner mood and temperament. It need not be motion, but the force that

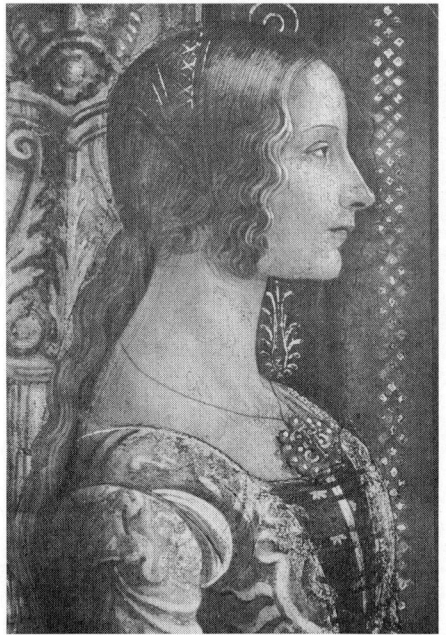

Figure 1. Ludovica Tornabuoni. *By* Ghirlandaio. Marie Novella, *Florence. This young woman gives the impression of mildness and gentle breeding.*

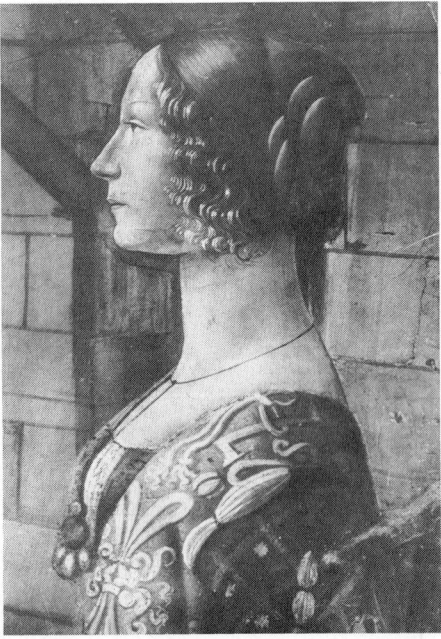

Figure 2. Giovanna Tornabuoni. *Detail from* The Visitation *by* Ghirlandaio. Marie Novella, *Florence. This portrait of a Renaissance aristocrat gives the impression of dignity, stately reserve, austerity, command, perhaps arrogance.*

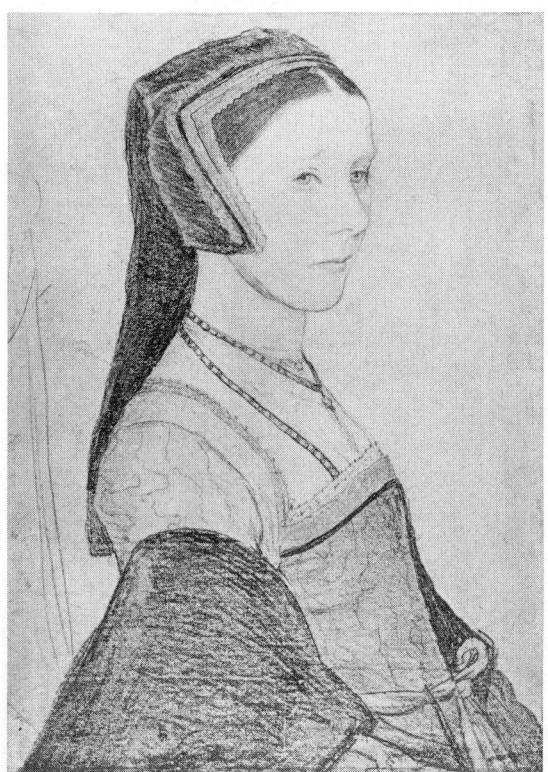

Figure 3. Anne Grisacre. *By* Hans Holbein. Windsor Castle.

we feel in every line and muscle—the tenseness of jaw that points to a sense of power, a sureness in the way of doing things, or conversely, an impression of naïve elusiveness. The two young aristocrats of the Italian Tornabuoni family manifest marked contrast in expression (Figures 1 and 2). Hans Holbein's portrait of *Anne Grisacre* depicts a gentle, sweet, demure, and slightly aloof young maiden of the sixteenth century (Figure 3).

In order that we may recognize, classify, and use these personal qualities as influencing factors or tools in the selection of apparel, we need some terms which will apply equally well in describing the overall effect of appearance in both individuals and costumes. The terms used by Miss Belle Northrup, formerly of Columbia University, for describing these opposing traits are *Yin* and *Yang*. They were found originally in ancient Chinese literature. These terms, while interesting in sound, are meaningless upon first hearing; at the same time they are easy to say, easy to remember, and they carry no undesirable connotation. To the Chinese, and hence to us, Yin means delicacy, softness, gentleness, fineness, fragility, exquisiteness, sensitiveness. All these traits imply feminine qualities. Yang is used to denote opposing traits such as sturdiness, firmness, strength, vigor, endurance. Yin aptly describes for us the exquisiteness of frost traceries in winter; and Yang, the sturdiness of the pine tree.

Individual Differences among Characters in History and Art

The embodiment of certain similar qualities may be recognized as we recall individuals depicted in history, literature, and the arts. There are those ladylike nineteenth century heroines, gentle, submissive, femininely alluring, whom we speak of patronizingly as Victorian. There is the great Elizabeth I of England who in her address to her officers before the attack of the Spanish Armada apologized for being "a weak woman." But she added, "I have the heart and stomach of a prince." There are also the many unknown aristocrats that reveal personality differences to us as we study canvases of the old masters.

Margot Fonteyn, contemporary English dancer and prima ballerina of The Royal Ballet, is known for her roles in *The Sleeping Beauty* and *Swan Lake*. She is dedicated to her work; it is almost a religion with her. "Off-stage, she retains the dignity associated with the many aristocratic parts she portrays, but there is no haughtiness, no coldness in this attitude, for her frequent smile is genuine and her laughing, mischievous eyes reveal a girl who likes nothing better than a joke, particularly when she herself is the butt of the joke." [2]

And there is Martha Graham, who "has made theatre a sacred place and has restored the dance to the position it once held as the expression of mankind's deepest thoughts and insights." She is "world famous and a classic figure in her own time. She belongs to that pitifully small group of the elect, who know no compromise and who hesitate at no sacrifice for their art." [3] Miss Graham's pioneering achievements in creative and dramatic dance express the forcefulness of a strong Yang personality.

Nature Expresses Opposing Qualities

We delight in the aesthetic charm of a fine flower garden in full bloom. The wonder of nature and the artistry of man merge to present an enchant-

---

[2] Walter Terry, *Star Performance,* Doubleday and Co., Inc., New York, 1954, p. 201.
[3] "The Martha Graham Season," Robert Sabin, *Dance Observer,* Vol. 29, No. 4, April 1962, pp. 53–54.

ing picture to behold. We realize that there are many scientific essentials involved, but do we recognize the semihuman factors? "Plants, like ourselves, have varying 'personalities,' although they cannot speak, hear, or see as we understand those faculties. Some of them are so vigorous and dominating that, without our equally forthright counteractions, they would soon crowd their weaker and less assertive neighbors to death. There are finicky ones, too, which sulk or succumb unless they receive the right amounts of water, heat, sunlight, or shade to which they have been accustomed." [4] We are impressed with opposing qualities as evidenced in nature. The delicate shape and color of the wood violet, the lacy leaf and the intriguing blossom of the bleeding heart, the daintiness and waxy whiteness of the lily-of-the-valley, all suggest to us the feminine or Yin attributes. In contrast to these we see the Shasta daisy with its fresh, clean-cut sturdiness, the robust zinnia, the vigorous sunflower, and the dramatic qualities of the calla lily, that reveal to us varying degrees of strength or forcefulness we call Yang.

The student of nature will recognize these qualities in birds, animals, and almost every natural object. You will find, however, that not all trees, flowers, and other living things can be fitted into these strongly opposing groups. Many objects of nature as well as individuals show a mingling of characteristics or express a combination of both qualities; we refer to these as intermediates. The fluctuation or the illusion of fluctuation given by the advancing and receding elements provide movement, and this is life. "When a proper balance has been reached, as in the ancient Yang-Yin symbol [Figure 4], it is impossible to say which is the negative and which is the positive element." [5] The pepper tree, with its gnarled sturdy structure, dainty leaf, and small red berry, exemplifies a composite of both Yang and Yin qualities. A similar combination may be seen in the iris. Its strong stems, stiff swordlike leaves, and deep green coloring denote Yang characteristics, while the delightfully fragile blossoms convey a feeling of Yin. Considering the above qualities from nature which express Yang or Yin, who would venture to say that one is more beautiful than the other—the violet, the calla lily, or the iris?

[4] Robert S. Lemmon and Charles L. Sherman, *Flowers of the World in Full Color*, Nelson Doubleday, Inc., New York, 1958, p. 183. (Reprinted by permission of Doubleday & Company, Inc.)
[5] Dorothy W. Riester, *Design for Flower Arrangers*, D. Van Nostrand Company, Inc., Princeton, N. J., 1959, p. 91.

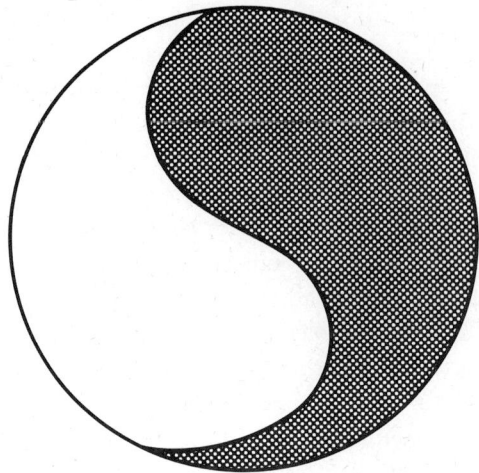

Figure 4. Yin-Yang symbol.

Evidences of Opposing Traits among Contemporary Women

Let us study these traits in some women of prominence and note some of the characteristics for which they are recognized. Dorothy Thompson, who was a journalist, lecturer, eminent authority on world affairs, and influential figure in American public life, had strong Yang qualities. These were exemplified in her leadership, drive, penetration, objectivity, and physical vitality. She was "possessed . . . of the gift of perpetual motion" [6] and so was at once exhilarating and exhausting.

Then there is Dorothy Shaver, former president of Lord and Taylor, a great New York retail store (Figure 5). Miss Shaver was the first woman in the history of the retail world to be elected to the presidency of a $50,000,000 corporation. She was recognized by the retail industry from the Atlantic to the Pacific for her merchandising foresight and vision. For this inspiring leadership and her numberless contributions to civic and national organizations, Miss Shaver received many awards. It was her belief that there is only one thing that keeps women from going ahead in business, and that is themselves. Her forceful and imaginative thinking has left its mark wherever fashion and creative design flourish.

That remarkable and admirable lady, Eleanor Roosevelt, was another indi-

---

[6] "Without Regrets," *Time,* Vol. 77, February 10, 1961, p. 66.

EXPRESSING PERSONALITY THROUGH COSTUME 53

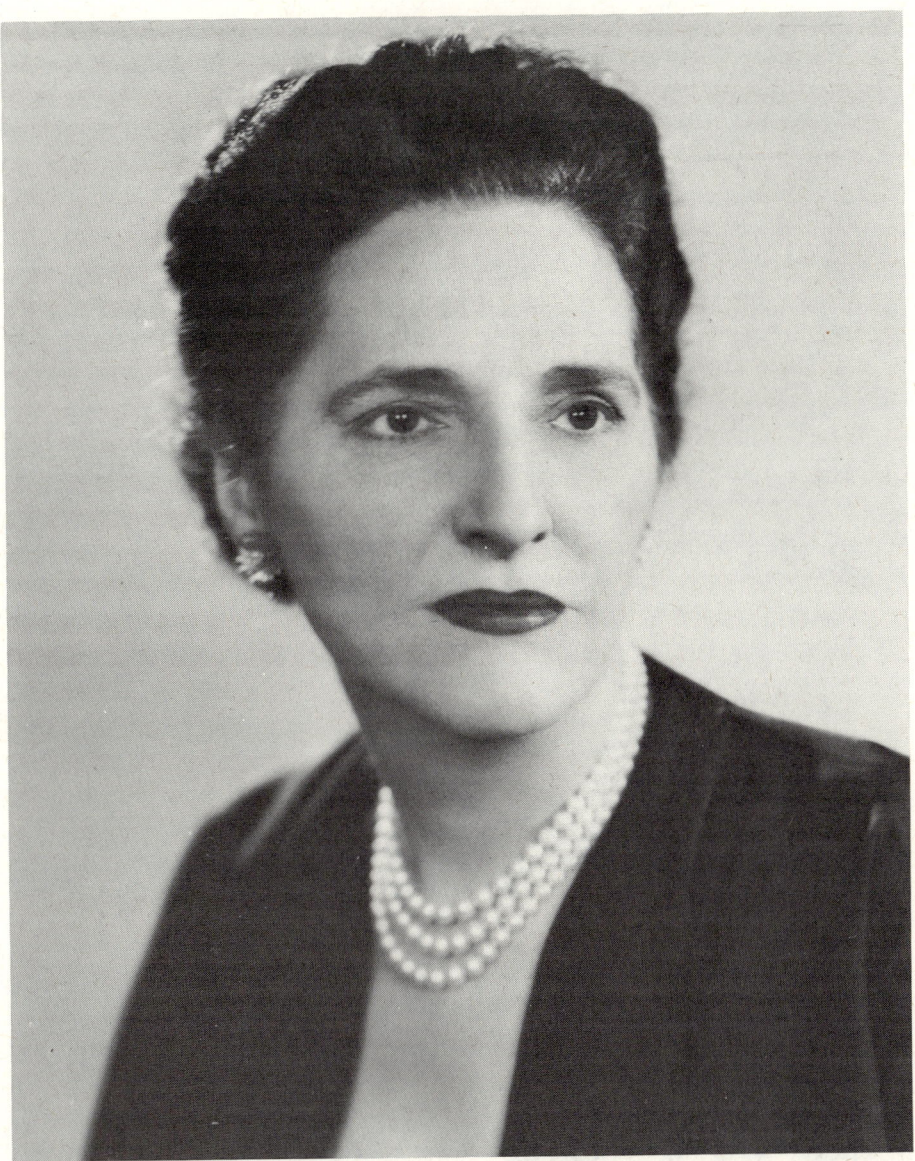

Figure 5. Dorothy Shaver. From this portrait one gains the impression of a forceful, compelling, objective mind, capable of great leadership and creative achievement. Courtesy of Lord & Taylor.

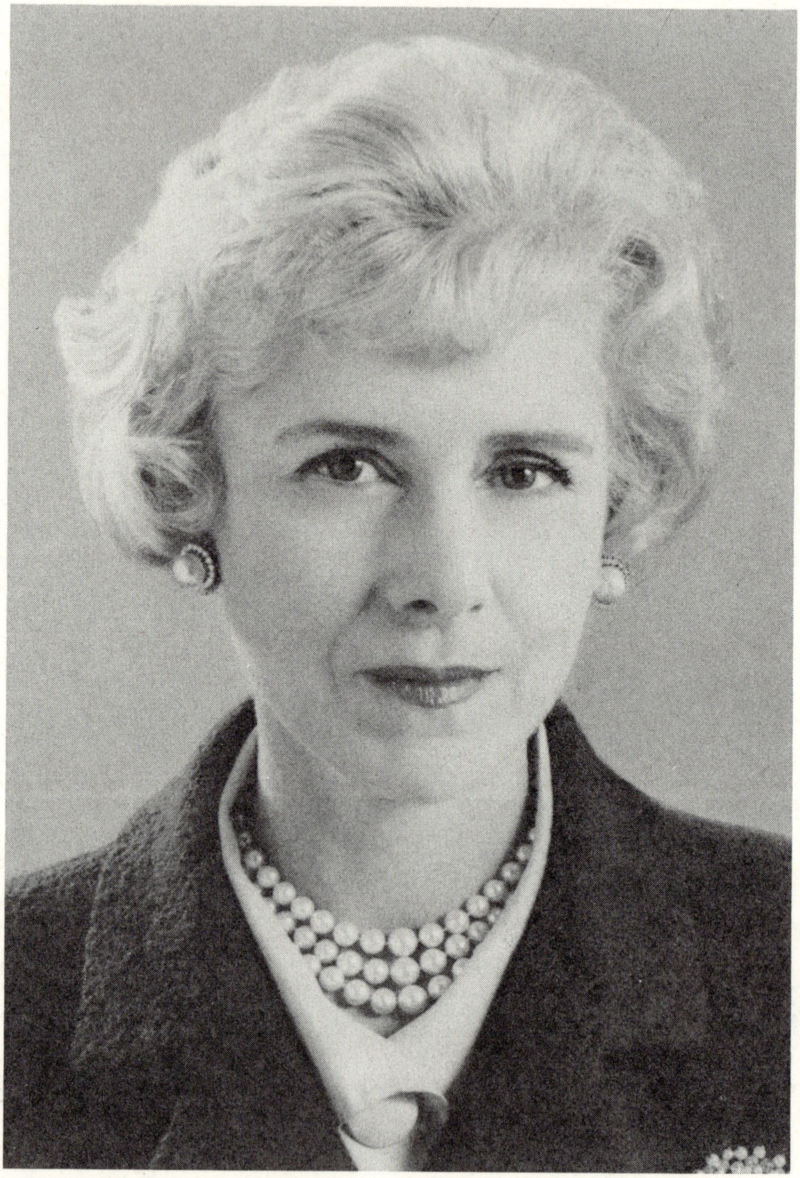

Figure 6. Clare Boothe Luce. A beautiful and talented woman who has gained distinction through her interest and understanding of national and international affairs. Courtesy of Mrs. Luce.

vidual with many forceful traits. From a tall, spindly, painfully shy girl, she developed into a fearless, direct, absolutely unself-conscious American woman whose energy was unflagging and who has been compared to a human dynamo. Her son described her as a "peripatetic spokesman for democracy, champion of the oppressed and underprivileged, and crusader for a thousand and one good causes." [7] Her own life, her own personality are typified by her words to the young, "Do not stop thinking of life as an adventure. You have no security unless you can live bravely, excitingly, and imaginatively; unless you can choose a challenge instead of a competence." [8]

Everywhere in professions and business we encounter successful women with marked Yang tendencies. Nevertheless, many of the finest women in public life today are those whose tendencies are inherently feminine or Yin but who possess sufficient force and drive to enable them to fill positions of great influence in business, the professions, and public life. Among these women we think of Clare Boothe Luce, who has managed a full life as author, playwright, congresswoman, and ambassador as well as being the wife of a famous editor. Newswriters have described her as a Beautiful American, a versatile woman, a headstrong person; but also as one with manners, one with information, and one with experience (Figure 6).

And then there is Great Britain's charming young monarch, Queen Elizabeth II, who exemplifies to a high degree a quality of femininity beautifully reflected in her devotion to family, combined with intuitive vision, tact, poise, understanding, and efficiency in discharging her responsibilities (Figure 7).

Another charming person in public life today is Queen Sirikit of Thailand. She is petite and womanly and has been described as one of the most delightful beauties in the world (Figure 8).

Similar characteristics may be recognized among women of all ages and stations in life.

Life Goals Reflected in Personal Qualities

There is a new freedom for women today and a feeling that "women, like men, should give their highest skills to a society which badly needs them." [9]

---

[7] "My Mother—Eleanor Roosevelt," James Roosevelt, *Good Housekeeping*, Vol. 150, May 1960, pp. 62–63. (Reprinted by permission.)
[8] "What Has Happened to the American Dream," Eleanor Roosevelt, *Atlantic*, Vol. 207, April 1961, pp. 46–50.
[9] "Femininity," Betty Hannah Hoffman, *Ladies Home Journal*, Vol. 79, No. 7, July–August, 1962, p. 56. (By special permission.)

56 *The Arts of Costume and Personal Appearance*

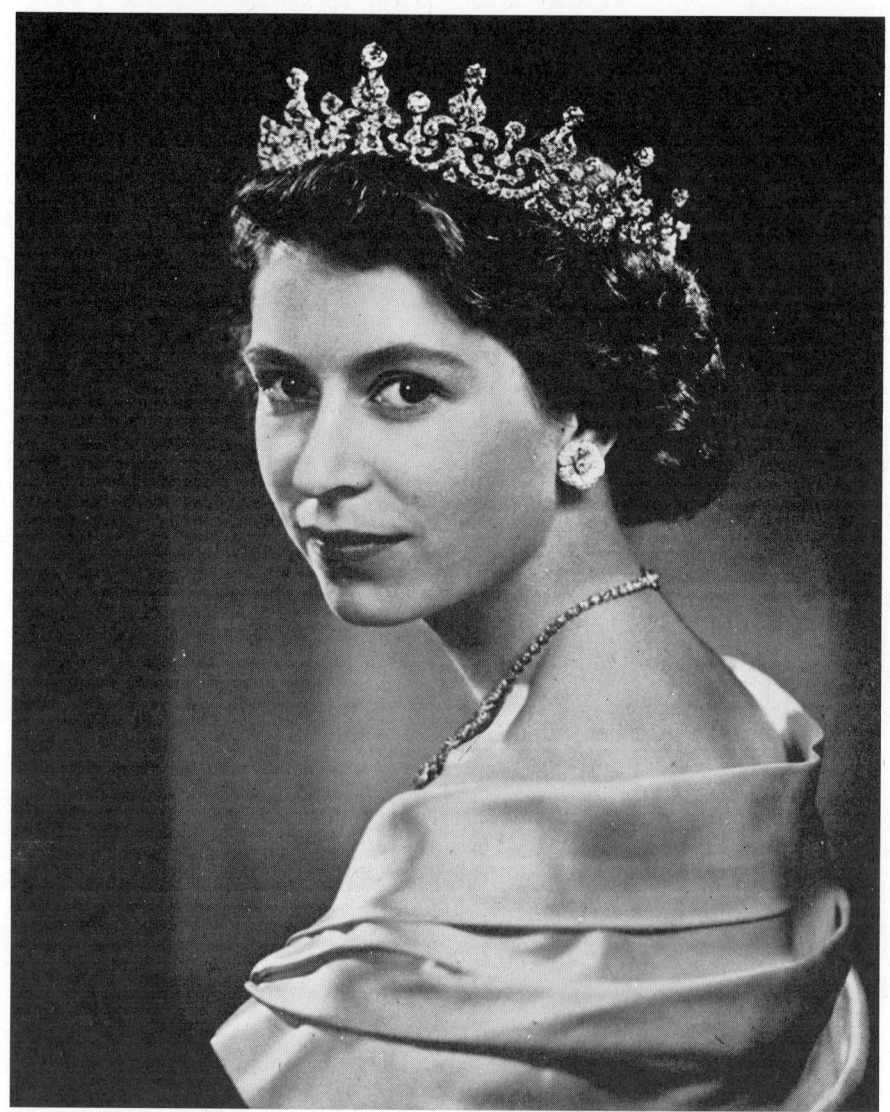

Figure 7. Elizabeth II. This portrait reflects the delightful feminine charm of Great Britain's Queen, which has endeared her to peoples of all countries. Courtesy of British Information Service.

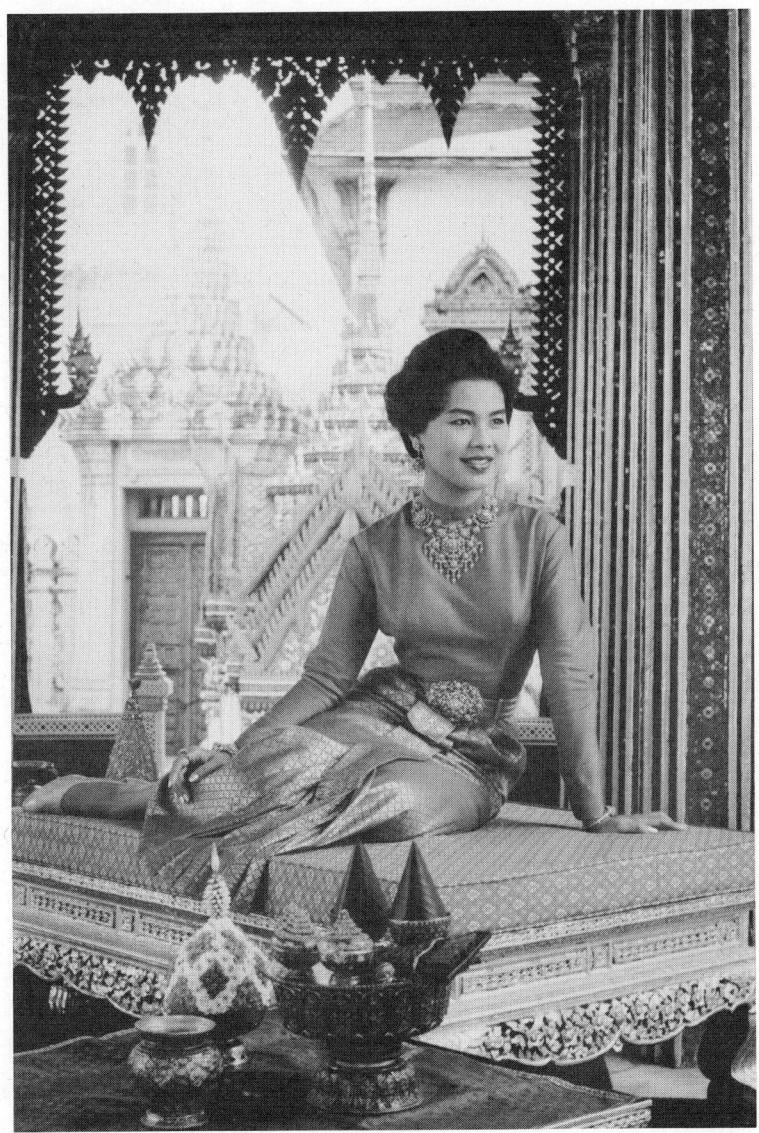

Figure 8. Sirikit. Her Majesty the Queen of Thailand. Courtesy of the Queen.

Woman wants this new freedom to help develop her capacities—both intellectual and emotional—to the fullest extent. In her desire for self-expression, however, she often becomes ill-natured and shrewish. When women are too intense in the pursuit of their goal, they lose the warmth and wholesome womanliness one has a right to expect in them, and become too self-sufficient, sometimes intolerant. "This need not be," says charming actress Arlene Francis. "I'm just beginning to see a Renaissance of femininity, which did not exist a few years ago. Now there is a new awareness on women's part that they don't have to push and strain. If a woman is aware that *first of all* she is a woman—then she can do anything without losing her femininity. . . ."[10] And being first of all a woman means that she is as little like a man as possible. Women must realize that men cannot accept women who do not accept themselves as feminine beings.

The secrets of Helen Hayes' success as a personality are her seemingly utter freedom from pride and egotism, her unassuming ingenuousness, her intuition and discernment. Being a star has never lessened her greatness as a personality nor her dedication to public service (Figure 9).

It is this warmth and emotional quality that has made us regard Katharine Cornell as one of the most charming of actresses. Theater-goers appreciated this quality; in empathy with her, found release from their own tense natures (Figure 10).

One of the delightful postwar personalities of stage and screen is Julie Harris (Figure 11). Her rise to prominence has been meteoric, and she is considered one of the "greats" in the theater today. Descriptive terms used by critics concerning Miss Harris include "enormous range," "incomparable sensibility," "subtle, elusive, poignant play of moods," "poetic and lovable," "wistful and tender." She is a small, slender person with blue eyes, reddish blond hair, and mobile features.

Anne Fogarty is another career woman, wife, and mother who reveals herself to us as a light, gay, artistic, feminine, but practical woman (Figure 12). Glamourous, feminine, and easy-to-wear clothes comprise the Anne Fogarty Look that has influenced the entire fashion world in but a few short years.

The above instances give brief glimpses of some of the outstanding attributes of a few notable contemporary women, and they may help us to see and appreciate the traits which tend to make one woman different from another. The analyses in Table 1 present some of these physical characteristics, in

[10] *Ibid.*, p. 57.

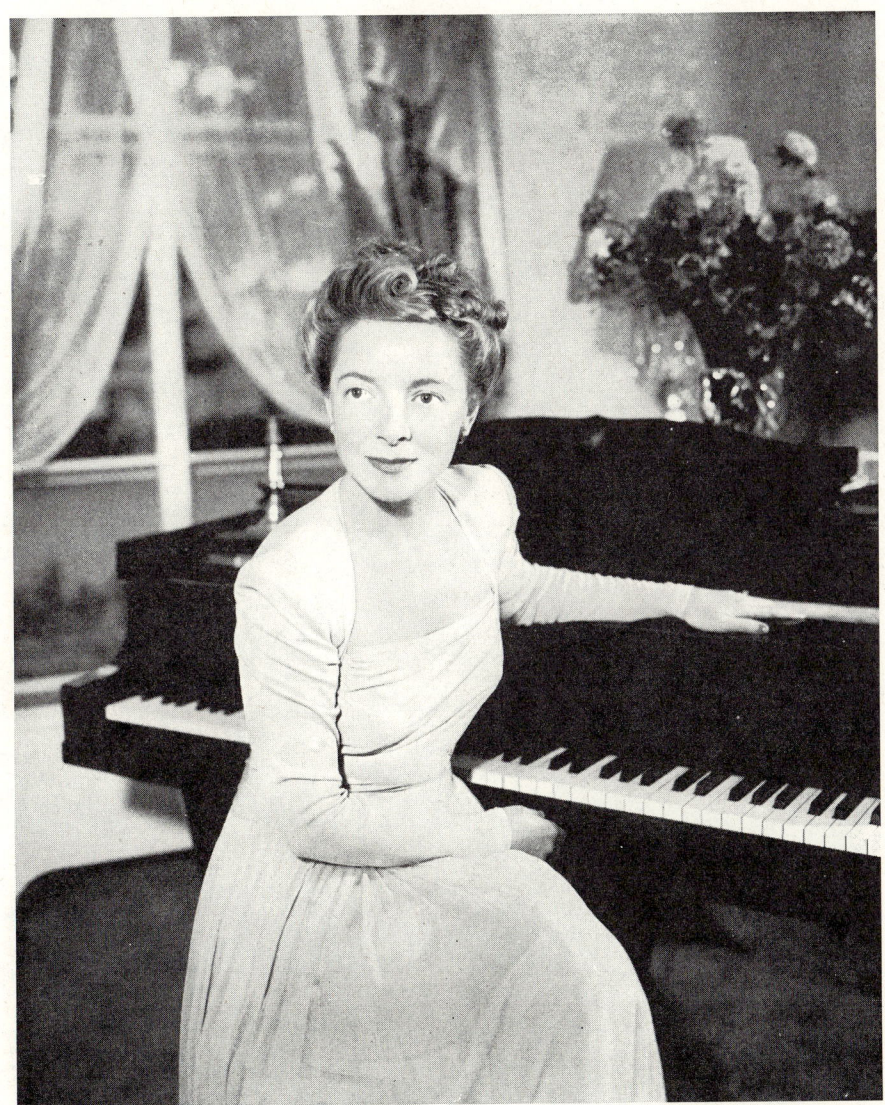

Figure 9. Helen Hayes in her Nyack home. Small, dainty, ingenuous-looking; a distinctly feminine personality of strong idealism. Courtesy of Miss Hayes.

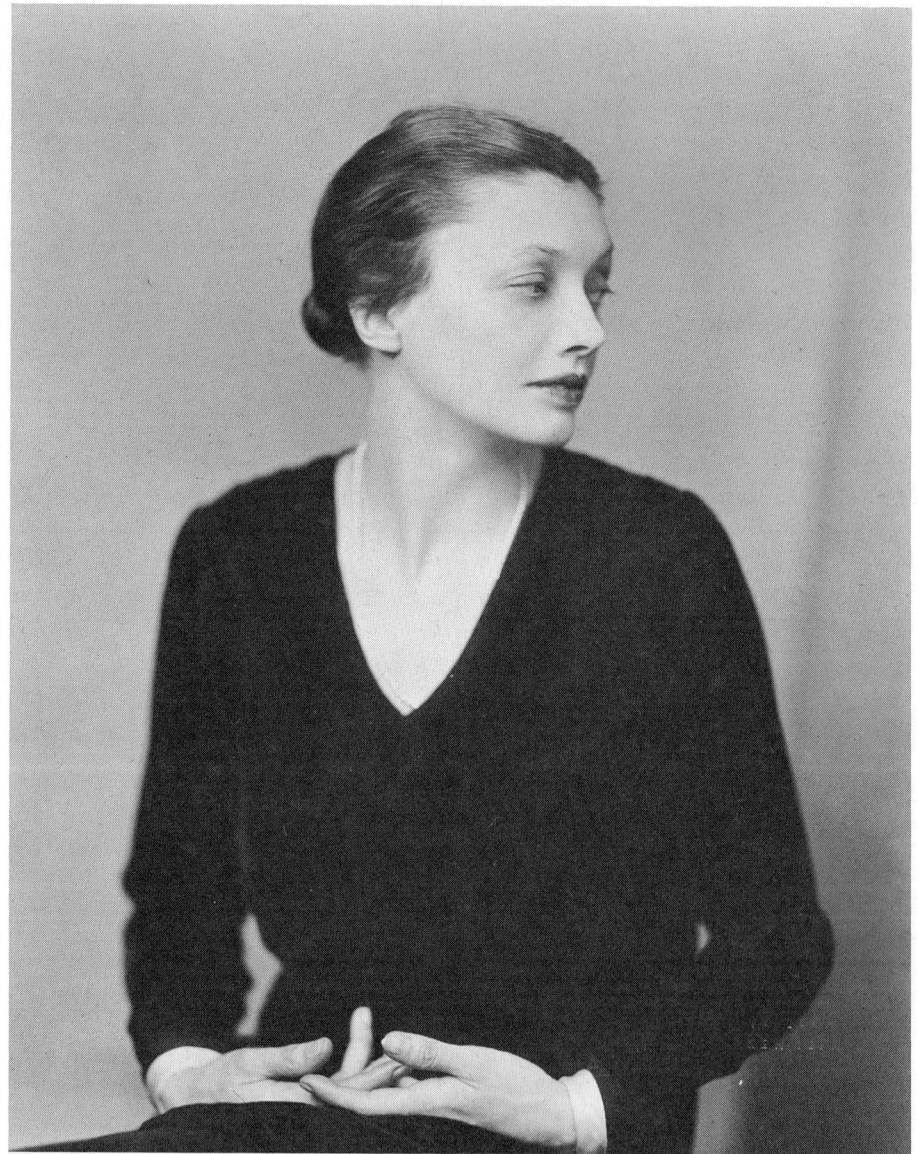

Figure 10. Katharine Cornell in a favorite portrait which makes its appeal through its pervading quality of grace, sincerity, and charm. Courtesy of Miss Cornell.

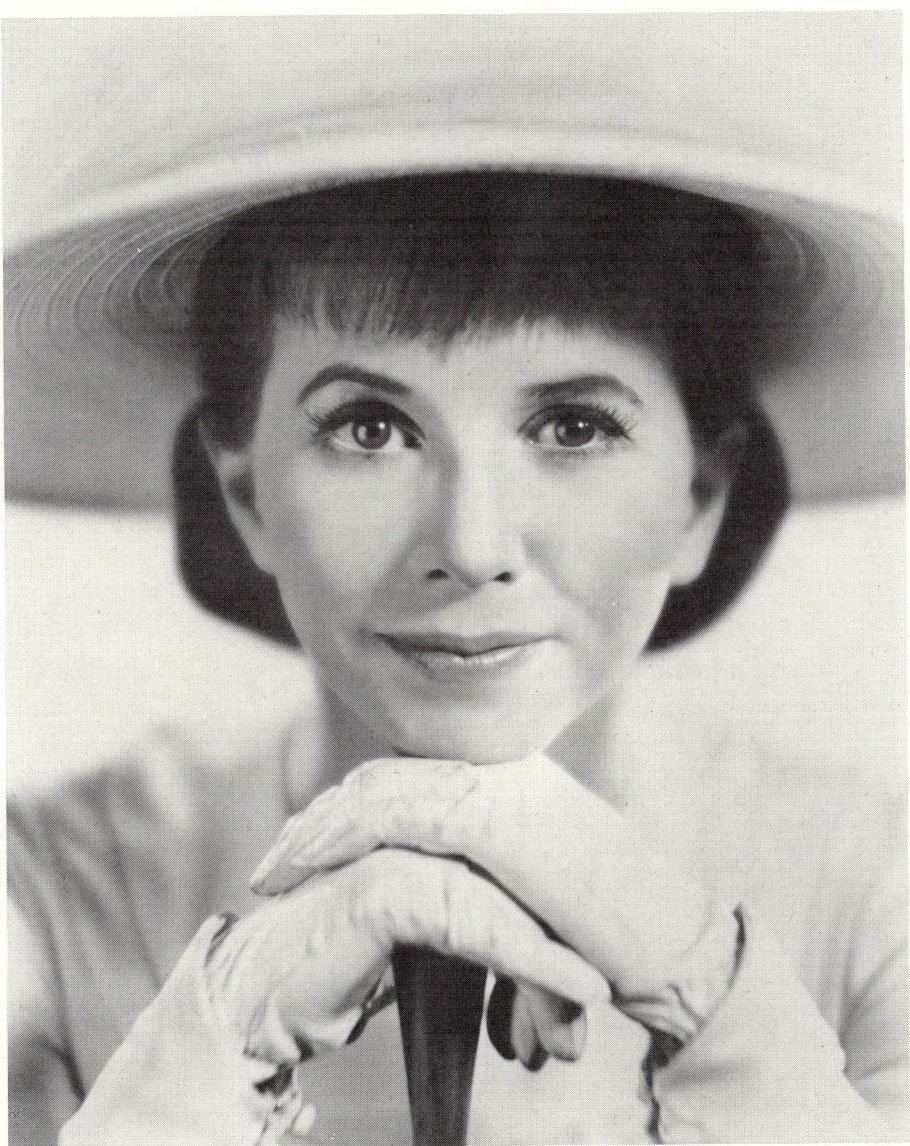

Figure 11. Julie Harris. Small, blue-eyed, unfreckled redhead with clear, pleasant and expressive features. Courtesy of Miss Harris.

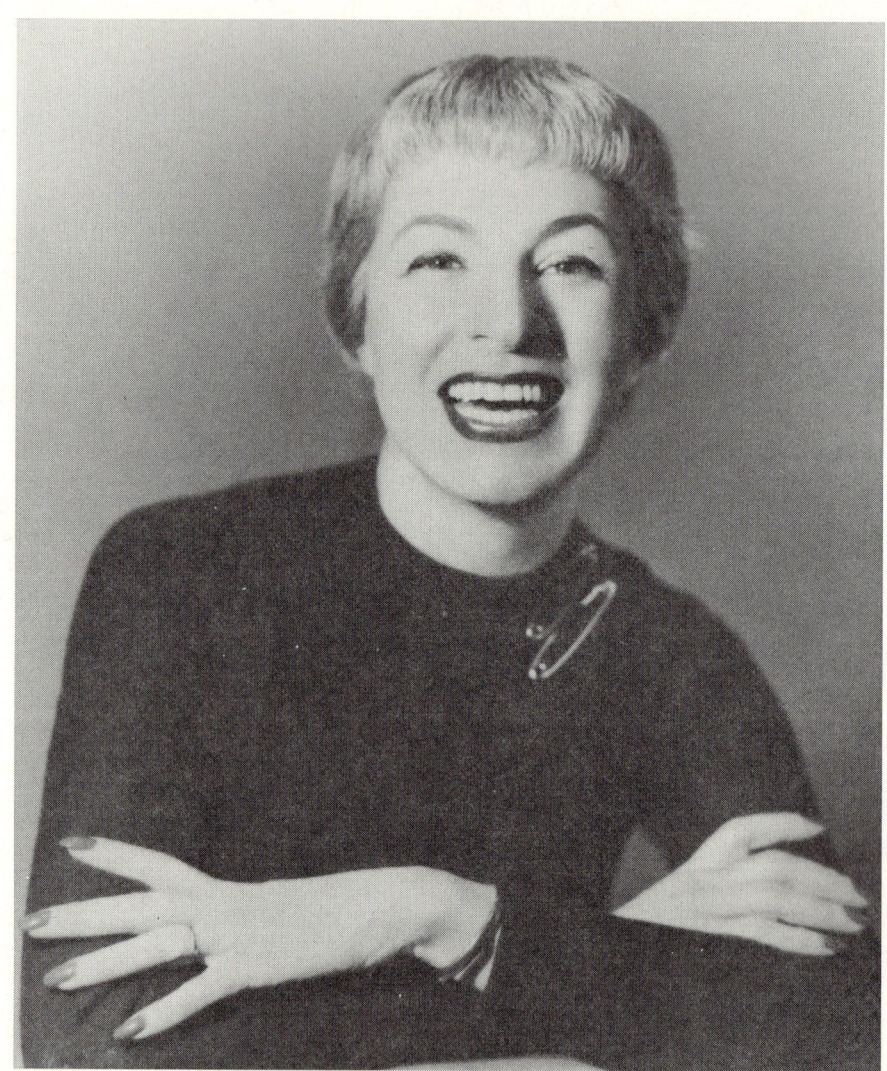

Figure 12. Anne Fogarty. Her talent for creating clothes so typically American has won her recognition throughout the fashion world. Courtesy of Miss Fogarty.

TABLE 1 PERSONAL CHARACTERISTICS AFFECTING COSTUME SELECTION

YANG
PHYSICAL ASPECTS

Body structure
Tall, large-scale, well-proportioned, erect, expressing strength, stateliness, forcefulness, vitality, and dynamic energy; large, clear-cut features.

Traits of movement
Firm, long vigorous stride, purposeful, legato, steady, and controlled.

Coloring
Vivid, warm, tending to be dark with strong contrast.

Skin
Rich, smooth, tending to be heavier in texture, sometimes coarse.

Hair
Straight or large loose waves, smooth, sleek.

Eyes
Large, long oval; dark eyebrows, sharply marked.

TEMPERAMENTAL ASPECTS
Self-sufficient, compelling, aggressive, dominating, decisive, reserved, desiring to lead and protect.

Objective
Analytical quality of mind.

Realistic
Recognition of conditions as they exist, with an attempt to modify them where improvement seems possible.

Sophisticated
Air of experience, knowing one's way about, ability to disguise or dramatize feelings.

YIN
PHYSICAL ASPECTS

Body structure
Petite, small-scale, well-proportioned, delicately formed, expressing daintiness, fragileness, and femininity; small dainty features.

Traits of movement
Light, airy, graceful, quick, staccato, impulsive.

Coloring
Delicate, cool, tending to be light with medium to slight contrast.

Skin
Delicately smooth, fresh, usually fine texture.

Hair
Soft, fluffy or curly, fine texture.

Eyes
Wide open, rounded; arched eyebrows.

TEMPERAMENTAL ASPECTS
Dependent, gentle, pliant, receptive, submissive, yielding, tactful, desiring to follow and to please.

Intuitive
Quick perception of truth without resort to reasoning.

Idealistic
Tendency to form ideals which may be difficult of realization.

Ingenuous
Natural, simple, naïve, unsophisticated, artless.

TABLE 2 YIN-YANG COSTUME CHARACTERISTICS

	QUALITIES OF DESIGN, COLOR, AND TEXTURE GIVING A YANG EFFECT	QUALITIES OF DESIGN, COLOR, AND TEXTURE GIVING A YIN EFFECT
LINES	Straight and restrained curves, usually used in a vertical movement. Long, unbroken, or having large sharp distinct breaks. Large, full, round curves.	Modified straight, restrained curves broken in such a way as to produce small detail. No unrelieved straight sharp lines. Full round curves.
SILHOUETTE	Straight and modified straight. Smooth, striking. Extremes of the bouffant for the young sophisticates.	Straight when modified by soft details. Bouffant. Short jackets. Boleros. Brief peplums.
SPACES	Large, bold. Unrelieved unbroken areas.	Smaller broken areas. Large areas broken by gathers, shirring, tucks, pleats, seaming, pockets.
SCALE	Individual sections of silhouette large in scale, as: large sleeves, collars, cuffs, yokes, torso jackets; large trimmings, as buttons, belts.	Small detail, such as dainty yokes, collars, and other trimming details; small buttons, bows, lace, cording.
FABRIC DESIGN AND TEXTURE	Large to medium size, exotic or conventionalized figures. Stripes and plaids.	Small scale allover conventionalized floral designs and geometric patterns which blend closely with backgrounds.
	Texture: Heavy, stiff, rough, rich, metallic, drapable, lustrous. Voluminous amounts of light-weight material.	Texture: Soft, pliable, fine, dull, crisp, sheer, napped, delicate.
COLOR AND VALUE CONTRAST	Strong contrasts in value. Dark, rich colors. Warm and warm-cool hues. Bright intensities.	Medium to close values. Medium to light colors. Cool and cool-warm hues. Soft grayed intensities.

their superlative form, that affect one's selection of costume. They are generic qualities which may be used to recount many of the opposing traits recognized in women of all ages.

As you study these characteristics which give the impression of Yang and Yin, it may help you to understand yourself better if you underline those which you feel best relate to you. It is likely that few of you will find that you embody exclusively the qualities expressed by either of the opposing groups. It is also likely that very few, if any, would have a great desire to be either Yin or Yang exclusively. This organization of traits may serve, however, as a guide in discerning certain outer manifestations of individual differences as they occur in varying degrees and combinations.

CONVEYING INDIVIDUALITY THROUGH COSTUME

The greatest use of such an appraisal of individual differences lies in the possibility it affords of relating these qualities to the character or style of costume. All manner of individual variations may be found among us. Some women express Yang characteristics through body structure and coloring, but are gentle and receptive in their responses; others may be dainty or even fragile in build but inclined to be dominating and decisive in their reactions. These many variables provide abundant opportunity for imagination and creative ability in the field of costume. The character or expressiveness of a costume depends upon the quality of line, the silhouette, the boldness or daintiness of detail, the texture, and the color or color combination, each element reflecting in its own way certain significant qualities of the wearer. In subsequent chapters we shall discuss some of the principles which should be observed in recognizing, understanding, and using the plastic elements of design in producing distinctive and expressive effects. In Table 2, opposing expressive effects are differentiated.

You will enjoy the following references which will help to broaden your understanding of people and of dressing to convey personal mood and expression.

Anne Fogarty, *Wife Dressing,* Julian Messner, Inc., New York, 1959.
Elizabeth Hawes, *It's Still Spinach,* Little, Brown and Company, Boston, 1954.
Edith Head, *The Dress Doctor,* Little, Brown and Company, Boston, 1959.

Anne Morrow Lindbergh, *Gift from the Sea,* Pantheon Books, Inc., New York, 1955. (A delightful book that may help the reader to understand herself a little better.)

Claire McCardell, *What Shall I Wear?,* Simon and Schuster, New York, 1956.

Exercises

1. Look up the meanings of the following traits and attempt to recognize these traits in people of your acquaintance: pliant, phlegmatic, objective, nurturing, ingenuous, direct, indirect, naïve, intuitive.
2. Study the members of your class and your associates for differences in personal expression.
3. Among men and women passing in a public place, attempt to identify physical and temperamental traits by appearance. Write an analysis of several whose physical or temperamental traits interest you.
4. Select photographs of women from magazines and analyze them for their Yin-Yang characteristics.

Five

Design Essentials for Good Costume

One who is learning the meaning of taste and distinction in costume must think of it as an art, understand what constitutes good design, and learn to distinguish real beauty and elegance from the tricky or eye-catching so frequently seen around us. We must view designs quite apart from personal preference, and test them by the same criteria we would use in judging a painting or a work of sculpture. We need familiarity with design principles, not as rigid laws to follow unerringly, but as guides. We must remember that these guides are the result of centuries of observation on the part of people of taste, and the beginner will find them the best basis for determining what will be agreeable to the sensitive observer.

All art is concerned with the organization of certain fundamental elements, called by some the *plastic elements,* because it is possible to manipulate them. The plastic elements are line, form, space, color, and texture. In order that we may grasp what we see when we are making selections of costume, it is necessary to think of each element individually so that we may better see how it fits into an organization, and determine wherein it makes the design pleasing or otherwise.

George Cox writes in his *Art for Amateurs and Students,* "We cannot

68   *The Arts of Costume and Personal Appearance*

say that one line is ugly and another beautiful, one space fine and another unsightly, until they belong to some definite organization, for everything depends upon the relative position and proportions of such lines and spaces within a composition, whether the frame be a building or a vase, a rug or a picture."[1] In a similar manner we judge the relationship of individual lines and spaces to each other and to the silhouette of the costume.

The classification of art terminology as outlined below may enable us to see the plastic elements in relation to the principles which determine the manner of their use. In this chapter we shall study those plastic elements which form the structure of any work of art, learn to recognize their different aspects, and by studying illustrations of masterpieces, come to recognize their use in costume.

BASIC ART TERMS

PLASTIC ELEMENTS	PRINCIPLES OF COMPOSITION	ATTAINMENT
Line	Balance	Harmony
Form	Proportion	
Space	Rhythm	
Color	Emphasis	
Texture		

LINE

A line joins two points. This is a very simple definition, and yet line wields an immense power within and about each one of us. Lines indicate the shape of things; they provide movement and direction; and they express attitudes and emotions. Line is the easiest, yet the most difficult element to learn to know; easy because we constantly abstract it from nature, and difficult because it is so subtle.

In nature we enjoy lines in the branching of trees, in the movement of fish through water, the contour of hills, the plumes of smoke, or the rhythm of dancing figures. In art we know them as the distinguishing element in fine etchings, in Japanese prints, or in the drawings of Botticelli, Holbein, or Leonardo da Vinci.

No other element is so important to good costume. All the great periods of fashion are distinguished by their line. Lines separate entire areas into

---

[1] George Cox, *Art for Amateurs and Students,* Doubleday, Doran & Co., New York, 1926, p. 16.

individual shapes and background spaces and are an important contributing factor in beauty of form.

Sometimes the creative designer best expresses his intention by giving his design a certain line quality, as in the robes of medieval figures, the portrait drawings of Ingres (Figures 1 and 2), or the draped evening gowns of today in which the fabric has the right weight or body. On the other hand the

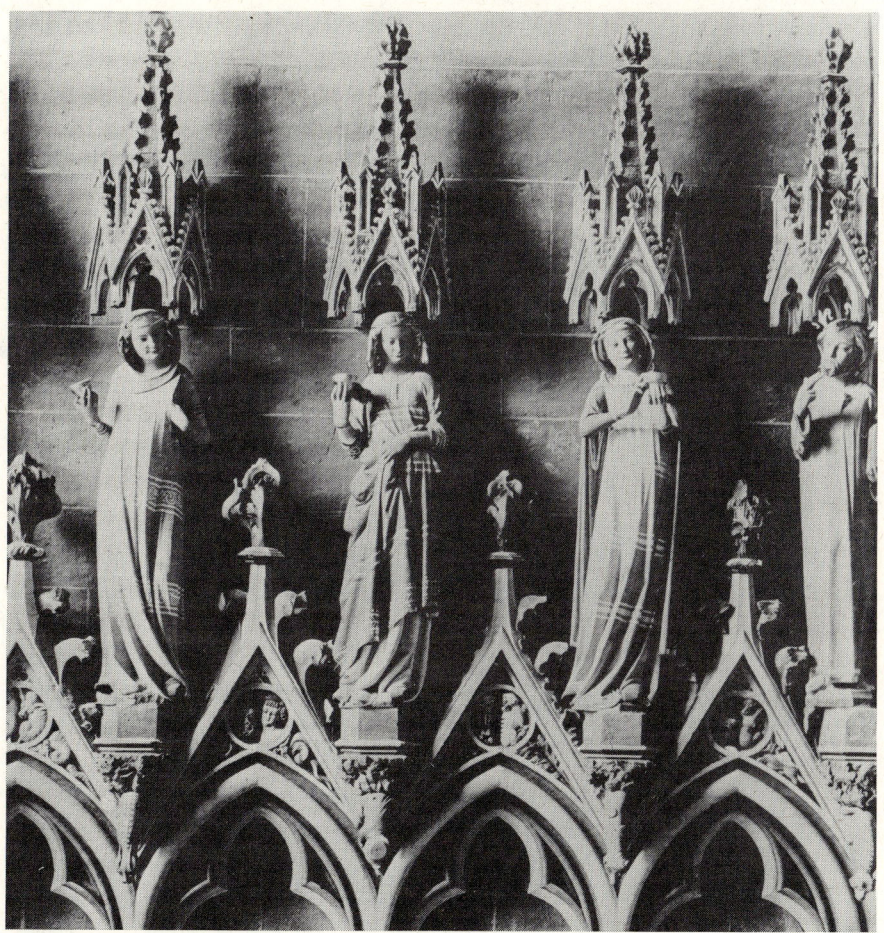

Figure 1. Fifteenth-century sculptured figures. Freiburg Cathedral. *Vertical upward-rising lines form the dominant structure of these medieval robed figures, but a more careful study reveals also groupings of horizontal lines, beautifully spaced.*

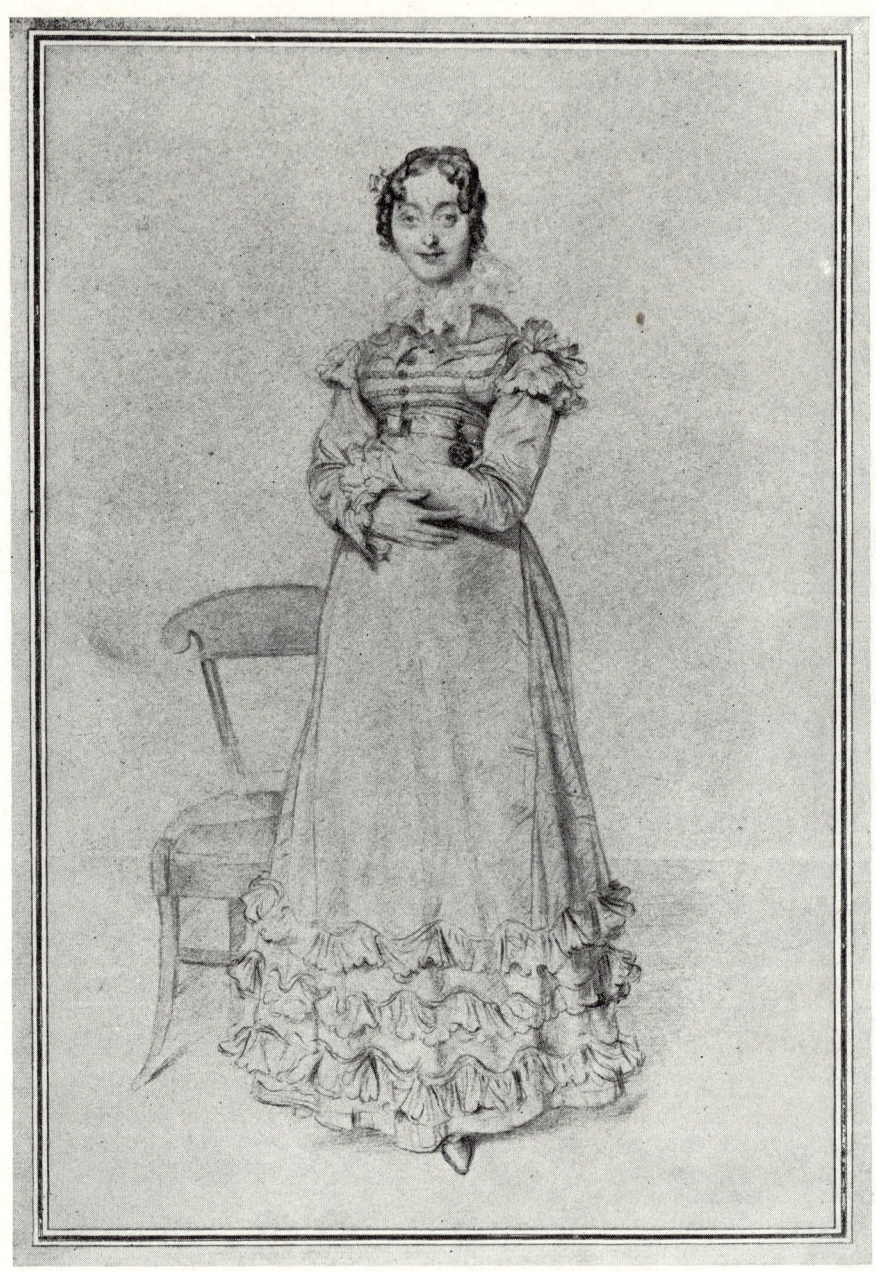

Figure 2. Madame Le Blanc. *By Jean Auguste Ingres, 1819. Ingres' portrait of a lady interests us for its delicate line quality. The simple vertical lines of the Empire gown are enriched by the horizontal movement of frills, and pastel-colored bows and belt contrast vivaciously with the clear, definite shape of the chair.*

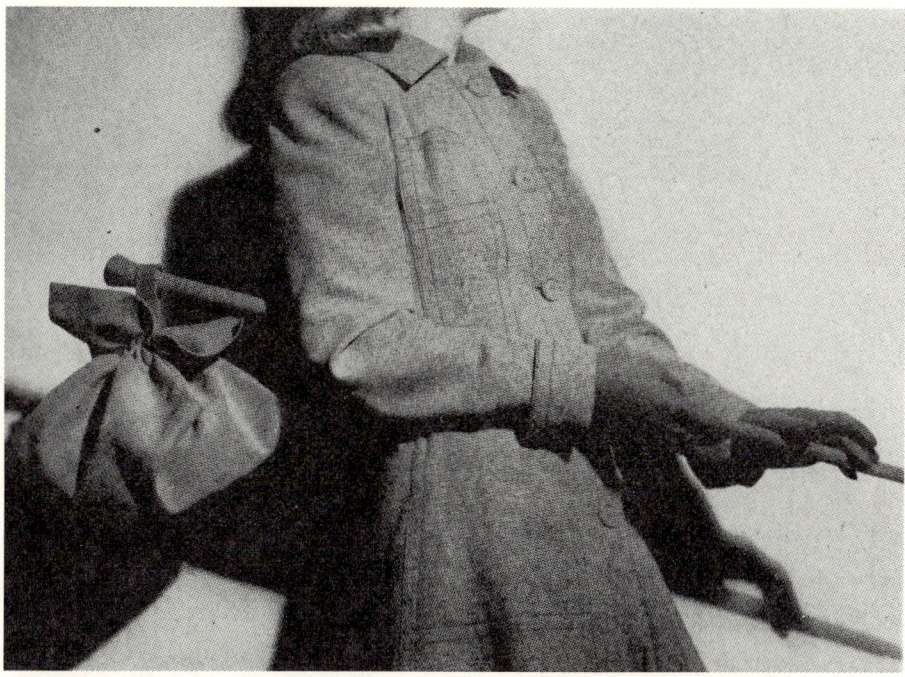

Figure 3. Trench coat. By Lucien Lelong. Courtesy of Harper's Bazaar. Cut on straight lines, this coat of gray flannel gains distinction by its simple structure outlined in machine stitching, expertly done.

designer may want his shapes to dominate his work; then he invents ways to accent his shapes whereby certain areas are outlined distinctly against their background.

Basically, there are two kinds of lines.

Straight lines form the basic structure of skyscrapers, contemporary furniture, and tailored street clothes worn by both men and women (Figure 3). These lines are rather stiff and severe; they suggest something impersonal, firm, and practical.

Curved lines are neither straight nor angular, but rounded to whatever degree desired. The degree to which they are rounded determines the kind of curve. We see restrained curves in the graceful stem of a flower, in trailing smoke, in the line direction which a football takes when kicked into the air, in the figures of ancient Chinese paintings, and in the undulating lines of a picture hat (Figures 4 and 5). Full, round curves are exemplified by the

72　*The Arts of Costume and Personal Appearance*

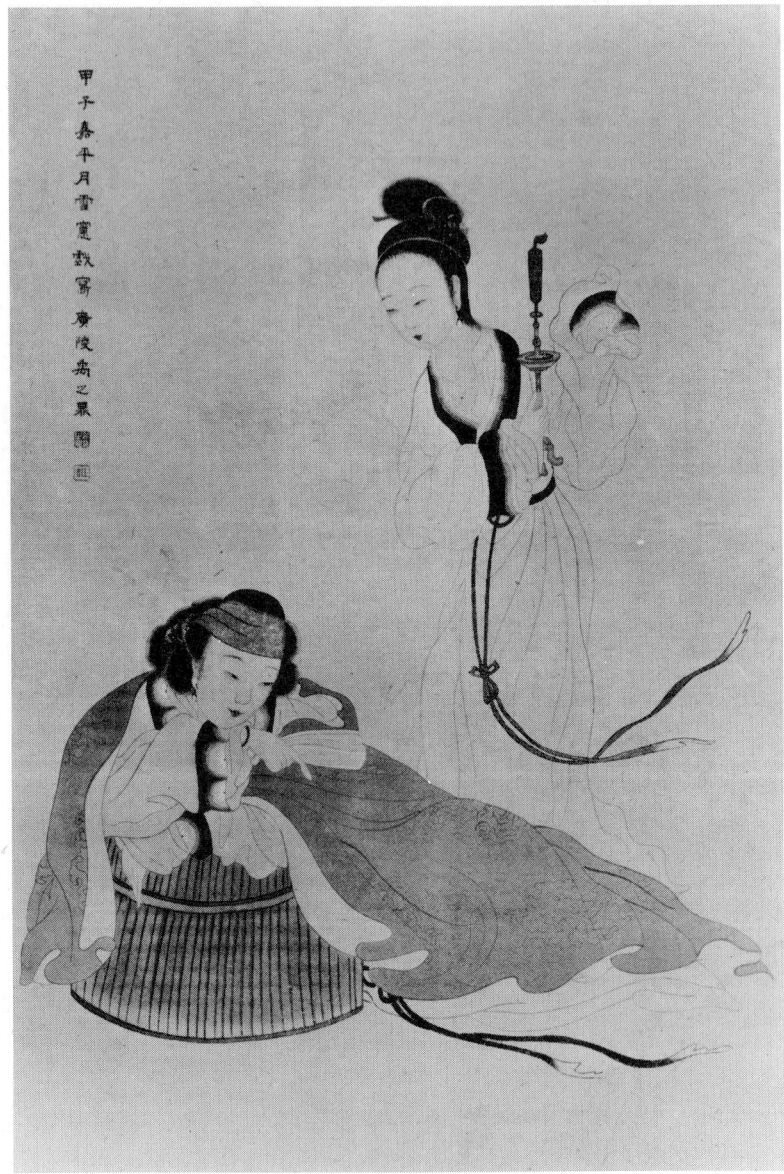

Figure 4. Maiden bringing a candle to her mistress. By Yü Chih-Ting, A.D. *1684. Courtesy of British Museum. The graceful, flowing quality of line in the gowns is emphasized by the intense blacks and the delicate orange and pale greenish blue of mantle and headband against quiet, restful background spaces.*

DESIGN ESSENTIALS FOR GOOD COSTUME 73

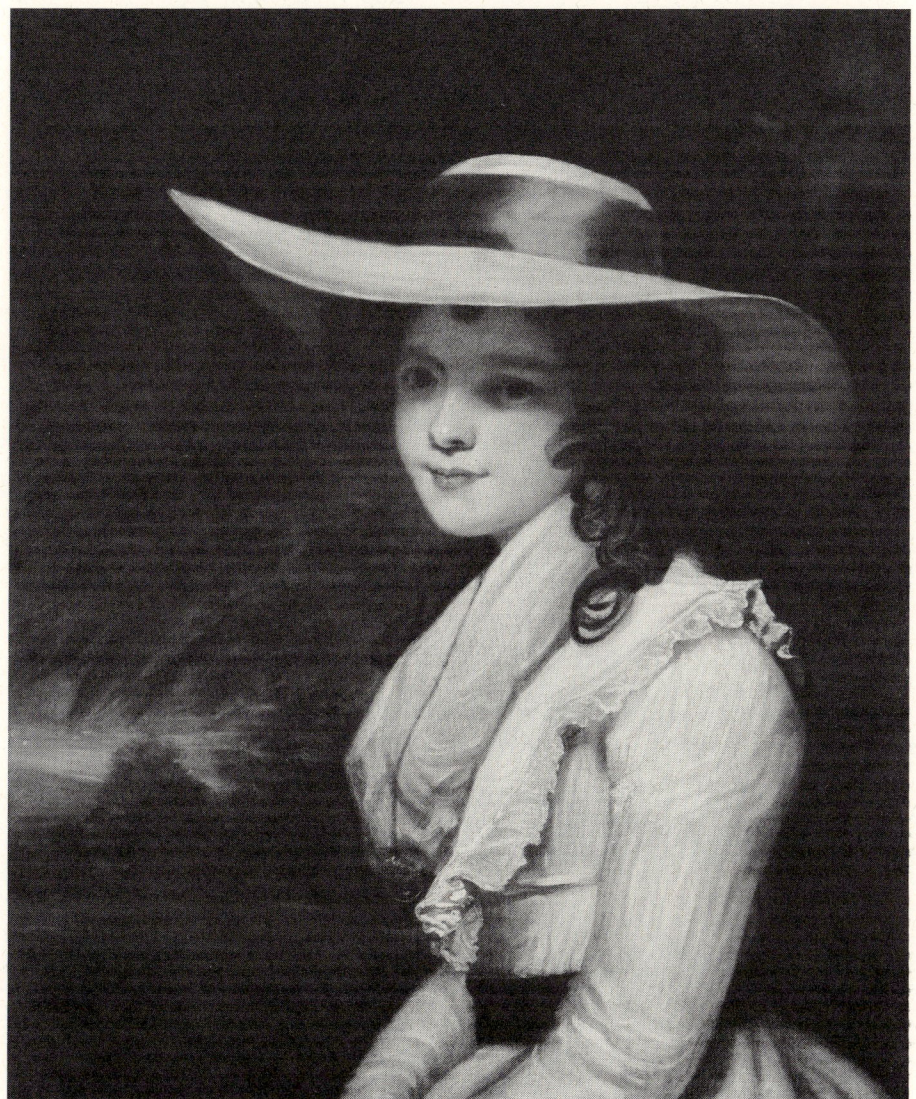

Figure 5. Lavinia Bingham, Countess of Spencer (*1762–1831*). *By* Sir Joshua Reynolds. *Courtesy of* Huntington Art Gallery, *San Marino, California.* The strong undulating line of the hat, contrasting with the softness of the rococo effect in hair and frilled fichu, so typical of English dress in the late eighteenth century, is the flattering line used in our contemporary capeline.

74   *The Arts of Costume and Personal Appearance*

buoyant, round, curved lines achieved when crisp material is made into flounces or handled in a full, bouffant manner (Figures 6, 7, and 8). They are also seen in the *S*-like curves of the baroque and rococo styles of the costume and interiors of France in the eighteenth century, when every line was a curve and every curve compound (Figures 8 and 9). Today these curved

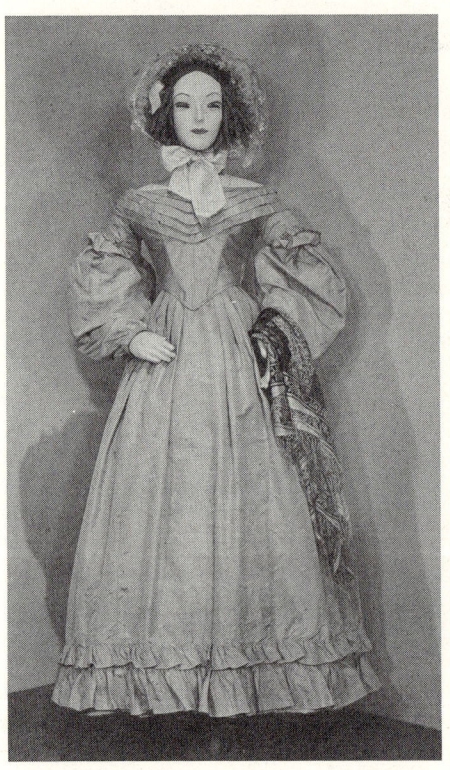 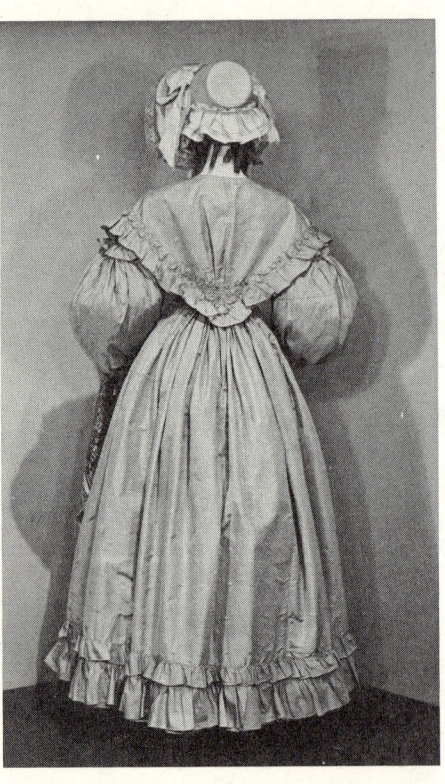

a   *b*

Figure 6. Gray-green sprigged silk visiting dress, American, 1830–1835. From the collection of Mrs. William W. Witherell. Exhibited at the Museum of Costume Art *in "A Cycle of American Dress, Part I, 1939." Courtesy of* Museum of Costume Art *and the owner. a. Front view. Horizontal line direction is typical of the nineteenth century Romantic period. In this example the boat-shaped neck, outlined by folds of taffeta, the wide bouffant sleeves, the ruffles at shoulder and hem, the hair parted in the center, all contribute to this kind of movement. b. Back view. The detachable cape deviates from the horizontal movement of the skirt and sleeves creating in diagonal movement a charming center of interest.*

DESIGN ESSENTIALS FOR GOOD COSTUME 75

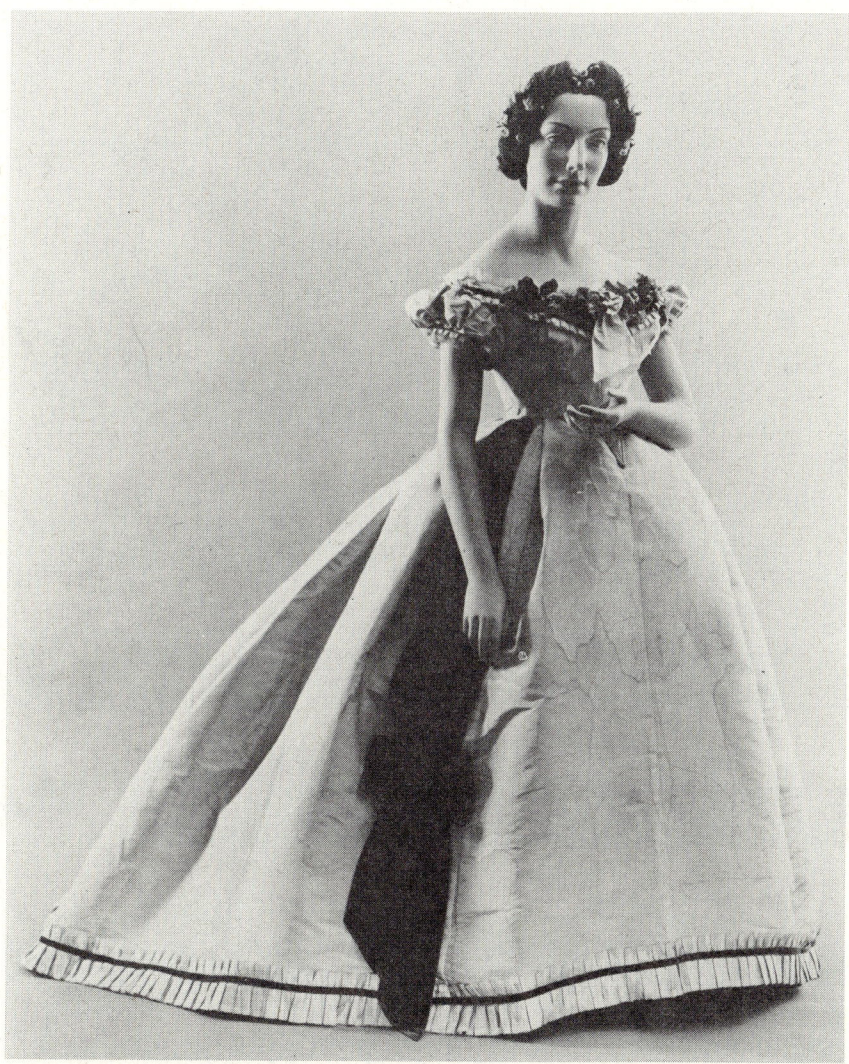

Figure 7. Ball dress of white moiré trimmed with turquoise-blue velvet. Probably American, 1861. Courtesy of Museum of the City of New York. Self-pleating held with bands of velvet outlines the horizontal structure of the skirt and décolletage, and forms the basic theme. This idea is further elaborated by an accent of velvet flowers at the bosom, and a wide sash of velvet leads the eye throughout the design.

76   The Arts of Costume and Personal Appearance

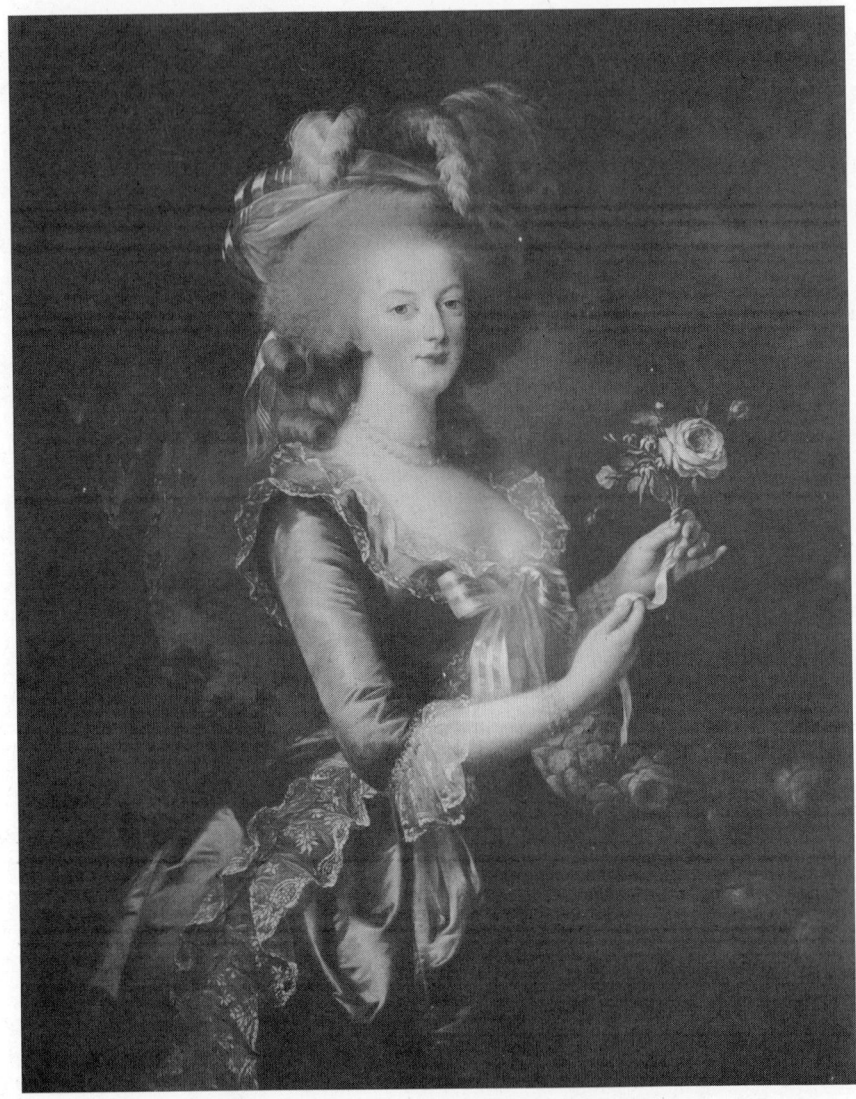

Figure 8. Marie Antoinette. *By* Elizabeth Le Brun. Alinari. *Rococo at its best. The restrained use of lace frills and ribbon bows used structurally gives a rich and beautiful effect frequently overdone in the age of the Louis.*

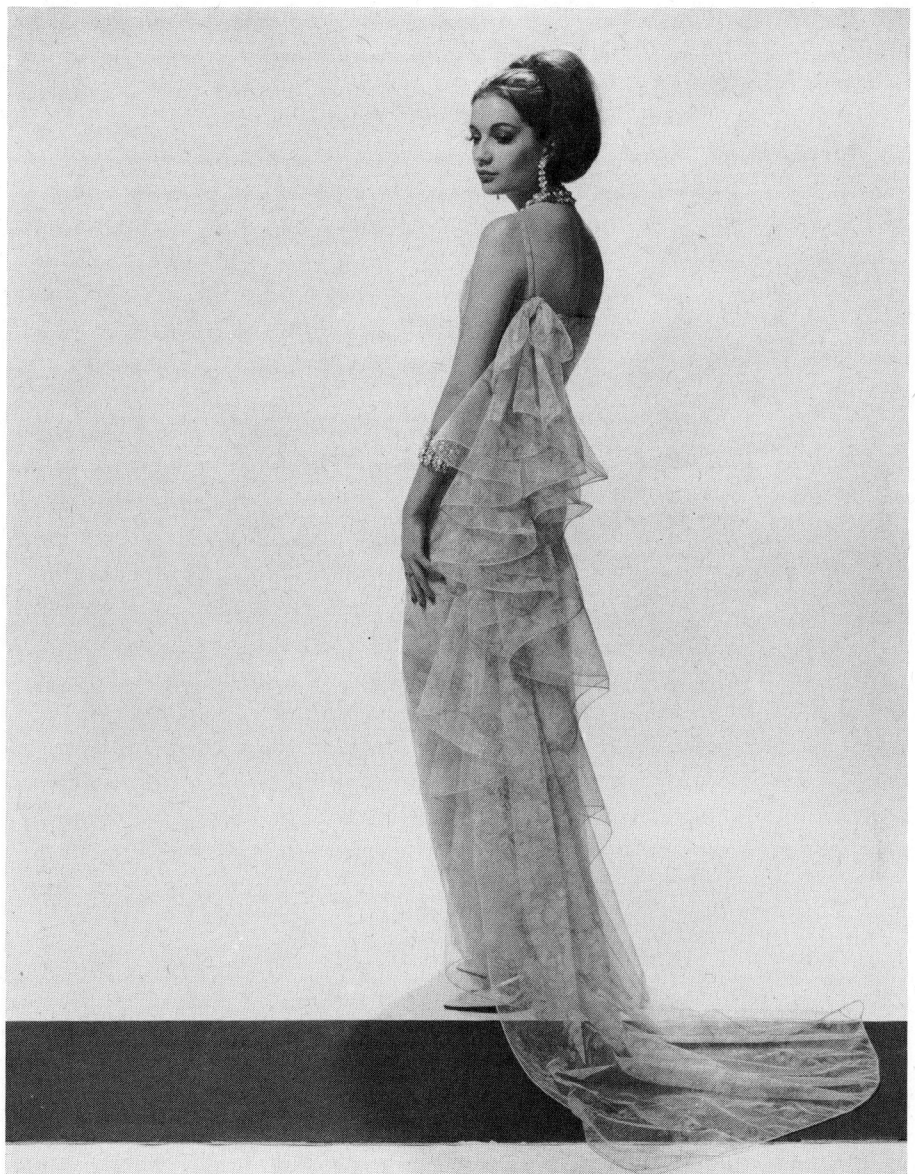

Figure 9. Blue printed evening gown by Christian Dior. Courtesy of L'Art et la Mode. Photograph by Georges Saad. A contemporary adaptation of eighteenth century rococo.

lines are particularly evident in allover embroidered linens or cottons, and in beaded embroidery on formal wear.

Line can cause the eye to move in any direction although it has only one dimension, that of length. There are three kinds of movement.

Vertical lines are those at right angles to the earth, or the position our bodies take as we stand. These lines manifest the feelings of poise, strength, stability, uprightness, or aspiration. Vertical lines may also create impressions of imposing grandeur, stateliness or austerity, or an impression of added height (Figures 1 and 10). Vertical line movement is the distinguishing feature of Gothic sculpture and painting (Figures 1 and 11). It is the movement we enjoy in redingote styles adapted from the First Empire mode, in pleated skirts, or in striped shirtings.

Horizontal lines are lines at rest. We associate them with repose, the calm of the horizon, or flat, quiet, resting waters. These lines suggest a sense of calm, serenity, gentleness, or an illusion of greater breadth (Figures 2 and 6). Horizontal line movement is readily recognized in the flounced skirts of Empress Eugenie's time, or in the wide, off-the-shoulder necklines of the Romantic period, or where striped materials are made up horizontally (Figure 7).

Diagonal lines may be described best by the body in motion. This line may at times seem unstable, but when properly used it can portray powerful movement and activity. Diagonal line movement when curved upward is forceful, animated, dynamic, and creates an impression of height. Curved downward, this movement is lifeless and depressing. Diagonal line movement is seen in surplice bodice closings, in chevron treatment of stripes, and in the placement of decorative design (Figure 6 and Figure 3 Chapter Six).

FORM AND SHAPE

One function of line is to define contours and to divide total areas into shapes or forms as well as spaces. In using the term shape, we mean the contour or outside characteristics of the object. There are various terms used for describing the contour; we say the pattern is square, oval, ovoid, triangular, or round. Form can be used synonymously with shape if we are speaking only of structure. Keep in mind, however, that form is often used in a larger sense in which it denotes a total organization—the external shape as well as the internal nature.

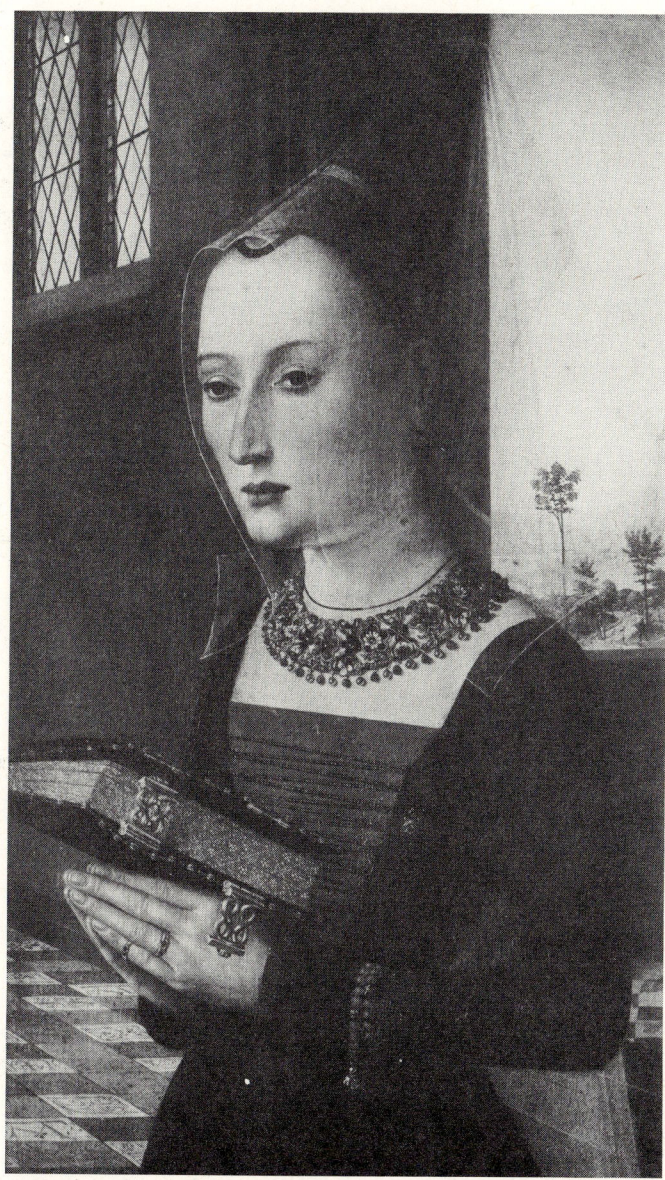

Figure 10. Maria Boneian. *By* Van der Goes. Alinari. *The dominant line movement in this medieval portrait is upward rising. There are aloofness and great refinement in her slender features and dress; the background of straight verticals repeats the dignity and austerity of the figure.*

80   *The Arts of Costume and Personal Appearance*

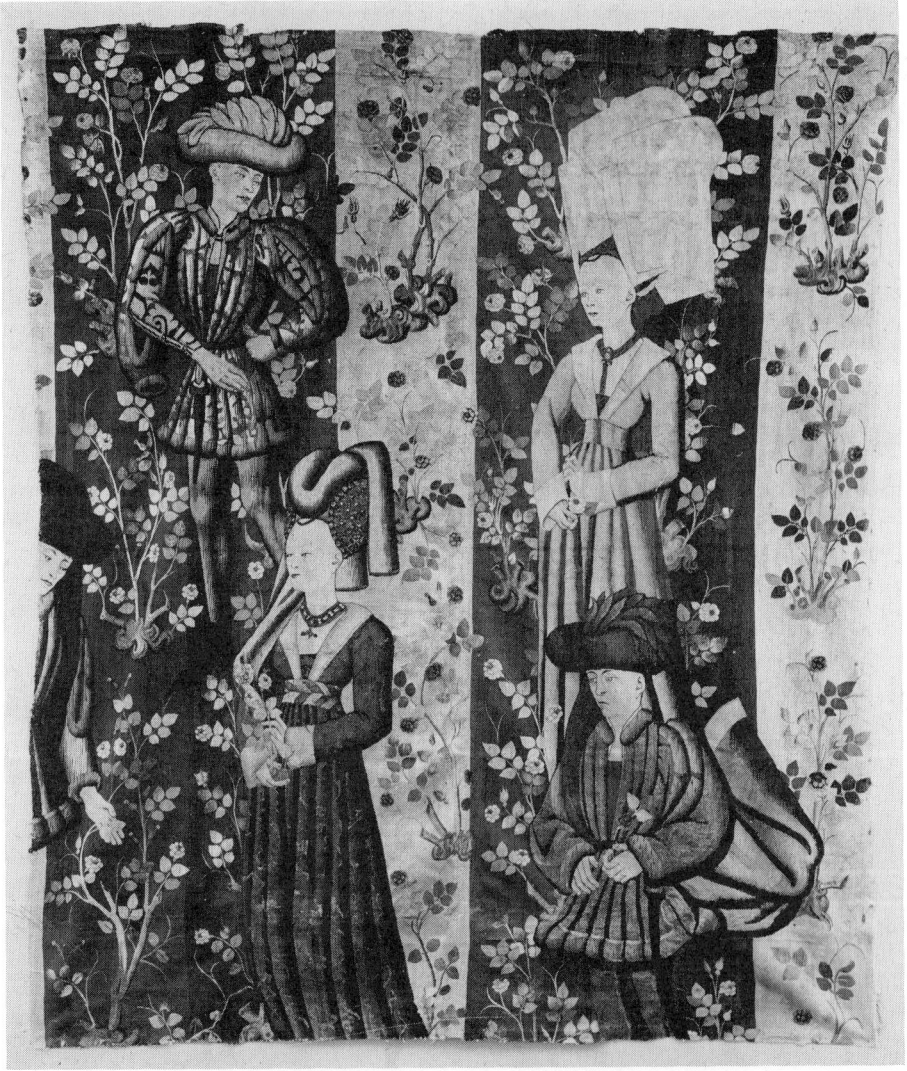

Figure 11. A Gothic tapestry, La Baillie des Roses *(French, fifteenth century). Courtesy of* Metropolitan Museum of Art. *These tall, slender men and women seem very stately and imposing in their strange headdresses and the organ pipe folds of their rich flowing robes. The lovely floral background, also upward-rising, lends a gayer note to the dignity of the festival.*

DESIGN ESSENTIALS FOR GOOD COSTUME   81

In our study of design we shall employ the terms form and shape synonymously, and think of them as being "positive" spaces.[2]

The silhouette, outline, or contour of an entire costume is often spoken of as its shape or form.

The individual parts which compose the silhouette and make up the structure are thought of as forms or shapes.

SPACE

The void or emptiness between forms or shapes may be defined as "negative" space.[3] Applied to costume, it is the background area on which individual shapes or decorative details are imposed. It is important to remember that the background areas are quite as important as the shapes imposed upon them. Thus the background space around a pocket or yoke or ornament becomes of equal importance with the shape itself (Figure 12). The same is true of the background against which the pattern of a silk print is imposed, or the spaces between a group of tucks.

Large, bold spaces against a plain, unrelieved background give impressions of forcefulness, the severe, the striking and dramatic, the sophisticated, or the masculine. Shapes and spaces, small in scale, where large surfaces are broken up considerably into small areas, suggest refinement, daintiness, and femininity. We feel this quality in fine pleating and flutings, and in prints with tiny flowerettes worn by very feminine women.

But our study of shapes and spacings is concerned most with infinite variations changing in character with the times. It is a necessity that the student of costume become observant of and sensitive to them everywhere. It is a part of education to gain acquaintance with the typical motifs of different times and lands. Medieval emblems, the crests of trade guilds, the ogival patterns of fifteenth century brocades, the contours of Directoire furniture, and the shapes of Greek vases should become etched in memory. One of the beautiful ogival shapes of the fifteenth century may be seen in the velvet used as a background for an Italian portrait bust (Figure 2 Chapter Six). The lovely flame motif (Figure 13) is one of ancient Persian origin. All about

---

[2] Wallace S. Baldinger, *The Visual Arts,* Holt, Rinehart and Winston, Inc., New York, 1960, p. 11.
[3] *Ibid.*

82   *The Arts of Costume and Personal Appearance*

us are shapes sharply silhouetted against their backgrounds—some of great distinction and others mediocre. It is part of our study to learn to recognize those that are significant.

Many attempts have been made to discover the most pleasing space divisions. The German student Zeising believed its secret to be in the Golden Section, found by dividing a line so that "the small segment has the same

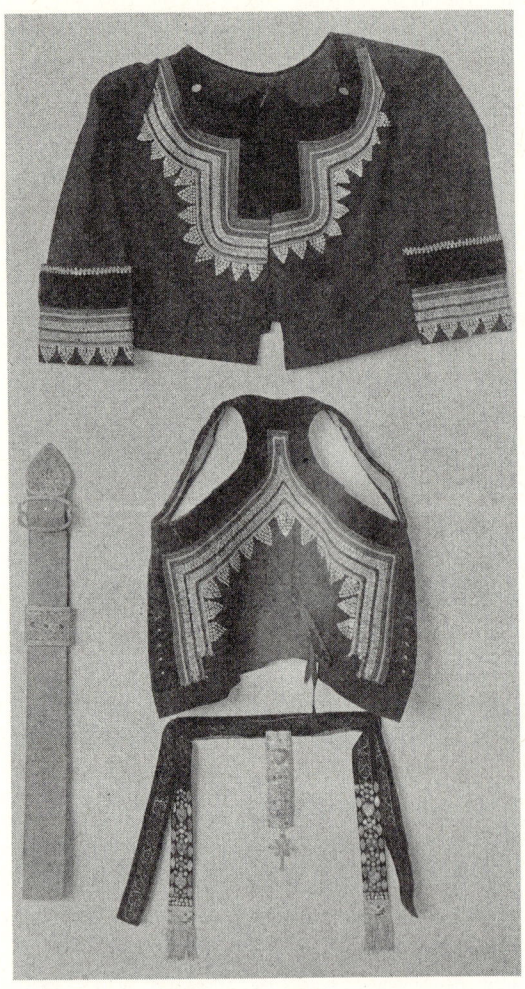

Figure 12. Breton coat, vest, and belt. Courtesy of Metropolitan Museum of Art. The peasant designer of these garments has made the shapes important by silhouetting black velvet facings sharply against their background in a rich beaded design.

relation to the large segment as the large one has to the whole." [4] Later students have written of the necessity to have the multiple parts unified by similarity of pattern groups, and by the introduction of some opposing element to hold attention and give relief and contrast. A great philosopher says in his work *Art as Experience,* "No whole is significant to us except that it is constituted of parts which have in themselves individuality and at the same time relationship to the whole." [5] The problem of the designer is always how close the relationship, how great the variety. Sir Francis Bacon in his essay "Of Beauty" wrote, "There is no excellent beauty that hath not some strangeness in the proportion." [6]

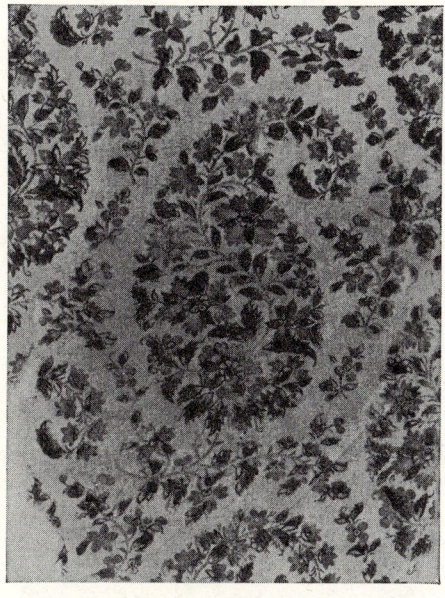

Figure 13. Persian flame or pine motif on a fragment of seventeenth century Persian cotton, memorable for its graceful shape.

COLOR

Light is the stimulus for the sensation of color, and it depends on the sense of sight as sound depends on the sense of hearing. If we could not see, color would not exist. This element will be studied more explicitly in Chapters Nine and Ten.

TEXTURE

Texture is the roughness or smoothness of fabric and is perceived as much by sight as by feel. In Chapter Seven you will find further discussion of the meaning of this design element.

---

[4] Albert R. Chandler, *Beauty and Human Nature,* D. Appleton-Century Co., New York, 1934, p. 33.
[5] John Dewey, *Art as Experience,* Minton, Balch & Company, New York, 1934, p. 204.
[6] Chandler, *op. cit.,* p. 51.

WHAT MAKES A BEAUTIFUL OR DISTINGUISHED DESIGN

Any design for a hat, dress, or suit is made up of its silhouette and the lines, shapes, and spaces which compose its structure. It is our problem now to examine individual elements of structure so that we may understand how they contribute to the making of a beautiful design.

Silhouettes

By half closing the eyes one can eliminate individual shapes and spaces and thereby readily reduce a design to its essential structure or skeleton for analysis. The silhouette of a costume is most important; it is what we see from a distance before details of structure or decoration are visible, and is responsible for first impressions.

To the uninitiated the different silhouettes which women have worn through the centuries seem myriad; actually, there are only three. Mrs. Young, in her book *Recurring Cycles of Fashion,* traces the three basic silhouettes and their variations from 1760 to 1937.[7] They comprise the straight or tubular, the bell-shaped or bouffant, and the bustle silhouette. Her study shows that these three basic silhouettes occur in the same order but once in a century (Figure 14). The changes which occur frequently are only those of texture, color, and minor detail of silhouette, which give the impression to the unobservant that fashion is fickle. The silhouette indicates whether our apparel is in the current mode or a relic of some past season. Since the silhouette of our clothes changes from season to season, and year to year, insight into the styles of silhouettes will enable one to tell almost the year or season when it was fashionable.

Individual Shapes within the Silhouette

The individual shapes and areas which go into costume defy classification, because they are based on abstract conception or are adaptations from nature in infinite variety. Geometric shapes of equal measure such as the square, the circle, and the triangle are static and without value for costume. Geometric shapes of unequal measure have a place in the structure of costume.

---

[7] Agnes Brooks Young, *Recurring Cycles of Fashion (1760–1937),* Harper and Brothers, New York, 1937, p. 22.

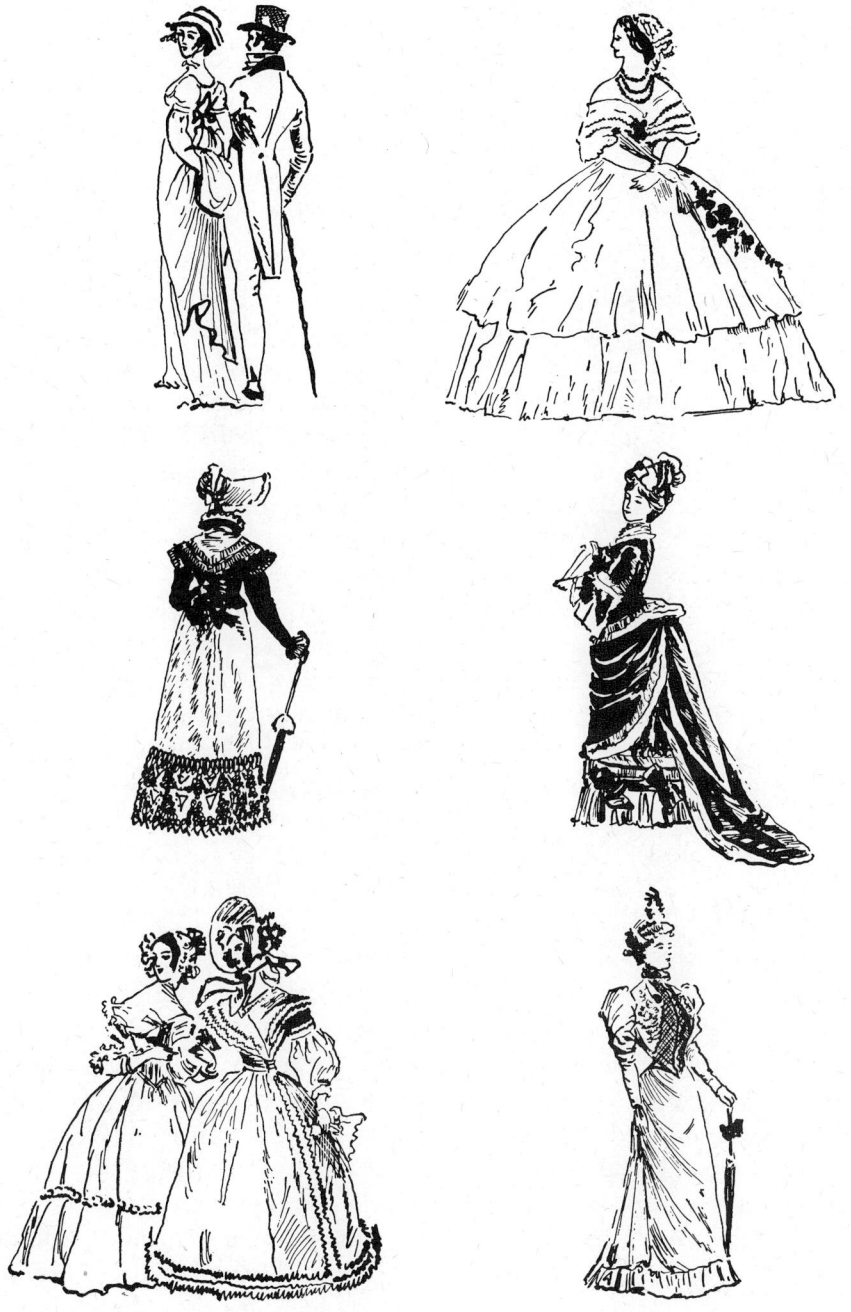

Figure 14. Typical stages in the evolution of nineteenth century costume, including the tube, the bell, and the bustle. From Uzanne's Fashions in Paris, 1797–1897. *Courtesy of Charles Scribner's Sons.*

The oblong is the most used form in all composition.
The oval possesses interest because of its variation.
The ovoid or egg-shaped form elicits more interest and subtlety than other geometric forms because of its constantly changing contour. The human head and the oval of the face are based on the ovoid.

The silhouette tells us a number of things about the shapes and spaces within it. We can tell the general style of the coiffure; whether the hat is small, fitting the head closely, or large and picturesque. We can tell whether the sleeves are long and close fitting or large and puffed; whether the waistline is high or low; whether the bodice is bloused or torso-revealing; whether the skirt is long and narrow or short and bouffant, and whether its hemline is even or irregular. We can tell, as well, if the shoes are broad and flat or have French heels and are pointed; whether the wearer gives the impression of a sleek, smooth, well-groomed person; or whether, on the other hand, her appearance is frumpy and unorganized.

On closer study of both the positive and negative areas within the silhouette, we will become aware of the fine relationship between the two. Either one wrongly used may make the other ineffective. It is important that each space and each shape contribute in some small way to make the whole costume pleasing. "The eye needs 'negative' spaces for rest from overstimulation or as contrast to the 'positive' shapes—even as the ear needs gaps of silence. Recognizing such need, the actor in reading his lines pauses for effect, and the musician in playing a composition stops for the 'rests'." [8]

Distinguished Line

Straight lines have in themselves little claim to beauty, because they are unvarying and static. Particularly in sharp fabrics, straight lines can be very severe and unflattering in effect; but they seldom appear unrelieved in costume, since they take on the curves of the body and its movements (Figure 15). Their severity is also lessened by soft fabrics, decorative edges, or curved lines introduced to give an effect less forceful or masculine.

The full, round curves of the circle, on the other hand—particularly in their small rococo forms and when used with little restraint—make for restlessness and weakness. But when employed with the restraint demanded in dress, full round curves may add a desirable note of enrichment and decorativeness.

Between the full round curve and the straight line are curves of great

[8] Baldinger, *loc. cit.*

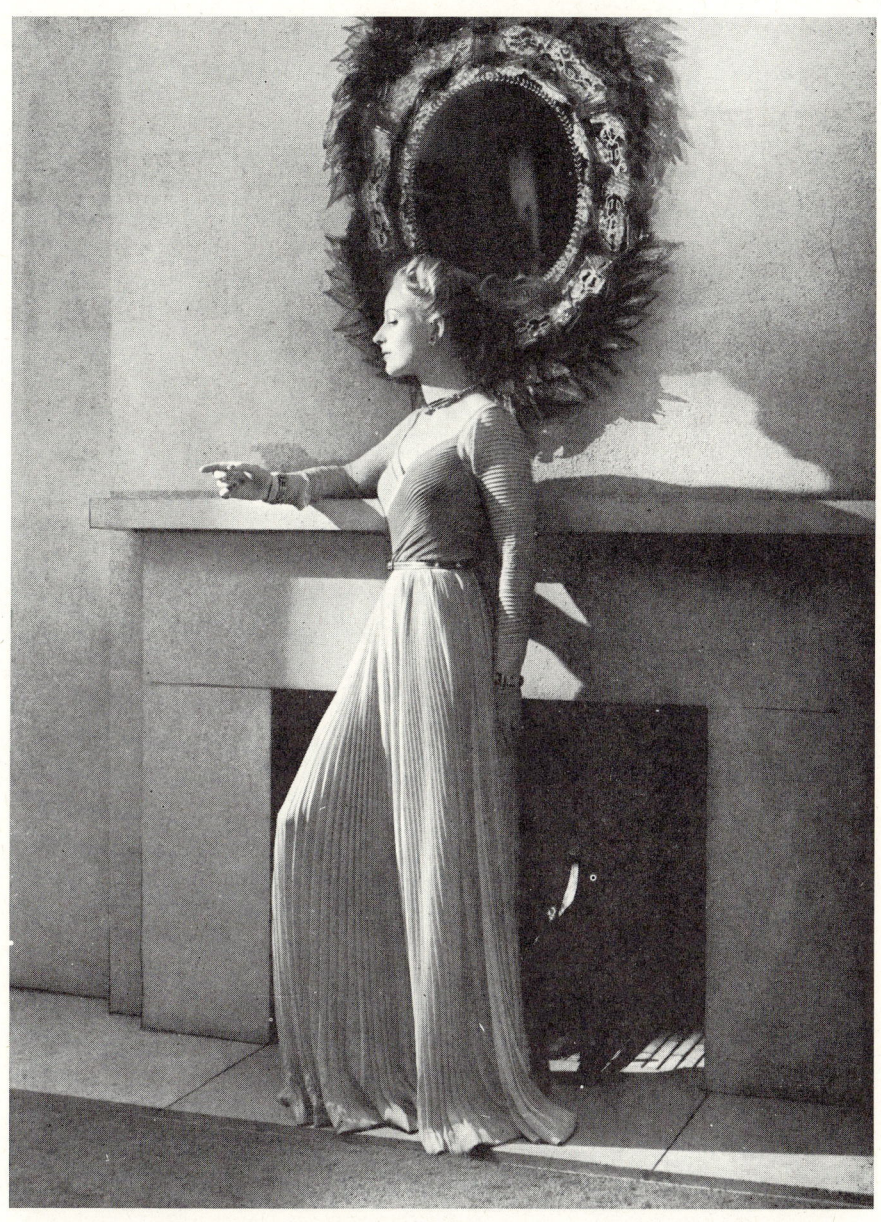

Figure 15. Evening gown. Maggy Rouff. Courtesy of Harper's Bazaar. *Perfection in this geranium-pink pleated crepe dinner gown, flowing gracefully with body lines and emphasizing points of body articulation. It satisfies the modern demand for elimination of every unnecessary detail and for a silhouette neither too revealing nor concealing.*

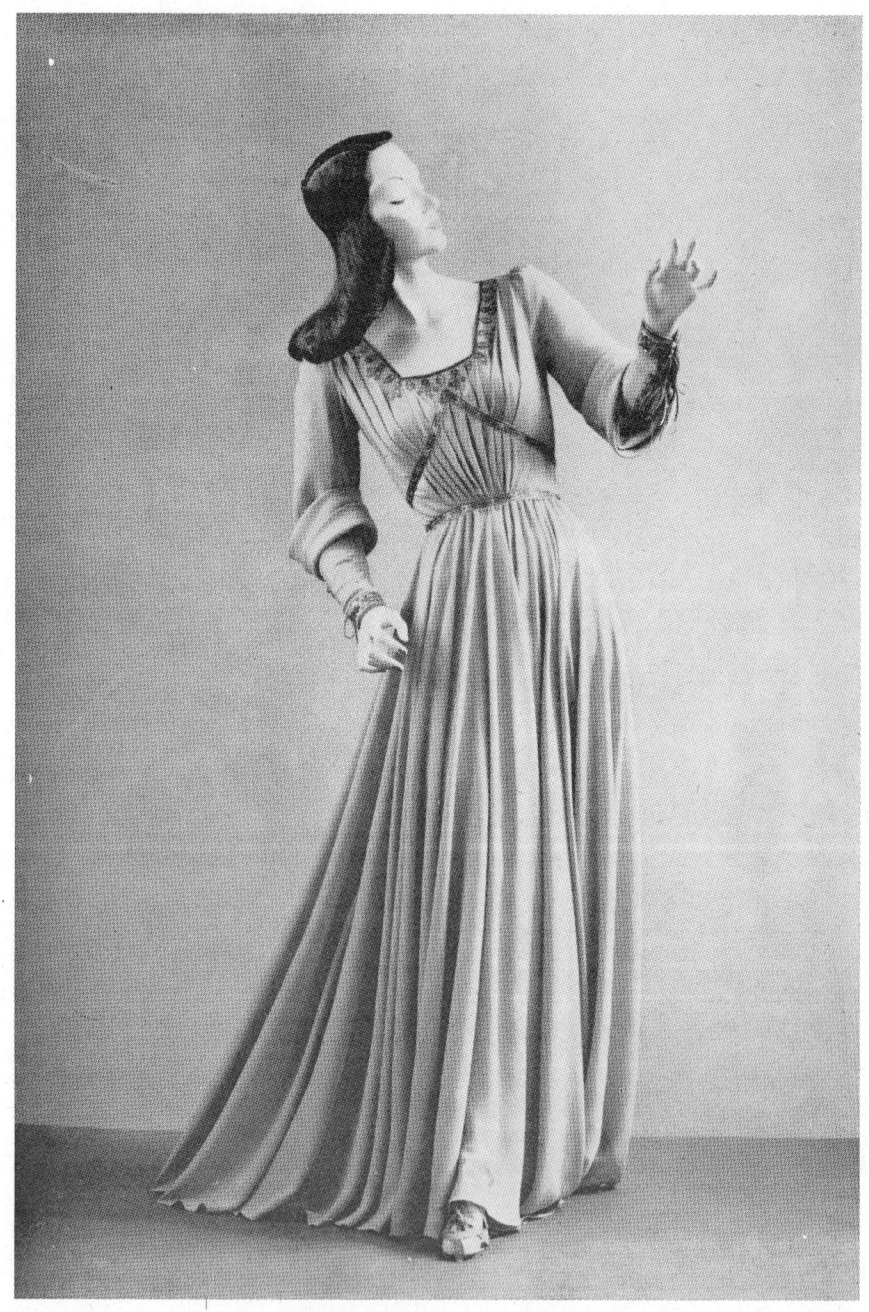

Figure 16. A distinguished dinner gown of mist-blue crepe in exuberant mood, inspired by Botticelli. Designed by Jessie Franklin Turner. Courtesy of Miss Turner and Metropolitan Museum of Art. Its restrained curves and folds are confined at structural points by bands of embroidery used with great artistry.

beauty usually found in the most distinguished costume. They are called restrained curves, because they are characterized by moderation. They vary constantly without varying too much; they are constantly tending to become straight (Figure 16). Ruskin calls this kind of line organic and infinite, because its construction implies the possibilities of continuation to infinity; it would never return upon itself though prolonged forever. Great pleasure comes to the eye from this line movement. We enjoy it in the flow of line in today's silk jersey evening gown or in the swirl of a dancer's scarf. Yet all curves and no straight lines are monotonous. Curves need the steadying influence of straight lines. Whistler, in his writings to artists, tells us that in the long curve of the narrow leaf connected by the straight tall stem, we learn "how grace is wedded to dignity, how strength enhances sweetness, that elegance may result" [9] (Figure 17).

Expressiveness of Lines, Spaces, and Shapes

Lines in costume, as in the major arts, should be studied from two aspects.

We may observe them intellectually; and by considering parts separately, we can better see how they function and how one part is related to another.

We may read into them meanings and expressions. Lines have power to speak as well as to depict, to create moods and states of mind, to arouse feelings and thoughts in the mind of the appreciative observer (Figure 18).

This expressiveness is the result of a process called *empathy*. For example, if we watch people skating or dancing or if we follow intently the actions at a ball game or a horse race, we may discover our bodies swaying to the rhythm of the players. We may not move visibly, but our feelings to some extent partake of those of the performers. We experience a kind of inner mimicry. In short, we put ourselves in the other person's place.

Likewise a kind of empathy is aroused by sounds, lines, and colors. The intelligent designer, as well as the one who selects, must understand empathy. This is the designer's means of communicating his moods, whether they be playful or quieting, exciting or alluring. This is the opportunity for one who selects and wears clothes to express her most agreeable traits, and to create

---

[9] George H. Opdyke, *Art and Nature Appreciation,* The Macmillan Co., New York, 1932, p. 406.

90   *The Arts of Costume and Personal Appearance*

in the sensitive observer moods and emotions in harmony with the purpose she intends.

But what are the evidences, the symbols, the motifs by which designs may impart emotion? The ancient Greeks and Chinese seem to have understood this language of the emotions. Suggested by the most common lines and

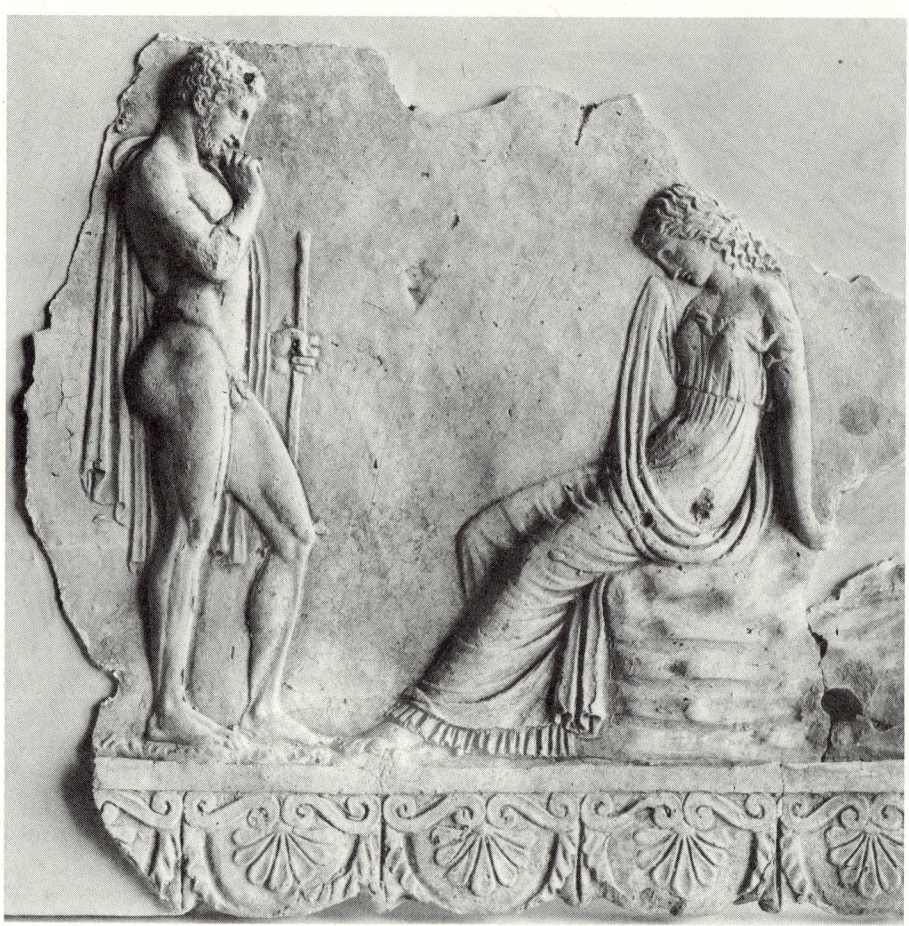

Figure 17. Farewell Scene between Theseus and Ariadne. *Classical terra cotta. Roman, first century* A.D. *Courtesy of Metropolitan Museum of Art. The full, rounded lines and the enchanting curves of Ariadne's robe are steadied by the restrained and forceful curves of the masculine Theseus, with their two movements so related that to disturb one line would interrupt the rhythm of all the others.*

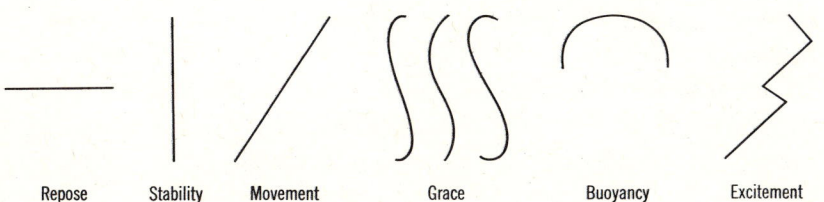

Figure 18. Symbols of expressionism: repose, stability, movement, grace, buoyancy, excitement.

forms in nature, their symbols stir in each of us the same emotions. We enjoy horizontal line movement because it suggests the repose and quiet calm of the horizon, or sleeping animals, or flat, quiet, resting waters. We respond to vertical shapes and areas because they revive in us the feeling of stability and grandeur, of tall cliffs and buildings, and people in perfect upright poise. We thrill to upward swirls and flowing drapery because it suggests vigorous plant growth or the fascination of rising flame.

Requirements of a Good Silhouette

One of the most important requirements of all art is that it conform to the law of unity with variety, or variety within unity. The silhouette must be judged by this law. Since the human body, when well proportioned, contains the most beautiful lines and forms of all created things, unity requires that we do not contradict its form; but variety demands that we enhance it with some variation from its contour. Thus the requirements of a good silhouette include the following:

> A good silhouette will be related to body structure. It will have emphasis at points of body articulation (Figures 15 and 16). It will emphasize good points and hide imperfections. It will have restraint and movement. A beautiful dress will never reveal all the lines of the feminine figure at one time, neither will it muffle its outlines as was done in the Middle Ages. In many past periods extenders such as crinolines, pads, and stomachers were fashionable. But these so-called improvements produced no beauty—only a broken, angular silhouette without grace or charm. A beautiful dress will reveal some parts of the anatomy, while others will be subtly concealed with graceful drapery or fullness. There will be balance between concealing and revealing; the wearer will be beautifully fused with her clothes.

A good silhouette will be composed of individual parts which have in themselves an interesting outline; it will have variety in its details. Perhaps the sleeves will have significance, or the hat will contribute importance. The resulting contour will be clear cut, and will have an individuality or a definiteness that gives it a certain style of its own (Figure 11 Chapter Six).

The silhouette must be in character with and reflect the spirit of the times for which it was designed. For instance, in the 1920's the ideal of the boyish silhouette was expressed by the slim legs in short skirts. Long skirts would have been inconsistent. During the early 1950's, emphasis was placed on femininity; the silhouette revealed smaller waists, curved bosoms, and graceful, flowing skirts consistent with that ideal (Figure 10 Chapter Three).

As we judge the silhouette by its conformity to the law of unity with variety, so must we judge lines, shapes, and spaces. The designer strives to achieve the most variety within unity, and one who recognizes and appreciates this kind of inventiveness in costume will demonstrate it in her own choices.

Another basic concept in the art world revolves around the harmony of form and function. By this we mean that inherent characteristics as well as external shape are in relation to the entire purpose of the composition and not merely for utility. Applying this to our study, the finest costume will be right for the person, for the time, and for the place. Clothes are utilitarian, but it is the combination of rightness for the occasion and tastefulness in design that produces a feeling of satisfaction in the wearer as well as in the observer. There are clothes with the primary goal of being aesthetically gratifying. Is this not a worthy purpose too?

The reader will be able to find many books dealing with the plastic elements and their application to all areas of living. The following references will broaden one's appreciation of design.

Donald M. Anderson, *Elements of Design,* Holt, Rinehart and Winston, Inc., New York, 1961.
Wallace S. Baldinger, *The Visual Arts,* Holt, Rinehart and Winston, Inc., New York, 1960.
Kenneth F. Bates, *Basic Design,* The World Publishing Company, New York, 1960.

Phillip C. Beam, *The Language of Art,* The Ronald Press Company, New York, 1958.

Ethel Jane Beitler and Bill C. Lockhart, *Design for You,* John Wiley & Sons, Inc., New York, 1961.

Ray Faulkner, Edwin Ziegfield and Gerald Hill, *Art Today,* Third Edition, Henry Holt and Company, New York, 1956.

Harriet and Vetta Goldstein, *Art in Everyday Life,* Fourth Edition, The Macmillan Company, New York, 1954.

Maitland Graves, *The Art of Color and Design,* Second Edition, McGraw-Hill Book Company, Inc., New York, 1951.

Robert Gillam Scott, *Design Fundamentals,* McGraw-Hill Book Company, Inc., New York, 1951.

Exercises

1. Study the lines, shapes, and space divisions in a collection of fine examples—paintings, prints, historic and contemporary costume. Try to identify the essential structure of each example by seeming to separate, through half-closed eyes, the lines and spaces that define structure and give direction.
2. Make lists of descriptive terms and phrases that explain characteristics of different kinds of line as well as movement. Do the same for shape, spacing, and silhouette. Consider the function of these elements and the emotional effect they produce on the beholder.
3. Study the lines of some fine Japanese prints and make a page of sketches of individual groups of lines, trying to catch their rhythmic qualities without reproducing the picture as a whole.
4. Study the silhouette changes in women's clothes since 1800 by examining some source books on costume. Select representative examples of different silhouette types; trace their outlines, ink in their surfaces, and estimate their values as good silhouettes.
5. Study today's fashions and make a report on significant features of silhouette in dresses, suits, coats, and millinery.
6. Study to determine whether the economic conditions of a country or the spirit of the times may be reflected in the silhouette of women's clothes.

Six

Principles of Composition

THE principles of composition are guides for the aesthetic use of the plastic elements studied in the previous chapter. Just as the plastic elements are the raw materials of any art work, so the principles of design—balance, proportion, rhythm, and emphasis—apply to any art whether fine or applied. These principles have been observed by artists in their aesthetic expressions through the ages. The fundamentals do not change but their application does, because the art of any age is an expression of the philosophy of those living at that time. The principles of composition have been called laws, but this term seems too rigid. Aesthetic expression cannot be regimented, or new creative statements become impossible. Rather than speaking of the elements of composition as laws, let us think of them as guides worthy of study; but once they are understood, interpret them with creativity. In any art work worthy of the name all the principles operate interrelatedly and lead to the ultimate goal of harmony. We shall study, however, each principle separately to better understand its contribution to beauty.

BALANCE

The first principle of composition, balance, is employed to satisfy the need for a sense of equilibrium, stability, and permanence. Balance is often de-

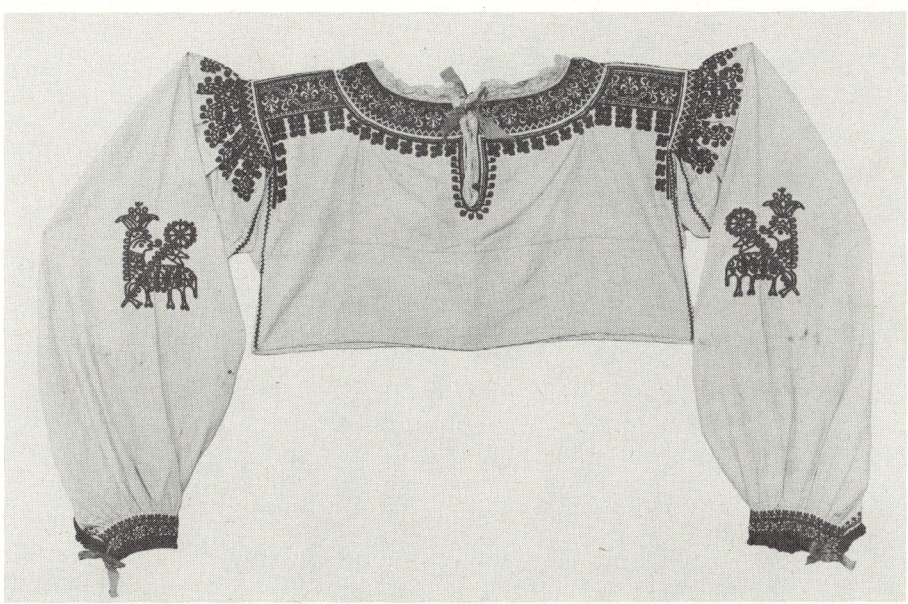

Figure 1. Spanish peasant blouse. Owned by Victoria and Albert Museum. *British Crown Copyright is strictly reserved. Bright green embroidery on oyster-white linen. A distinguished use of decorative design structurally placed and symmetrically balanced.*

fined as rest or repose. The feeling of repose is achieved through the illusion that the elements about the center of a composition are equal in their power of attraction. Balance may be accomplished in several ways. Easiest to understand and to use is *formal* or *bisymmetric balance*. When the objects or details on either side of an imaginary line through the center of a composition are identical, and each identical item is equally spaced from that center line, formal balance results (Figure 1). Frequently formal balance is illustrated by the seesaw on which two children of identical weight are seated equidistant from the center or fulcrum. Also included in the formal balance category are arrangements where the major components on either side of the center are almost mirror images, and only minor details are not exact duplicates (Figure 2). Formal balance with these slight deviations from symmetry may be distinguished by the use of the terms *obvious balance* or *approximate symmetry*. Bisymmetric balance tends to be static or passive, rather than dynamic; however, interesting shapes may give an active, moving

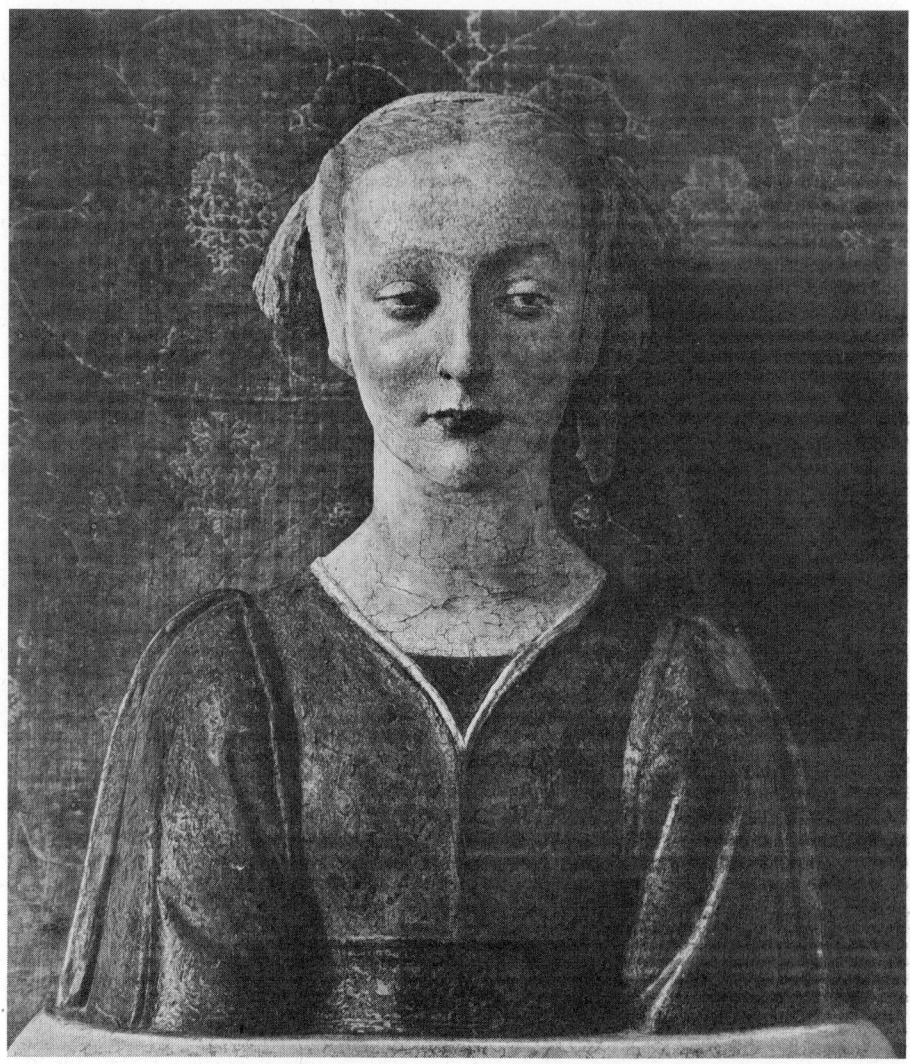

Figure 2. Bust of a Young Woman. *Florentine School. Louvre. The two sides of this portrait bust are in bisymmetric balance with the exception of the small detail of the headdress. Quite in the modern manner is the beautifully shaped neckline and the drapery of the headdress. The Renaissance fabric background has significance in its simple elegant motifs.*

quality to the arrangement. Feelings of dignity, stateliness, or regalness result from its use. Mechanically formal balance is easy to achieve, but interest is dependent upon sensitive space relationships which in turn give the composition rhythmic movement.

Another kind of balance is that termed *informal* or *asymmetric,* in which the two sides of the composition are not identical. Our sense of equilibrium is satisfied when the objects on the two sides of the design give the feeling of equality (Figure 3). Let us return again to the illustration of the seesaw. Two children of unequal weight require that the heavier move closer to the center or fulcrum to balance the lighter child seated at the end of the board. Asymmetric or *occult balance* in design is not a matter of actual weight, but one of the power of visual attraction. Through interest of unusual shape, a small area may be more emphatic and balance a larger but less commanding area. Color, line, texture, or surface pattern of significance also may exert unusual attraction and appear to balance larger masses of less significance. A grouping of smaller details into a unit will add commanding importance to the group. Informal balance is active and dynamic. It creates the impression of spontaneity, freedom of movement, the casual, and the unusual and reflects the feeling of our time. Because the means of achieving asymmetric equilibrium are less obvious, the eye is aroused to curiosity and explores the arrangement. The means of achieving informal balance are infinite and subtle. The designer is free to express himself more creatively. At the same time greater skill and sensitivity are required, and the eye must be trained to recognize a restful design.

Costume design makes use of both these aspects of balance. While formal balance is seen more frequently in clothing, asymmetry is demonstrated in fashions with a side closing where large areas on one side balance small, significant features on the other. Asymmetry may be found in diagonal drapery that directs the eye to a distant, culminating point of emphasis. A design may be structurally bisymmetric yet seem to require an important ornament, such as a clip, placed to one side of the neckline.

Perpendicular balance is demonstrated in the use of a dark skirt and a light blouse (Figure 10 Chapter Twelve). One's feeling of need for more weight in the lower than in the upper half of the costume is satisfied; but the proportions of the blouse and skirt areas also must be considered carefully in achieving a sense of vertical balance. It is evident in a costume where the more important design features occur in the bodice, and the more simple but larger skirt area balances it.

98   *The Arts of Costume and Personal Appearance*

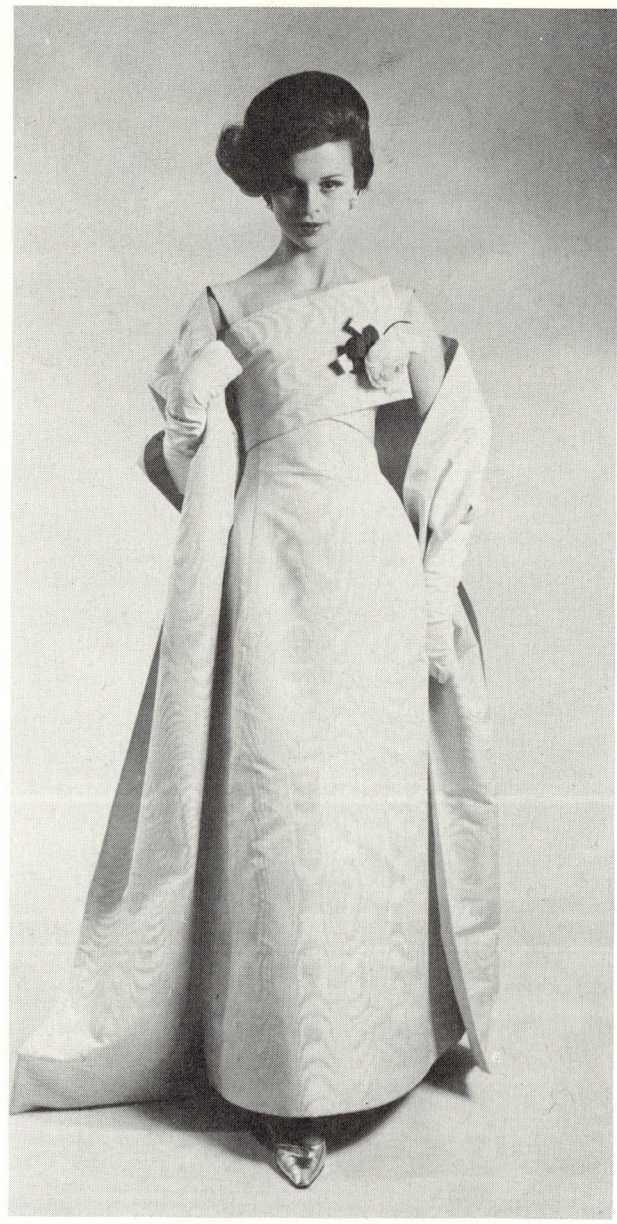

Figure 3. Pink moiré evening gown by Christian Dior. Courtesy of L'Officiel. Photograph by Ph. Pottier. The dominant diagonal line of the bodice generates the design of this gown which illustrates asymmetric balance.

Radial balance results from the control of opposing attractions around a central point. In a simple form, the design is balanced vertically and horizontally on two intersecting lines. More often the designs are balanced on a greater number of lines originating from a central point, like the spokes of a wheel. Frequently there is a feeling of movement around the center; frequently too, the center of the composition attracts attention. Radial balance is seldom used in costume except in surface patterns such as those of a printed fabric or in pieces of jewelry.

PROPORTION AND SCALE

Proportion, also called the law of relationships, is the pleasing relation of all parts of a design to each other and of these parts to the whole composition. It is the relationship of height, width, and the surrounding space in two-dimensional art; in three-dimensional design, the factor of depth is added. Design is not judged by any one of these isolated factors; but when they are combined, we become conscious of relationships and evaluate them. Proportions are originated when the designer uses lines to define silhouettes, and the space within the form subsequently is divided into shapes by details. The more sensitive the designer to fine proportions, the more ingenuity he will use in attaining them in any article of apparel. Another important aspect of proportion is that of creating optical illusions. Through the division of space, a semblance of change is produced; illusions are created which are important in minimizing or camouflaging figure irregularities.

Pleasing proportion is neither too obvious nor too difficult for the eye to perceive. The too evident ratio of 1 to 1 or of 1 to 2, as seen in the spacing of primitive art or in the work of beginners, does not satisfy our more cultivated perceptions. The eye too easily measures these obvious ratios and dismisses them without exploration. By contrast, the proportions found in Greek art and architecture, so frequently referred to as fine examples, are approximately 2 to 3 or 3 to 5. These too are mathematical ratios, but the relationship is not so obvious. The eye becomes intrigued, and explores the intricacies of the more subtle dimensions.

Scholars for many years have been fascinated by the timeless beauty of Greek proportions, and have worked out rather intricate mathematical formulas and pedantic theories; and when reduced to round numbers, they approximate the 2 to 3 and 3 to 5 ratios stated above. From this has evolved

100 *The Arts of Costume and Personal Appearance*

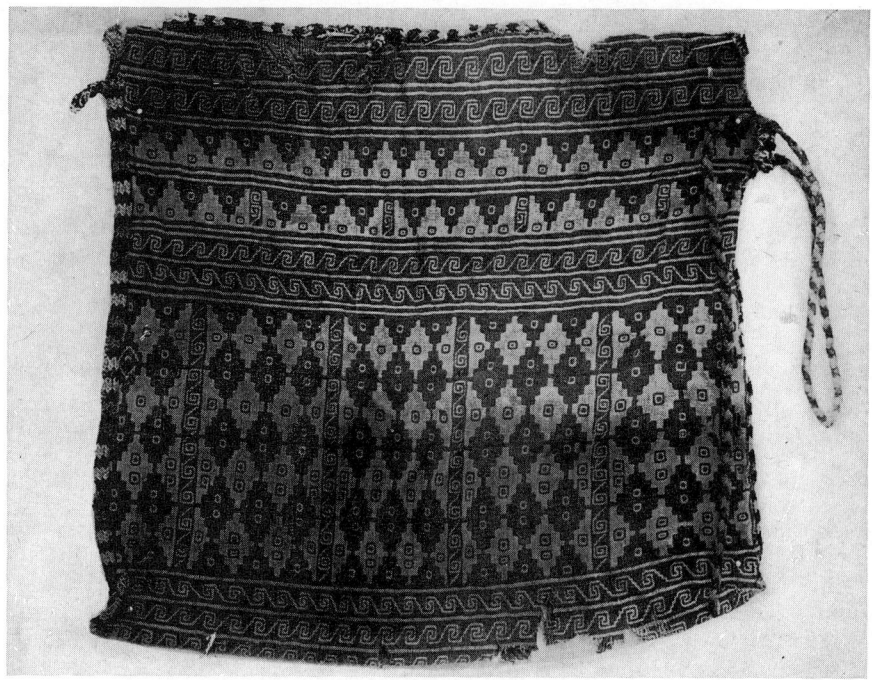

Figure 4. Peruvian bag. Courtesy of American Museum of Natural History. The fine proportions of this piece of double cloth weaving in brown and white cotton are indicative of sensitivity to space relations in a prehistoric people, comparable in a measure to that of the ancient Greeks.

the guide for dividing a space into two parts by making the division somewhere between the one-half and the one-third points. For our purposes we will consider one of the conclusions, the Rule of the Golden Section already mentioned in Chapter Five, which states that beautiful proportion results when "the smaller part is [approximately] to the larger as the larger is to the sum of both, i.e., $3:5::5:8$ or $5:8::8:13$."[1] In the division of a line labelled AB at point C, the relationship would be expressed as $AC:CB::CB:AB$. The same relationship can be extended to the height, width, and depth dimensions of solids.

Yet the finest things in any of the arts are surely the product of feeling and trained judgment, not of mathematics (Figure 4). It is possible to

[1] George H. Opdyke, *Art and Nature Appreciation,* The Macmillan Company, New York, 1932, p. 528.

express mathematical relations that are numerically correct but too complex to be felt. Further, proportions should be used to fit the purpose; the design should not be forced to fit a mathematical formula. Proportion is an expression of the times, as our concepts of proportion change with alterations in silhouette and details of costume. Finally so subtle an art as that of costume must rely on a trained sense of proportion.

One aspect of proportion has to do with the relationship of sizes of separate objects to each other and of the sizes of the separate parts within, and is called *scale*. Our sense of harmony demands that when articles of apparel are worn together there must not be too great a difference in size relationship to the wearer, nor should the articles differ too greatly in size from each other. All parts of an ensemble—the purse, the hat, the jewelry, the fur scarf—regardless of occasion, must be in scale with the wearer and the separate parts related to each other. Individual sections of a garment such as sleeves, pockets, collar, trimming details, motifs, or surface patterns must all be related to the size of the wearer and to each other (Figure 16 Chapter Five).

Let us see wherein proportion, scale, and spacing in costume are a matter of a feeling for consistency. It is through this sensitivity of relationships that undesirable figure proportions may be altered, creating the illusion of perfection (Figures 2 to 9 Chapter Twelve). Problems like the following are constantly demanding solutions in the designing or assembling of costume.

The spacing of borders, bands, and tucks that form integral parts of a design.
The proportion of the tiers of a wide, spreading skirt in relation to each other and to the whole skirt length.
The right relationship of the length of the jacket to the skirt and to the proportions of the figure.
The flare of a full coat to the build of the wearer.
The apparent width of shoulders in relation to the waistline, to the skirt width, and to the height.
The length of skirt in relation to the height of the wearer and to the proportions of her calves and feet.
The size and arrangement of a row of buttons with respect to each other, to the opening edge, and to the person wearing them.
The proportion of the crown and brim of a hat to the wearer's face and figure.

The hair style in relation to the proportion of head and features.

The breaking of space vertically, horizontally, or diagonally through placement of details of construction or trimming to create an illusion of greater perfection in figure proportions.

The proportion of darks against lights in an ensemble of several tones and colors.

The proportion of intense color used with a less intense color.

The suggested bulk of fabric textures in proportion to the figure.

The solution of problems of this kind, when worked out by the sensitive individual, becomes something very personal and creative. The trained judgment which recognizes fine proportion is not gained in a day. Study enables us to be quicker to see and to feel, and it leads us to be open-minded to new conceptions and new relationships as they present themselves to us in a constantly changing world of art and fashion.

RHYTHM

Rhythm or *continuity* is an essential instrument in the hands of the costume designer, because it is through rhythm that he gives his design movement. We evaluate his work to some extent by the way he is able to achieve this feeling. Many treat rhythm as a kind of measured repetition, but in this volume we take the view that fine rhythm is hardly something which can be measured. Rather, it is a movement which comes to the senses as a result of the particular way the designer manages his lines, spaces, colors, and textures in giving direction. Not all movement, however, is rhythmic. Rhythm is a regular and organized movement, actual or implied, leading the eye easily along a connected or suggested pathway through a composition in a series of expectations and fulfillments. Through the regularity and organization of elements our sense of anticipation is fulfilled; chaos is avoided. Rhythm leads the eye throughout a costume and enables it to travel with ease and power. It carries the eye smoothly along interesting pathways, permits it to tarry here and there, and finally leads it back to the main center of interest.

Let us look first at some isolated methods by which the designer may achieve rhythm. One means of attaining this design principle is through *repetition*. In its simplest expression, the repetition is regular and uniform;

this may be likened to the ticking of a clock, the drip of water, a picket fence. Frequently, unless skillfully handled, incessant repetition may be monotonous and uninteresting and goes unnoticed. It may be soothing through monotony, as is the practice of counting sheep; or it may become annoying, irritating, exasperating. In fine costume we see it used with discretion: the repeated motif of a lace edging (Figure 12 Chapter Five) or the crisp pleats of a skirt. In textile patterns we find regularity in the repeat of motifs; and when prints are properly designed, they become so subtle as to be a background.

Repetition becomes more interesting when the element of variation or alternation (*harmonic repetition*) is introduced. In its most simple form there are two elements alternating, as in the egg and dart motif of Greek art. There is repetition of some forms and spaces, but subtle changes in other parts of the design (Figure 1 Chapter Five). Immediately the possibilities of numerous arrangements of three, four, or more elements repeated in an orderly sequence become apparent.

Progression or *gradation* is another means of gaining rhythm. In this more dynamic form a transition between two opposing elements is made through an orderly sequence of gradually increasing or decreasing steps. This form of rhythm is seen in the ever widening concentric ripples from a pebble tossed into still water. Movement may be generated in a simple composition through the increase of elements such as lines or shapes in an orderly manner. The value scale, Table 1 Chapter Eight, is an orderly, regular graduation from white to black or black to white. After studying color, other such scales, as bright to dull or dull to bright, may be made. The color wheel exemplifies gradations by means of a common hue, such as green through the steps of green, green green-yellow, yellow-green, yellow yellow-green to yellow.

A fourth means of accomplishing rhythm is through *continuous line movement*. The line need not literally be connected, but the intervals between the components are small enough for the eye to easily bridge the gap and encompass the total sweep of pattern. In nature we observe this line movement in wind-bent trees, a range of mountains in the distance, and the winding of a brook. We see continuous line movement in Japanese prints and Chinese drawings (Figure 5, Figure 4 Chapter Five, Figures 1 and 5 Chapter Eight), in Greek art (Figure 17 Chapter Five) and in paintings (Figure 6).

Radiation, another method of obtaining organized movement, originates from a central point. It is evident in the patterns of snow flakes, the arrange-

104   *The Arts of Costume and Personal Appearance*

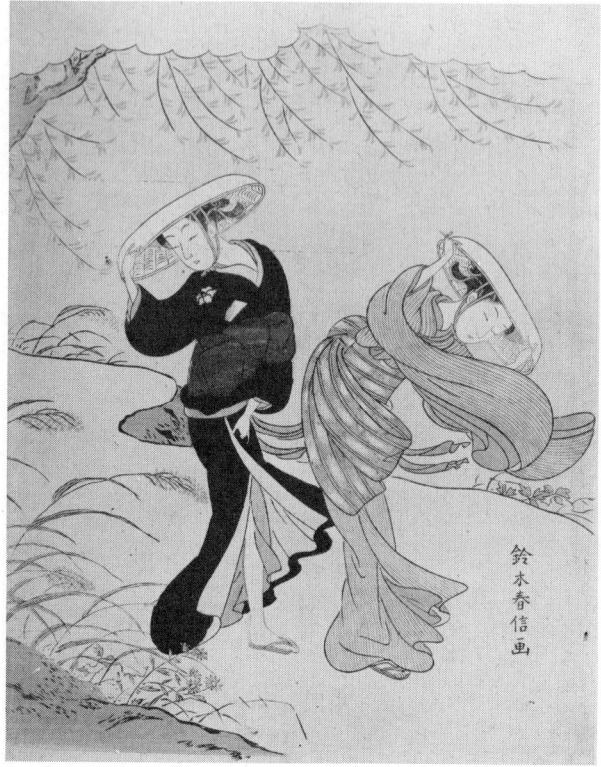

Figure 5. Two Women in a Spring Breeze. By Harunobu *(1720–1770)*. *Courtesy of* Boston Museum of Fine Arts. *One enjoys the vigorous sweep of line made by wind-blown kimonos, and the jolly exuberant movement of the leaves and grasses.*

ment of petals in some flowers, the swirl of many sea shells, or circles emanating from a pebble tossed into water. Movement through radiation is not frequently encountered in costume, but is confined more often to small notes such as the design of jewelry or applied decoration (Figure 7).

The final concept of rhythm is that of continuous, related movement (*occult movement*). This form presents the most exciting possibilities, involving the subtle relationships of all elements—space, form, line, texture, and color—in the production of a rhythmic pattern in the total costume. At this level of development there is a freer interpretation of repetition, progression, and line movement. One rhythmic element must be dominant,

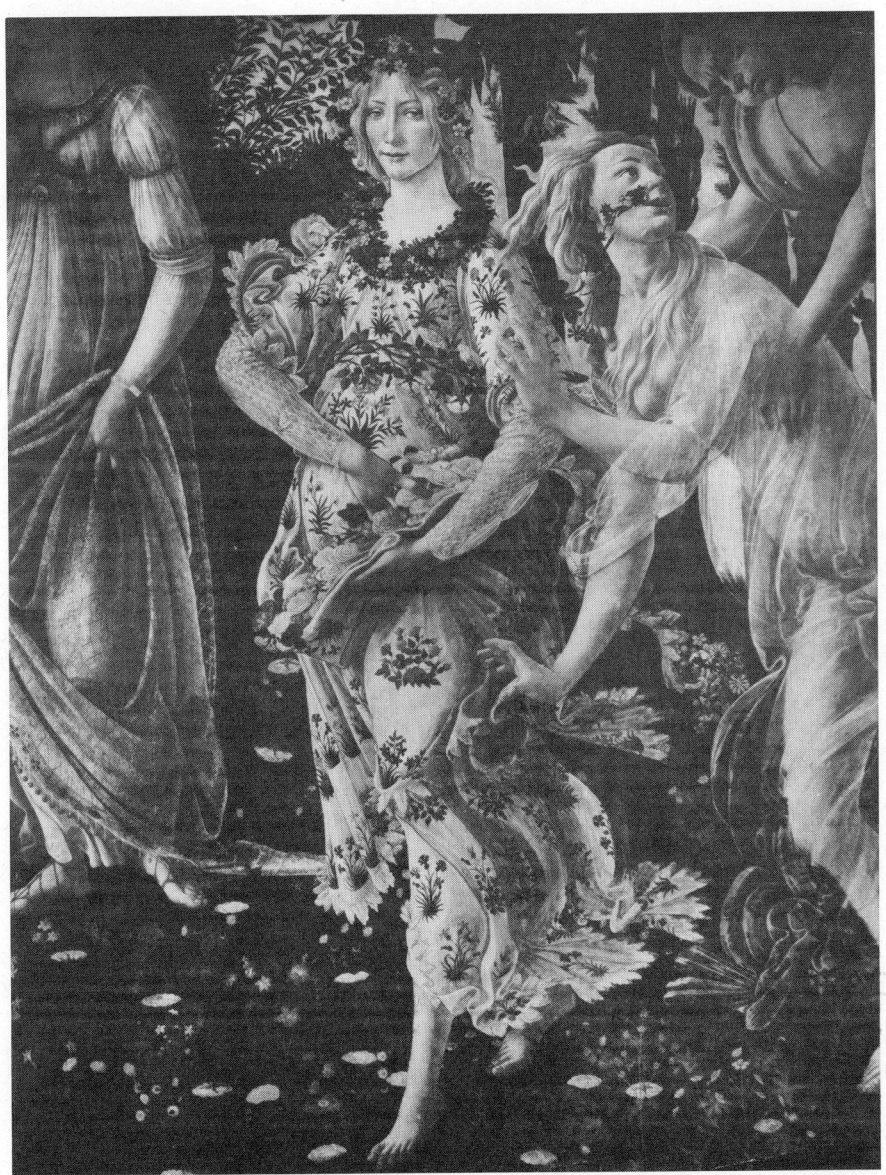

Figure 6. Primavera. By Botticelli. *The embodiment of springtime is felt in the tapestrylike background, in the floral wreaths, the buoyancy and animation of gossamer draperies, and the pose of the lovely Flora, goddess of spring.*

106　*The Arts of Costume and Personal Appearance*

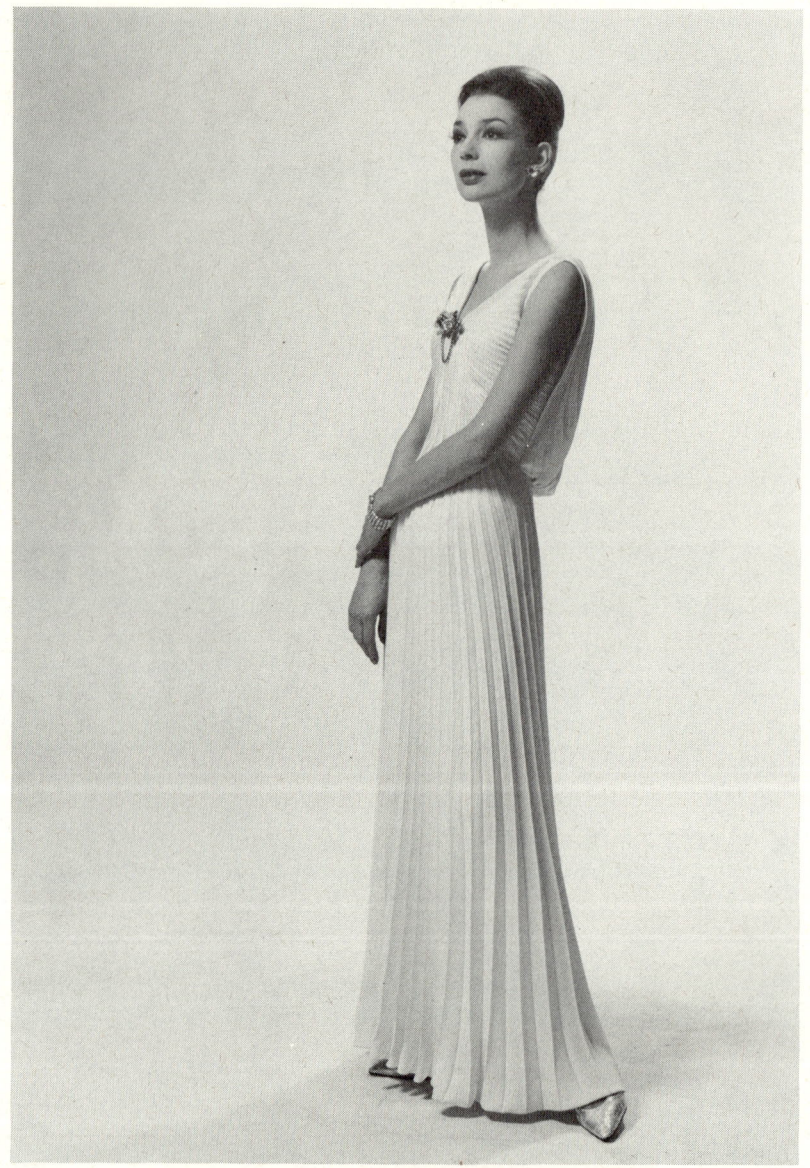

Figure 7. White crepe gown by Miguel Ferreras. Courtesy of L'Art et la Mode. Photograph by Georges Saad. An unusual use of rhythm by radiation is seen in the bodice. Rhythm by gradation is illustrated in the fan-pleated skirt.

and it is in this aspect that fine costume design resembles great painting or musical composition. Mature design is thus experienced.

The dominant line of the garment is repeated elsewhere with variation, important shapes are echoed, and the main textural theme is strengthened when similar characteristics are found in accessories, such as hat, bag, or shoes. Rhythm is seen in fine color where values progress from dark to light or from one hue to its neighbors. It is also found where a series of spaces is approximated in another part of a design.

Rhythm is the mainspring of fine costume and is expressed in the liquid flow of line in Greek drapery and in the limp folds of silk jersey or crepe in evening gowns created by our great designers (Figure 8). We feel it in the undulating lines of a picture hat as it dips in relation to the head and shoulders (Figure 5 Chapter Five, Figures 3 and 5 Chapter Thirteen), in the exuberant movement of costume worn by European peasants (Figure 9), or in the quick and animated motion of the straight lines in a pleated skirt. Rhythm is present in the arrangement of braids and sequins on contemporary costume and in the horizontal placement of trimming on full skirts of peasant influence. Well designed dark-and-light patterns as found in fine printed textiles exhibit rhythmic movement (Figure 10).

Rhythm is also one of the artist's ways of expressing mood and controlling intent. His rhythm may be vigorous and exuberant (Figure 1); or slow, stately, and majestic (Figure 11 Chapter Five); or gay and exciting (Figure 9); or tranquil and dignified (Figure 10 Chapter Five). Sometimes it is implied or subtle, but the sense of movement must be felt. The great works of art of every time reveal those forms of rhythm which express the temperament of the people. Dressing to express mood demands always the search for the right movement.

Let us study and enjoy rhythm intellectually and emotionally. Learn to see in fine costume the fluidity of line as a fusion or melting of one surface into another, each element so dependent on another for its existence that the whole becomes alive and moving. The student of costume must acquaint herself with various forms of rhythm. Museums and libraries everywhere have for your study many fine examples of rhythm in Japanese prints, early Chinese paintings, medieval textiles and embroideries, drawings by Holbein and Dürer, Gothic sculpture, Italian Renaissance painting, portraits by David and Ingres, and contemporary sculpture.

108 *The Arts of Costume and Personal Appearance*

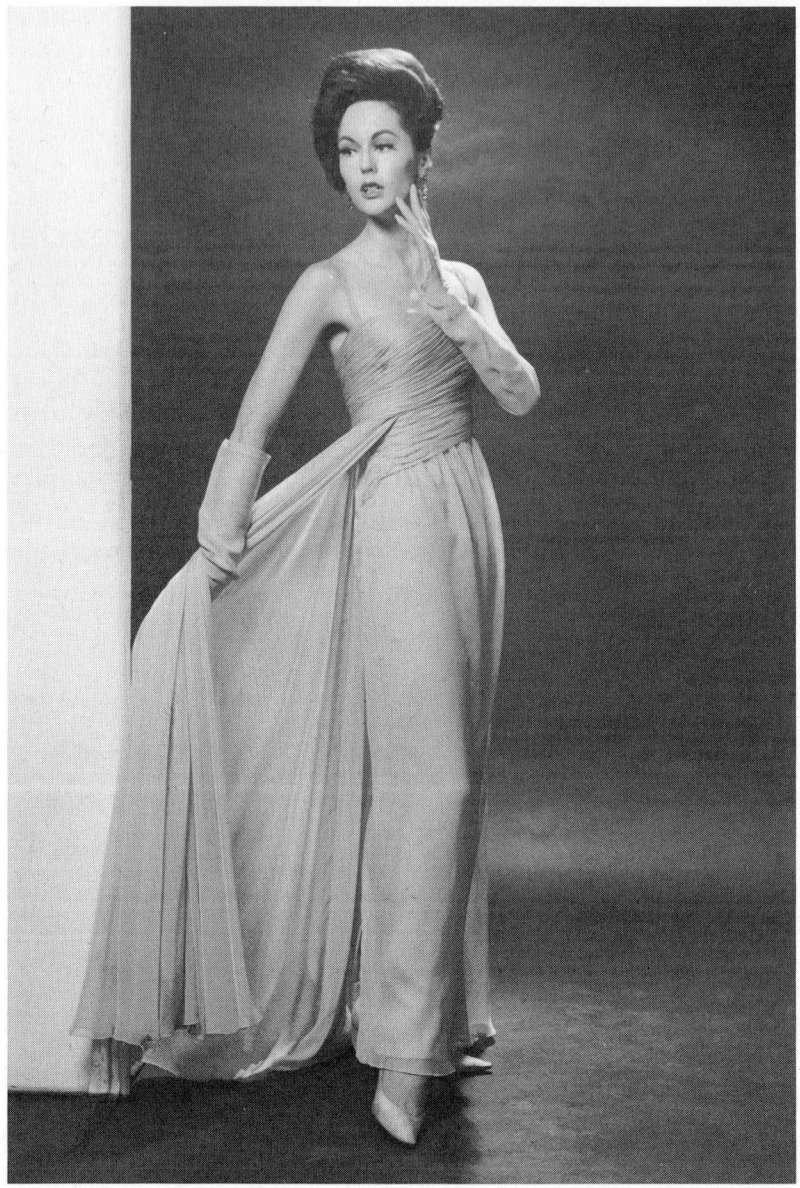

Figure 8. Mauve mousseline de soie evening gown by Jacques Heim. Courtesy of L'Art et la Mode. Photograph by Georges Saad. Beautiful rhythm achieved through continuity of line produced by skillful draping is seen in this gown of Grecian inspiration.

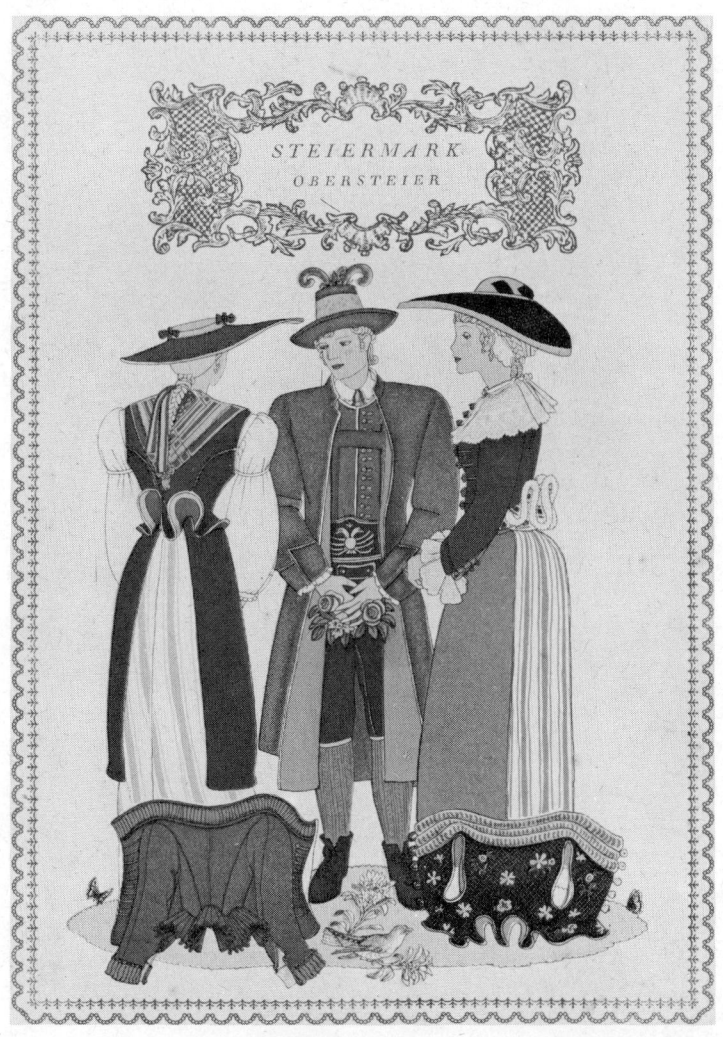

Figure 9. Tyrolean costume from Trachten der Alpenlander *by Hammerstein. Herbert R. Verlog, Vienna. Costumes such as these are the source of the popular dirndl. Strength, gaiety, and exuberance in frills and feathers, pleatings, and embroidered flowers. A study of the cut of these garments reveals rich inventiveness.*

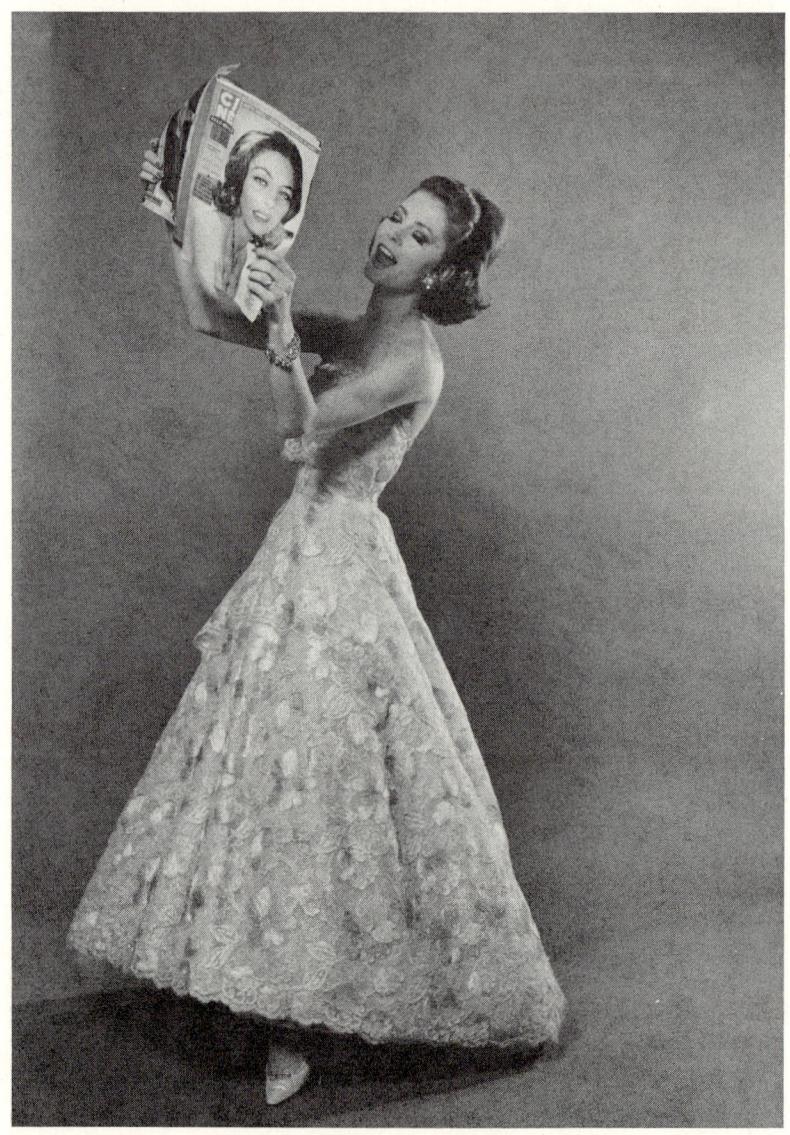

Figure 10. White lace re-embroidered in pink by Carven. Courtesy of L'Art et la Mode. Photograph by Georges Saad. Subtle gradation of values and careful spacing of the design produce a rhythmic pattern in the lace. Structural lines of garments should be kept to a minimum when fabric of lovely pattern is used.

EMPHASIS

The principle of emphasis or *dominance-subordination* leads the eye easily to the most important part of a design, then to the subordinate areas in order of their significance, and back again to the main center of interest. The principle of dominance-subordination is employed by the designer when he is concerned with giving proper emphasis to the parts of his work and to the whole. It is a fundamental principle running through all the arts—literary, musical, and visual. This principle demands that interest be achieved by holding and releasing attention.

In painting the artist focuses attention on his leading figures and subordinates the others. He gives them the most important position, the strongest color, the sharpest contrast, or the most unusual arrangement of line and, at the same time, subordinates the less important.

Emphasis properly used in costume design results in the statement of the major theme through the selection of a center of interest. The theme is supported by repetition in subordinated areas or minor centers. At the same time rhythm is generated through the organization of the elements of costume in their sequence of importance: thus order is brought to costume through emphasis. The eye can see and retain just so much. Too much elaboration results in chaos; too little interest, in monotony. The costume designer must first decide what is to be the major theme, and second, where the emphasis is to be placed. Then he must select from the multitude of means of creating emphasis the device he is going to employ. Emphasis may be created in these ways:

Certain lines and shapes are made more significant than the rest (Figure 16 Chapter Five).

Unusual shapes or details may attract the eye (Figure 10 Chapter Five).

Elements which in themselves may not be emphatic are grouped to gain importance and become a center of interest (Figure 12 Chapter Five).

Contrast readily generates emphasis, whether it is contrast of hue, value, or intensity or of line, shape, size, or texture (Figures 2 and 4 Chapter Eight).

Boldness of size or contrast command attention (Figure 12).

In distinctive designs, the structural lines in themselves are creative, and the originality and interest of line generates the center of interest (Figure 11).

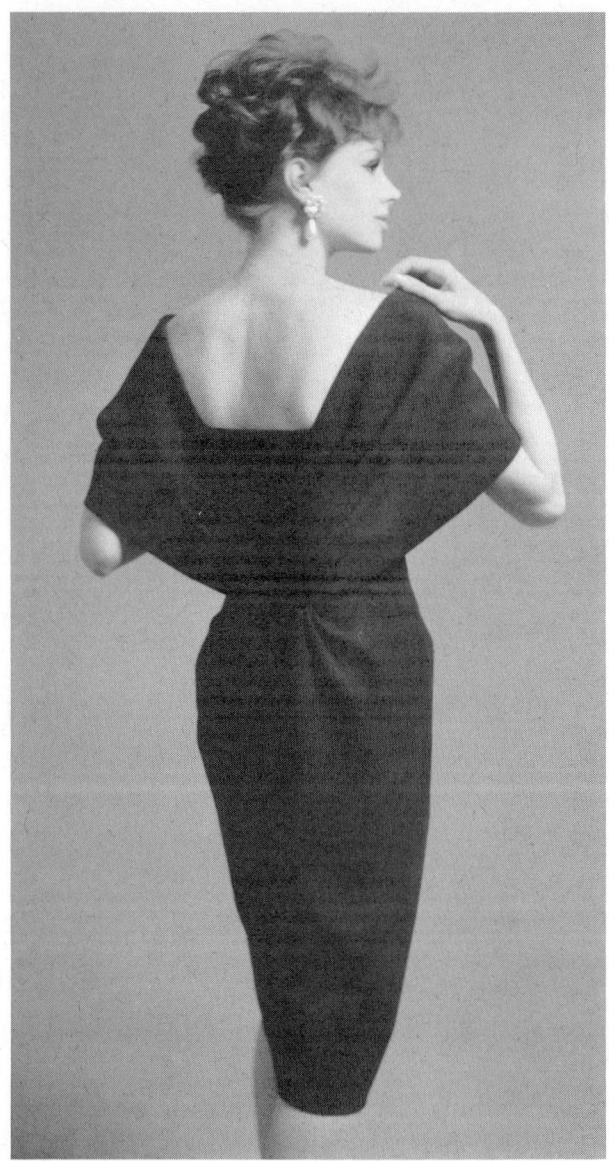

Figure 11. A late day dress executed in black crepe by Jean Patou. Courtesy of L'Officiel. Photograph by Ph. Pottier. The dominant idea of the dress is the gracious movement in the draped décolleté. The theme of suppleness is confirmed throughout the design. The center of interest originates from the structural design.

PRINCIPLES OF COMPOSITION 113

The addition of decoration becomes a focus of attention. Decoration should be applied at structural points to strengthen them (Figure 1).

Movement or rhythm is produced through leading lines, or through a series of accents each more important than the last, leading the eye finally to the culminating point of interest (Figure 10 Chapter Five).

Sufficient background space lends emphasis to a significant detail (Figure 4 Chapter Eight)

Limiting of dominant elements to an appropriate number is an essential of emphasis since its real value lies in economy of use (Figure 3).

The designer will select one means of obtaining emphasis (Figure 11), and perhaps will use others to a lesser extent. Whatever character of accent or shape is decided upon for one part of a design, it will be repeated in some related manner in other parts; and by this means subordination-dominance is gained. It is not obtained when sharp or dominating emphasis is used with little design interest in other parts of the costume to support it, for example, a large, ornate clip worn on a dress without structural significance. Accessories should be related to the creative structure of clothing and strengthen the design idea. Nor is dominance-subordination present without the ordering of the centers of interest in the proper sequence of importance. Without discipline costume may have too many features demanding attention. This could result from the overuse of accessories or from the use of competing textures, colors, shapes or forms, or lines. An example might be a heavy wool sport coat in a large, bold plaid with which a circular leather purse was carried. A lapel pin, earrings, bracelet, ring, necklace, and flower trimmed hat are all interesting in themselves but confusing when combined. Several ideas or centers of interest are competing, and no part is dominant. Costume should be subordinated to the wearer, as it is a background for the expression of the individual.

UNITY

Refer once again to the chart of "Basic Art Terms" at the beginning of Chapter Five. From this organizational plan it will be seen that unity or harmony is the resulting attribute of any work of art when the plastic elements have been used according to all the principles of design—balance, proportion, rhythm, and emphasis—in the expression of a concept. The skill of the designer lies in maintaining unity or harmony, but at the same time introducing variety to arouse interest. Unity is not an isolated entity, but results from the integration of all design principles (Figure 12).

Beautiful costume results from a well-developed idea or theme. Perhaps "idea" will be better understood if we think of a theme in music. Many great musical compositions are elaborations of one or a few themes. Beethoven's *Fifth Symphony* in C minor is built on a few themes developed through differences of orchestration, rhythm, harmony, and key level. When good costume is built around one theme, each part, although significant in itself, is a variation of the basic theme. The fabrics, trimmings, every line, shape, and detail must be a part of the idea itself (Figure 12).

Furthermore, there must be something in the idea to stimulate an interest. It is the sensitivity and experience of the outstanding designer which permits him to create new expressions. We do not find pleasure in the accustomed or the usual. We enjoy that which requires a new effort on our part. Our problem is ever to train the eye to distinguish the significant and creative from the commonplace or banal. A good idea may be suggested to the designer by the spirit of the occasion or the wearer's personal traits. Sometimes it is suggested by a beautiful fabric (Figure 10) or an unusual combination of fabrics. It may be developed from a clever shape or from some decorative detail that can be elaborated. In an important dinner gown, there is a beautiful movement of corded shirring across the shoulders, and the fullness of the garment generated by this detail is confined at the waistline with a simple cord. Here the goddess-like gown, with long close-fitted sleeves, simple but significantly designed in white silk jersey, is a background for the owner's beautiful topaz jewelry.

The basic idea or theme, then, is sounded in the major center of interest, and variations on the main theme are to be noted in subordinate, minor centers of interest. The consumer is a designer, in that through assembling a costume she is creating a background for herself as the theme or center of interest, and is expressing her individual personality through use of becoming color, lines, shapes, and textures in accordance with the principles of design. Each completed costume ensemble becomes a new expression and gives satisfaction to the human desire to continually create and conceive a new unity which is beautiful.

The references following Chapter Five will be helpful in broadening the scope of your understanding of the principles of design.

PRINCIPLES OF COMPOSITION 115

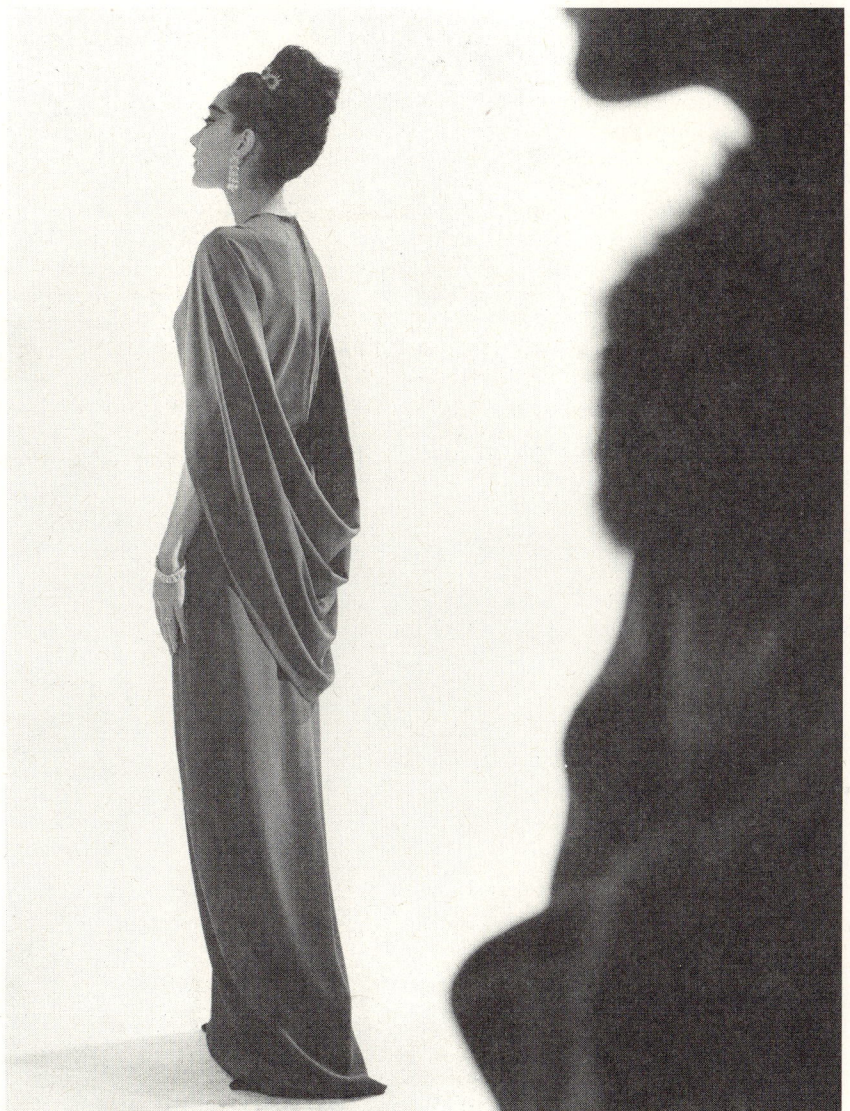

Figure 12. A crepe dinner gown by Mme. Alix Grès. Courtesy of L'Art et la Mode. Photograph by Georges Saad. A unified, creative inspiration which expresses a Yang personality. The dominant theme is supported by related attenuated lines, fabric of the proper weight, the coiffure, and the accessories.

Exercises

1. Select costumes which illustrate each type of balance or symmetry.
2. Collect plaid and striped materials which illustrate fine proportion.
3. Study current fashion sources to find costumes with good decorative design related to dress structure.
4. Select one distinguished evening gown illustrating subordination-dominance.
5. Make a collection of costume accessories such as shoes, bags, gloves, belts, jewelry, and millinery in which the structure has significance. At the same time the decoration should be restrained, emphasize structure, and be well suited to its function.
6. Find a costume design which you believe is an outstanding example of a center of interest originating from interesting structural lines.
7. Select a few complete ensembles that you feel have fine rhythmic movement and analyze the total ensemble to learn how the person assembling the costume achieved this rhythmic movement.
8. Select a few complete costume ensembles that illustrate unity of the entire costume theme.

Seven

Texture and Texture Combination

WHEN selecting clothes the average woman is apt to be influenced by color and line, although for her a more important consideration should be the fabric. Perfect design and color will be disappointing in an inappropriate or unbecoming texture.

The new fabrics appearing season after season inspire changes of fashion. The feel of the new textures, the play of light and shadow over fabric surfaces, the creation of new weaves and finishes, all inspire the intelligent designer to create new silhouettes. In a similar manner, those who select clothes for themselves and those whose profession involves advising others in their selections will gain real pleasure from sensitivity to the feel and draping quality and surface interest of textures. Whether our problem is the simplest article of apparel or the coordination of a complete ensemble, there will be greater beauty and satisfaction when textures have been skillfully chosen and combined.

TEXTURE DEFINED

The word *texture* comes from a Latin root meaning to weave, but as a borrowed term it is used today to mean the surface appearance and feel of all sorts of materials. Van Dyke in his *Art for Art's Sake* remarks that to English-speaking peoples line and form usually have more meaning than color and texture; and that we enjoy them at the expense of the more sensuous experiences gained through color and texture, which he calls *substance*.[1] It is with this essential nature of materials that we are concerned. Seeing, feeling, and hearing all play a part in our recognition of texture. The eye sees a fabric as bright or dull, light or dark, thick or thin, and on through a myriad of fine distinctions. On the other hand, with eyes closed as fabric is handled, we receive a mental picture of the surface contour, and will discover textures that are rough or smooth, coarse or fine, heavy or light, crisp or limp. And as some fabric surfaces touch one another, we are also conscious of sound, for example, in the characteristic *scroop* of silk.

Jakway writes that texture is often the most significant quality possessed by many objects. Line and color are in themselves "impersonal attributes," and "become individualized" through texture interest; and without texture, "decoration would be meaningless and beauty impossible." By texture variation "the dead gloom of black, the glare of white, are relieved and endowed with life and animation, as the heat of red, the cold of blue, and the brilliance of yellow are tempered by texture."[2]

Van Dyke, writing for painters, emphasizes the character or "vivid expression" given to painting by those who have the technical skill to render effects through texture. His description of the problem of the artist in rendering varied textures on canvas may help to open our eyes more fully to the possibilities of texture interest in costume.

> Suppose a woman dressed in yellow tulle. . . . The fabric is loosely woven, reflects no light of importance, is semi-transparent, gauzy, cloud-like. Suppose her wearing yellow ribbons. . . . One side of the ribbon shows a silk surface, closely woven, but reflecting little light, and dull in coloring; the reverse side shows perhaps a satin surface—glossy, bright in color—reflecting a great deal more light than the silk side. Suppose her wearing some gold ornaments; the metal is hard, compact, metallic, polished, shining with light. Suppose lastly, the woman herself has yellow hair; it is not a woven nor a metallic surface, but a mass of fine lines which, seen as a mass, is dull in parts and has some sheen in others; is light, wavy, fluffy, elastic. Here are five different materials not strongly distinguished by their coloring . . . yet distinctly five different materials by virtue of their light-reflecting surfaces. . . .

[1] John C. Van Dyke, *Art for Art's Sake,* Charles Scribner's Sons, New York, 1917, p. 214.
[2] Bernard Jakway, *Principles of Interior Decoration,* The Macmillan Co., New York, 1922, pp. 70–71.

Consider the great difference between the flesh of her arm and the glove below it; between the ivory of her fan and the rose at her waist; between the shining leather of her slippers and the floor she stands upon.[3]

Contrasting textures have been combined eminently well in the illustration of a distinguished costume, the work of one of America's most creative designers (Figure 1). There is a timelessness in the beauty of such a costume, which was designed in 1942 for the Metropolitan Museum's *Renaissance in Fashion*.

An appreciation of texture comes about through cultivation and association. Roughness and smoothness, softness and pliability, used functionally, give us aesthetic satisfaction. The trained eye of the designer is responsive to textures or stuffs that drape and tailor, pleat and ruffle, slenderize and cling, or stand away from the figure. She is concerned not only with surface appearance but also with those characteristics of weight which govern the kinds of edges and folds that fabrics take when manipulated. The fabric maker calls these qualities *hand,* a term he uses to cover their feel, body, weight, and fall.

TEXTURE IS IMPORTANT

This chapter introduces us to the study of textures in relation to their surface interest and to their use, as governed by the way they respond to manipulation. People who appreciate textures are usually acquainted with all kinds of materials. They are able to recognize the qualities of different materials by appearance and handling. They can usually tell the type of fiber of which they are composed; they appreciate differences in them which result from the way they are manufactured and finished; and they also have a certain judgment and taste concerning their best use.

To work professionally with fabrics, from the standpoint of construction or of selection, it is important to know what each will do in the hands of the dressmaker, how every different material falls when cut, as well as what effect it will have on the appearance and feeling of the individual who is to wear it. Furthermore, knowing the skill and effort which go into the making of a piece of beautiful silk or woolen or a bit of fine lace, a person will handle it with respect and a thrill of delight.

The mechanization of all our industries, which began with the Industrial Revolution and seems to have speeded up enormously since the Second World

---

[3] Van Dyke, *op. cit.,* p. 216.

120   *The Arts of Costume and Personal Appearance*

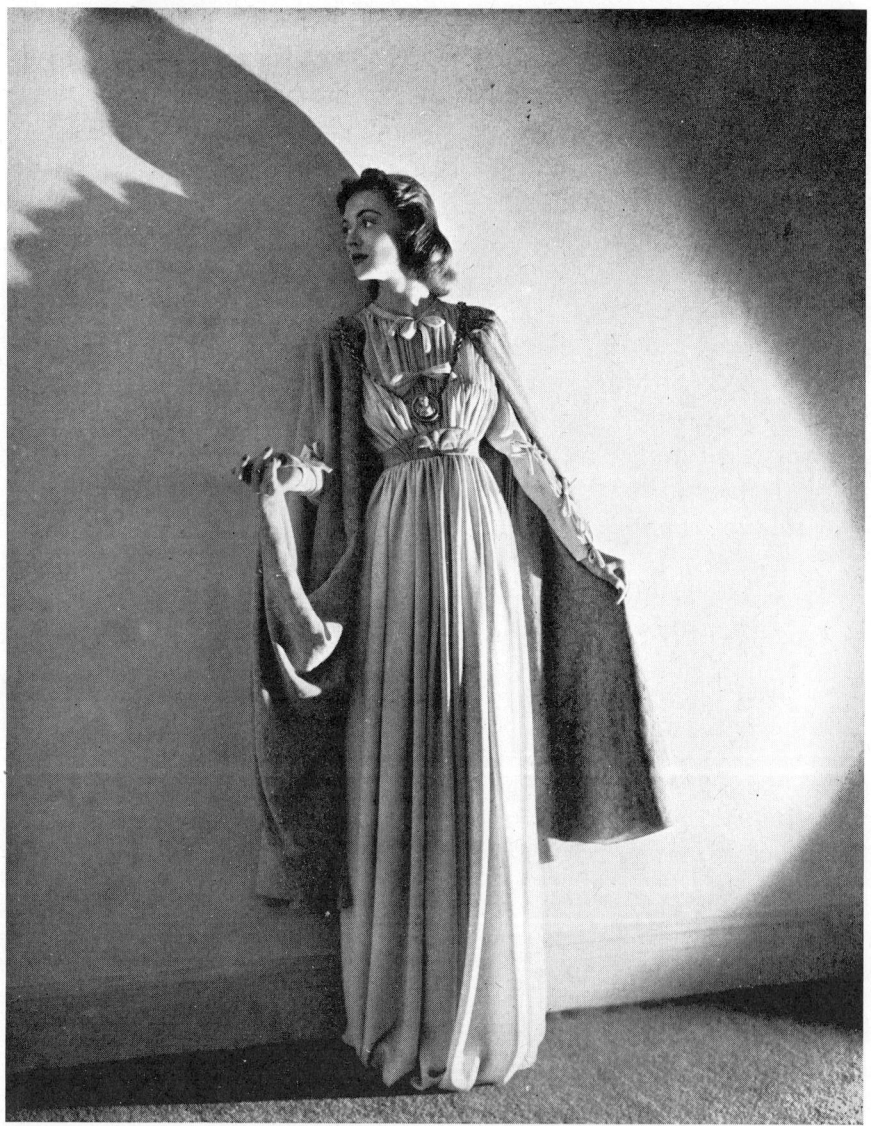

Figure 1. Valentina chose Celanese Creative Fabrics for this magnificent dinner ensemble designed for the Metropolitan Museum of Art's exhibit, Renaissance in Fashion, *in 1942. The gown is of white crepe, fastened with small self bows in the manner of early Renaissance fashions. Over it is a cape of Forstmann's beige wool lined with gold brocade and held in place by an antique gold chain. Flame-colored slippers. Courtesy of Madame Valentina and Celanese Corporation of America.*

War, has taken more and more of the chance for creativeness and originality out of our lives. Americans are criticized for being spectators and listeners rather than actors in all sorts of activities, from sports to musical performances. One well-known sociologist deplores this tendency; she feels that the strength of this country stems from the pioneers who learned to work with their hands, to know the materials they worked with, and to be independent and creative.

All of the plastic elements and principles of design should be considered and an attempt made to apply them when planning, developing, and completing an aesthetically pleasing costume. Anni Albers charmingly expresses her thoughts on designing from the point of view of a hand weaver.

Designing has become more and more an intellectual performance. . . . It deals no longer directly with the medium but vicariously. To restore to the designer the . . . *direct* experience of a medium is . . . as I see it, a justification for crafts today. . . . It means taking, for instance, the working material into the hand, learning by working it of its obedience and its resistance, its potency and its weakness, its charm and dullness. . . . We learn to respect material in working it.

Civilization seems in general to estrange men from materials, that is, from materials in their original form. . . . One person is rarely involved in the whole course of manufacture, often knowing only the finished product. But if we want to get from materials the sense of directness, the adventure of being close to the stuff the world is made of, we have to go back to the material itself, to its original state, and from there on partake in its stages of change.

Weaving is an example of a craft which is many-sided. Besides surface qualities, such as rough and smooth, dull and shiny, hard and soft, it also includes color, and as the dominating element, texture, which is the result of the construction of weaves. Like any craft, it may end in producing useful objects, or it may rise to the level of art.[4]

TEXTURE AND LIGHT

Maitland Graves' comments on texture interest in the arts in general are quite as true of texture in costume.

Texture is visual as well as tactile. That is, texture is perceived by our eyes as well as by our sense of touch, because wet or glossy surfaces reflect more light than dry, dull, or matt surfaces, and rough surfaces absorb light more unevenly and to a greater extent than smooth surfaces. Thus by association of visual experiences with tactile experiences, things look, as well as feel, wet or dry, rough or smooth. Also, because

---

[4] Anni Albers, *On Designing,* Pelango Press, New Haven, 1959, pp. 6, 33, 50, 52.

texture affects light absorption and reflectance—that is, color—texture and color are directly related. For example, the same color may appear different when wet, dry, rough and smooth.

Because of these visual aspects, texture is as important a design element as shape, size, and color in the visual arts.[5]

Textures may be divided into several classes:

Those that absorb the light and are consequently dull-surfaced, because of the character of their raw materials, rough yarns, fabric construction, or finish, as moss crepe or a rough cotton suiting.

Those that reflect the light and are lustrous, because of the luster and smoothness of their raw materials, or the smoothness of the yarns or the weave, as satin; or because of the kind of finish, as glazed chintz.

Those that both reflect and absorb light, as pile materials. Let us study a piece of faille crepe with a reading glass and note the luster of those yarns that catch the light and the dullness of those in the shadows. Or study a piece of satin and note the luster of the long floats with few shadows throughout their entire length, reflecting so much light that they fairly dilute their own color, making the fabric seem lighter than it actually is. Compare it with a piece of velvet of the same hue. Every thread of the velvet pile is casting a little shadow on its neighbor, so that the reflection on the surface of the velvet is limited to the tips of the pile. Notice how much richer the velvet seems than the satin, even though there is no color difference. The velvet intensifies its own color by multiple reflection, because the light falling onto the velvet is reflected from fiber to fiber, picking up with each reflection a little more color, whereas in its folds the color appears even richer and deeper.

TEXTURES AND TOUCH

In certain European countries in times past the development of the sense of touch was considered so important to education that children of twelve or fourteen were put in classes, then blindfolded and led to tables on which were placed mixed piles of all manner of materials encountered in furnishing homes or making clothing: feathers, straws, braids, wood, bone, lace, porce-

---

[5] Maitland Graves, *Art in Color and Design,* Second Edition, McGraw-Hill Book Company, New York, 1951, p. 221.

lain, cottons, silks, metals. The children were then asked to assemble by feel those which they considered texturally harmonious. Afterwards they compared what had been chosen by feel with what they would choose by sight and were thus led to sense texture relationships. Perhaps this emphasis in their schools explains the fine craftsmanship shown in both fabric and fashion creation in European countries.

"We examine the textural environment," says Donald Anderson, "for information and pleasure. We seem to require variations in the field for our own well-being . . . and can only imagine a world of identical surfaces as some kind of torture. As presently constituted we might not be able to exist in such a world." [6]

Young people today in the United States seem to lack this tactile sense, but it must be emphasized that one who works professionally with colors and fabrics will not go far without it.

Each of the textile fibers has inherent properties which help to determine the appearance and feel of the finished fabric. Thus we must come to know something of the full, soft fuzziness of cotton before it is processed; the cool, sleek, hard, inelastic feel of flax or linen; the softness, warmth, and elasticity of high grade wool. We must know, too, the soft sheen and smooth, warm, pliant feel of a skein of raw silk; the duller, rough feel of wild silk; the metallic sheen and slipperiness of bright man-made fibers; and the dull opaqueness of delustered or pigmented ones.

MANUFACTURE AFFECTS TEXTURE

By modern spinning processes these different fibers may be converted into yarns of a thousand varieties in size and nature. They may be spun into yarns of undreamed-of fineness and delicacy, or made into large, coarse, irregular yarns of many types. Sometimes they are merely carded to straighten the fibers, the loose, short ends producing a fuzzy appearance; or the combing process may be used to separate out all the short ends, leaving a smooth, thready appearance in the finished fabric.

Other yarns, such as reeled silk and many of the man-made fibers, are used in the form of filaments of indefinite length, with no short fibers to form a fuzzy effect, so that the fabrics made from them may be very smooth

---

[6] Donald Anderson, *Elements of Design,* Holt, Rinehart and Winston, New York, 1961, p. 121.

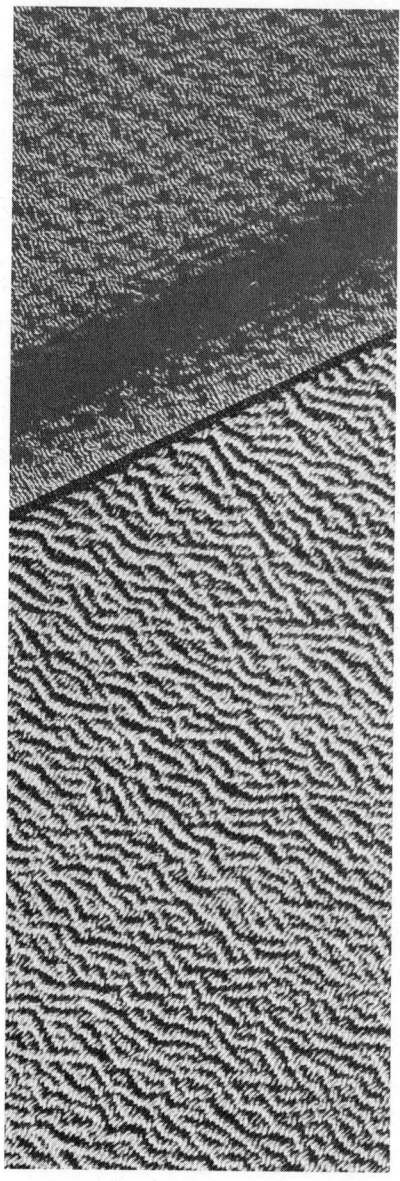 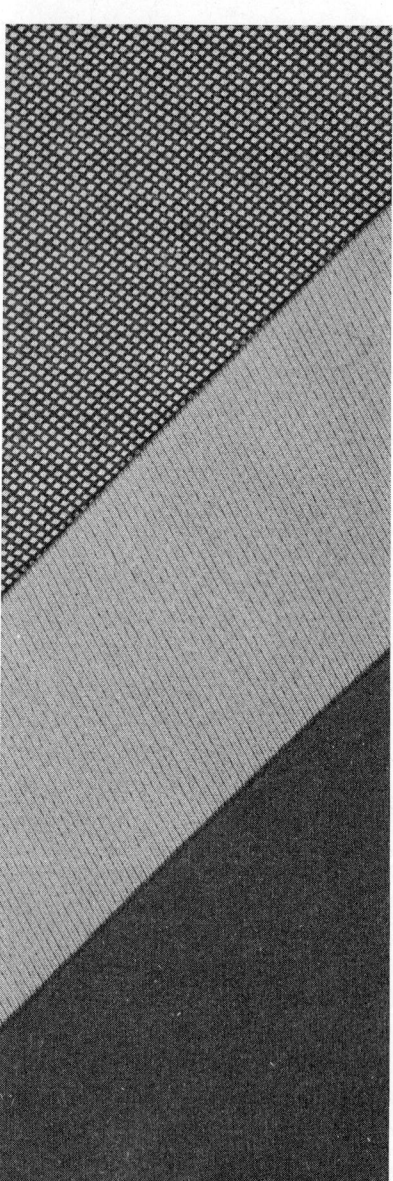

Figure 2. Rough crepes which have relatively high twist, causing surface irregularities which both reflect and absorb light. Courtesy of International Silk Association.

Figure 3. Worsted fabrics of combed yarns and hard surface, lending themselves to fine tailoring.

and shiny. Some yarns are twisted barely enough to hold the fibers together in strands, when soft, drapable materials are desired; other yarns are dull, and form a more or less pebbly or rough surface, depending on the size, tension, and twist of the yarns (Figure 2). Combed yarns in a firm, close weave form the clear finish characteristic of fine worsteds, and make a strong, hard-feeling fabric suited to tailoring (Figure 3).

In addition to the numberless ways of changing the character of fibers and yarns, great variation results from the processes used in constructing them into fabrics, and finally from the finishing treatments which different cloths undergo. A detailed discussion of modern fibers, weaves, and finishes is not within the scope of this book, but in Appendix C we have attempted to describe a number of standard materials, chosen from the galaxy of our contemporary world of fabrics, furs, and leathers, considering those factors in their appearance and hand which influence their possible draping and tailoring qualities. Even among standard fabrics quality plays an important role, for any type distinguished by its pliability or resilience tends to be less so when of a poor grade. Scientists have developed a scale for describing the hand of fabrics, as shown in the chart of "Terms Relating to Hand of Fabrics," developed by a joint committee of the American Association of Textile Chemists and Colorists and Committee D-13 of the American Society for Testing Materials.

In addition to standard well-known textures there are at our disposal innumerable fabrics which may be classed as novelties, in which the weaver has run in little bits of furry wool, a lustrous thread, tufts of cotton, or a fleck of gold to add interest or sparkle and to stimulate the imagination of the clothes designer. And then there is the entire range of trimmings, contributing richly to decoration. There is the smooth, sleek flow of line in fringes, the play of light and dark in lustrous braids against handsome worsteds. The trained eye appreciates the soft, refined polish of fine bone, plastic, or wooden buttons on napped woolens, the satiny sheen of black soleil felt against grosgrain or velvet, and the texture interest of certain straws such as milan, paillasson, and crocheted braids. The designer must be acquainted with the scintillating quality of rhinestones, the iridescence of sequins, the opalescence of good pearls, and the soft, pearl-like glazes of certain porcelains and metals used in today's costume jewelry. She must know the suitability of exquisitely delicate Chantilly and the rich, flower-patterned Venetian laces in texture combinations. All these she should come to know and enjoy, even though she may not possess them as her own.

TERMS RELATING TO HAND OF FABRICS*

PHYSICAL PROPERTY	EXPLANATORY PHRASE	TERMS TO BE USED IN DESCRIBING RANGE OF CORRESPONDING COMPONENT OF HAND
Flexibility	Ease of bending	Pliable (high) to stiff (low)
Compressibility	Ease of squeezing	Soft (high) to hard (low)
Extensibility	Ease of stretching	Stretchy (high) to non-stretchy (low)
Resilience	Ability to recover from deformation	Springy (high) to limp (low); resilience may be flexural, compressional, extensional, or torsional
Density	Weight per unit volume (based on measurement of thickness† and fabric weight)	Compact (high) to open (low)
Surface Contour	Divergence of the surface from planeness	Rough (high) to smooth (low)
Surface Friction	Resistance to slipping offered by the surface	Harsh (high) to slippery (low)
Thermal Character	Apparent difference in temperature of the fabric and the skin of the observer touching it	Cool (high) to warm (low)

* From ASTM *Standards on Textile Materials,* Standard D-123, American Society for Testing Materials, 1916 Race Street, Philadelphia 3, Pa., October 1962, p. 57.
† Thickness measurements and weight are made in accordance with the procedures described in the ASTM method for specific fabrics.

THE RIGHT TEXTURE

In order to dress beautifully one should grasp every means of knowing the fabrics of today: how they feel and respond to manipulation; what silhouettes can be made from them; the kinds of seams and dressmaker finishes they will take; which to choose for country clothes, and town and evening fashions; how to combine them appropriately. Use imagination to adapt untried materials to costume uses.

The designer must understand the importance of *grain* in the material, the way the lengthwise and crosswise yarns must lie in the garment to give the effect she visualizes. Dior said, "I learned the importance of this principle—the most essential one in dressmaking . . . the *direction* of a material. A dress may be a success or a complete failure, depending on whether or not one has known how to direct the natural movement of the cloth, which one must always obey. . . . Fabric not only expresses a designer's dreams but also stimulates his own ideas. . . . Many a dress of mine is born of the fabric alone. . . . One must be able to resist temptations and avoid the traps of too beautiful a material, which by its very beauty sometimes makes it impossible to use."[7]

Another test of one's skill is selecting the right fabric to create illusions, express temperament, and flatter complexions. There will always be needed that fine shade of difference that is right for a particular individual. Will a crepe of a degree less heavy than faille better express the mood? Will the merest sheen be more flattering than one entirely dull, though receding? What weight and fineness of tweed will be entirely right for this individual to wear?

TEXTURE INFLUENCES THE SILHOUETTE

It will be recalled that silhouettes class themselves into three types and their modifications: the tubular, the bell, and the bustle. But from the standpoint of texture and the manner of manipulation, silhouettes may be classified in a different manner:

Tailored Silhouettes
   1. Severely tailored or formal
   2. Soft-tailored or dressmaker-tailored
Draped Silhouettes
   1. Straight-draped or soft-hanging
   2. Bias-draped
   3. Crisp
      a. Circular cut
      b. Full bouffant
      c. Bustle

Clothing of the earliest types from various parts of the world can be classified under one or another of these silhouette types. The tailored type comes

---

[7] Christian Dior, *Talking About Fashion*, G. P. Putnam's Sons, New York, 1954, pp. 23, 34, 35.

from northern regions, and is associated with the use of furs and the invention of the eyed needle. In caves of the paleolithic age in France, needles made of mammoth ivory have been found, fine enough to sew a tailor-made garment of today.

The draped garment originated in warmer regions of the world; the graceful folds of the garments in Greek statues and the sari as draped in many different styles in various parts of India show the timeless beauty in this use of lovely fabric. These garments were not cut and sewn, but were draped or pleated and held in place by a knot of the fabric or a jeweled clasp.

Texture and Tailored Silhouettes

The formal, tailored silhouette is best represented by the man-tailored suit. It demands firm but pliable sleek-looking materials, which are at their best made up in designs that have plain, flat surfaces and sharp edges, and for which perfection in cut and excellent workmanship are necessities. These materials must respond well to outside stitching and pressing and must resist wrinkling. Fabrics which work up well in coats and suits on these severely tailored lines are dry-feeling worsteds and twills, heavy tweeds and wool broadcloths, the stiffer moirés and bengalines, crease-resistant dress linens, piqués, and sharkskins. Denims and other heavy cotton suitings, such as gabardines, failles, ottomans, and "transitional" cottons, have recently been used by leading designers, tailored as carefully as worsteds. Firm interfacings are usually used in these tailored costumes, enhancing the firmness of the outer material.

We can draw no hard-and-fast dividing line between this type of tailored garment and the following one.

The soft, dressmaker-tailored silhouette depends less on perfect tailoring and detail than on individuality and a soft, graceful effect. It may be a molded type of suit, following the contours of the body, but with less precise detail and interfacing than the tailored suit. Or it may be a suit or dress-jacket ensemble of the casual, straight-line Chanel type. This silhouette may be made successfully in a wide variety of fabrics that fall in soft lines and look well in flat surfaces. We may choose from such textures as feather-weight tweeds, corded worsteds, surah or silk serge (Figure 4), shantungs, faille crepes, checked and plaid ginghams, and medium-weight cotton suitings. Soft napped and textured woolens (Figure 5) lend themselves to the dressmaker type of tailoring, in contrast to the worsteds (Figure 3).

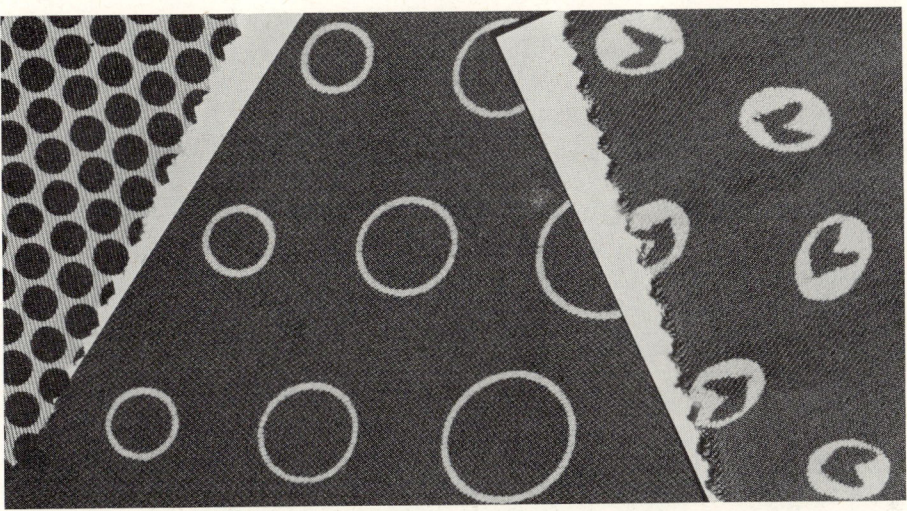

Figure 4. Printed twilled silks (surahs) for soft-tailored street dresses and blouses. Courtesy of International Silk Association. Left, black dots on greenish gold; center, white circles on green; right, white figures on wine red.

Texture and Draped Silhouettes

The straight-draped, soft-hanging silhouette is one that depends on soft material which hangs naturally in straight, vertical folds. Texture interest is added by the use of gathers, shirring, smocking, or dart tucks. Interest is also obtained when unpressed pleats are allowed to fall softly from shoulder to waistline or from hip to hem in flat, firm, nonbulky materials. The material must be heavy enough to fall close to the body.

Many materials handle well in these soft, heavy folds; the character of the folds themselves depends on the body of the material. Often a material such as voile or batiste would have little texture interest when used on flat surfaces, but gains distinction when its surfaces are broken into small tucks and straight-hanging folds. Chiffon, georgette, jersey, crepe, and crepe-back satin hang in a similar way (Figure 1), but may be pleated as well (Figure 15 Chapter Five). Soft gingham and chambray, challis, and sheer wool crepe take somewhat crisper folds and may be used in full gathered skirts adapted from Tyrolean costume. Jerseys of silk, wool, or man-made fibers lend themselves to small folds and to draping in a soft, clinging fashion. These fabrics are adaptable to daytime dresses and, in white or pastels, to

130   *The Arts of Costume and Personal Appearance*

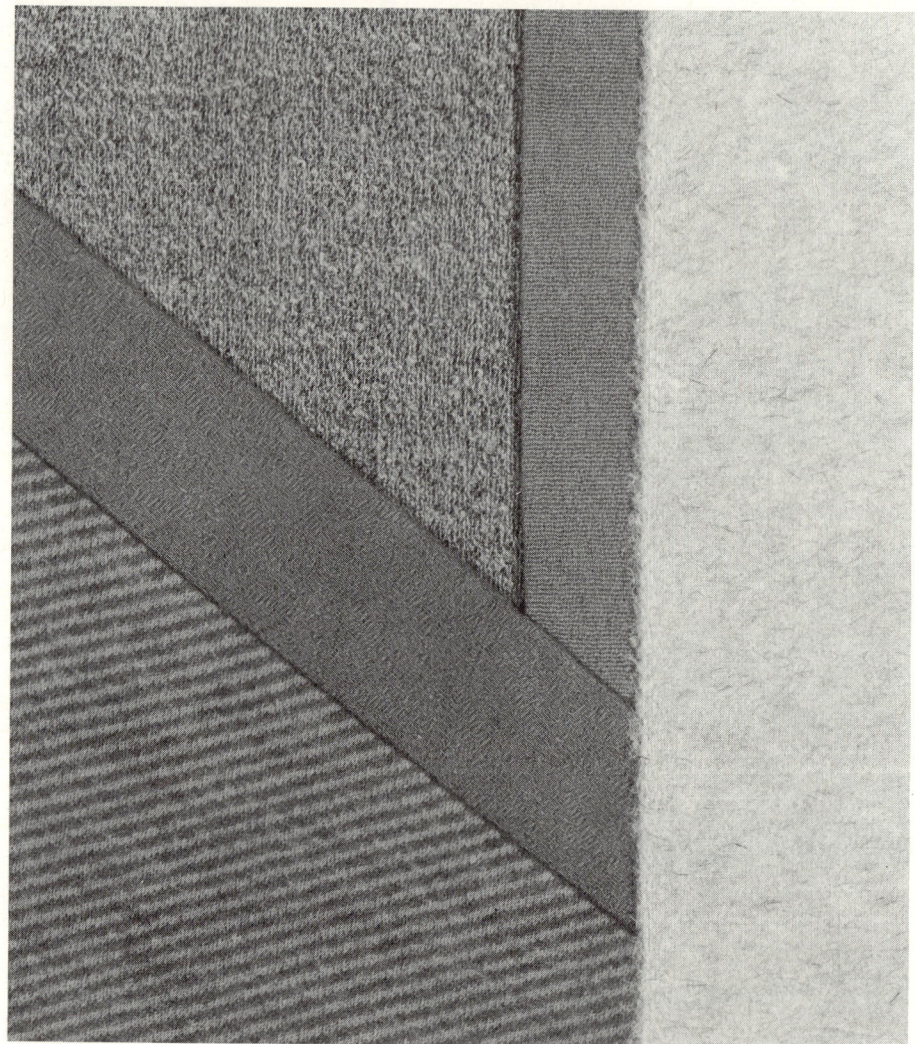

Figure 5. Soft and spongy textured woolens, in bouclé, jersey, crepe, and fleece fabrics.

evening types. Sheer wool (Figure 6) in an open weave is shown here in an afternoon or informal evening dress. It is graceful and feminine in its soft-hanging fullness.

The bias-draped silhouette, suggested by the Indian sari and by an asymmetric type of draping in sophisticated afternoon and evening gowns, offers

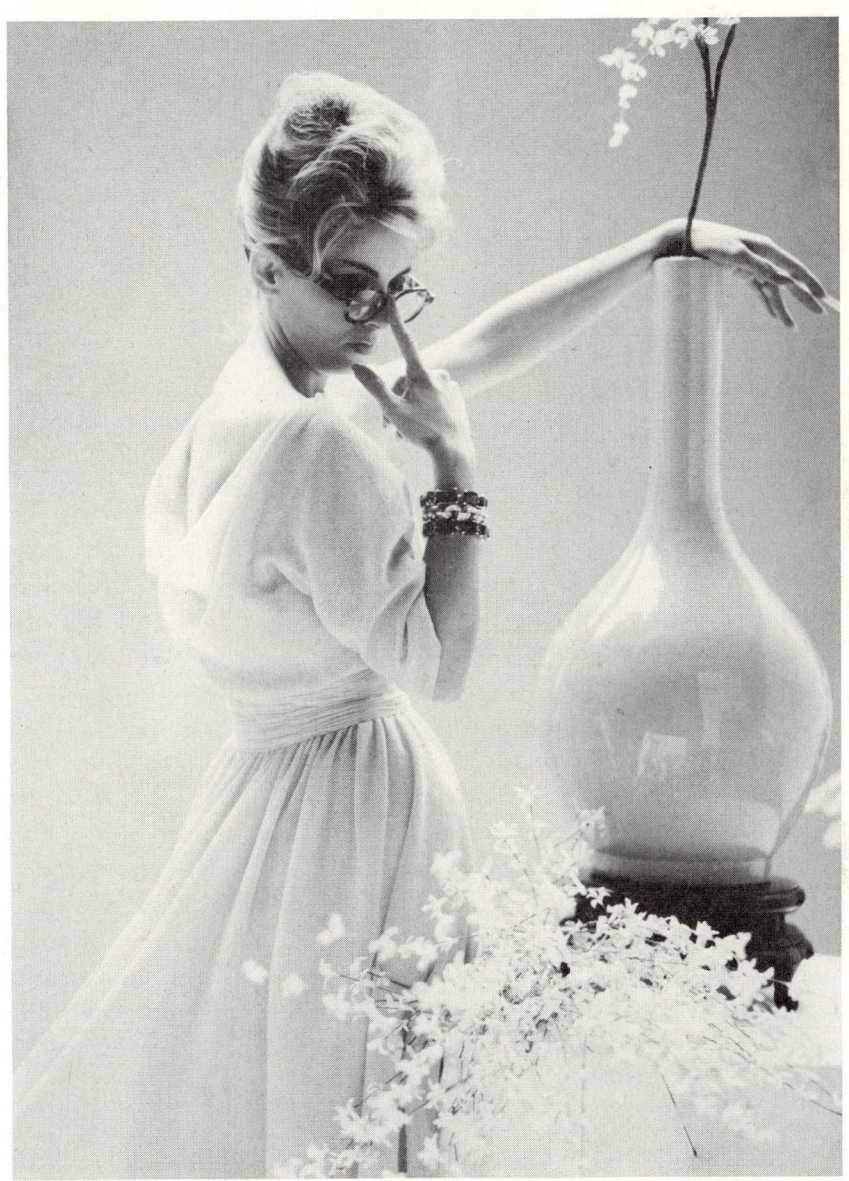

Figure 6. The sheerest of wools in a leno weave lends itself to soft draping. Courtesy of the Wool Bureau, Inc.

scope for creative skill. It requires material with beautiful, rich highlights or dull matte surfaces to give the effect wanted. In any case, the fabric must be adaptable to manipulation on the bias grain and yet must possess a body that produces beautiful curves in an infinite number of ways. The skillful dressmaker does this kind of draping on a dress form or a mannequin, rather than with flat patterns. Suitable textures are heavy rich crepes, crepe-back satins, soft moirés and failles, chiffon velvets, semisheer brocades, and lamés. The lovely sheer jerseys also adapt themselves well to drapery of this kind, because their liquid fall permits the creating of effects like those found in Greek sculpture.

The crisp silhouette stands away from the figure and requires crisp or stiff fabrics to produce a bouffant effect (Figure 7). This is accomplished either by cutting on the circular or by gathering. The silhouette in which the "stand alone" quality in the material produces a bouffant effect would be a straight-hanging silhouette in a soft fabric.

Circular or *flared silhouettes* require materials which are crisp but have the kind of texture interest to look well when seen in fairly large unbroken areas. Suitable materials are Lyons-type velvets, peau de soie, failles, stiffened laces, stiff taffetas, and brocaded lamés (Figures 8 and 9). Other materials, such as organdy, dotted Swiss, organza, stiffened net, piqué, and linen, are also made into these flared or circular silhouettes.

Some materials have sufficient body to permit cutting on the circular for street length garments. These include firm woolens, felt, faille, linen, cotton satins and ottomans, piqués, denims, and similar weaves in the man-made fibers and blends.

Full bouffant silhouettes are produced when crisp or transparent materials are gathered or pleated, ruffled or tiered, with fullness beginning at the waistline, in contrast to the circular or gored skirt, where the fullness increases toward the lower edge of the skirt. Suitable fabrics are stiffened net or marquisette, tulle, organdy, taffeta, moiré, peau de soie or organza (Figure 10). An interesting contrast in which the very texture, sheen, and cut of the garments forms an appropriate expression of the differences in the personalities of two women, one mature and sophisticated, the other demure and ingénue, is illustrated in portraits by Ingres and Winterhalter (Figures 11 and 12). The couturiers who designed the costumes and the artists who painted the portraits may be credited with the happy association of costume and personality.

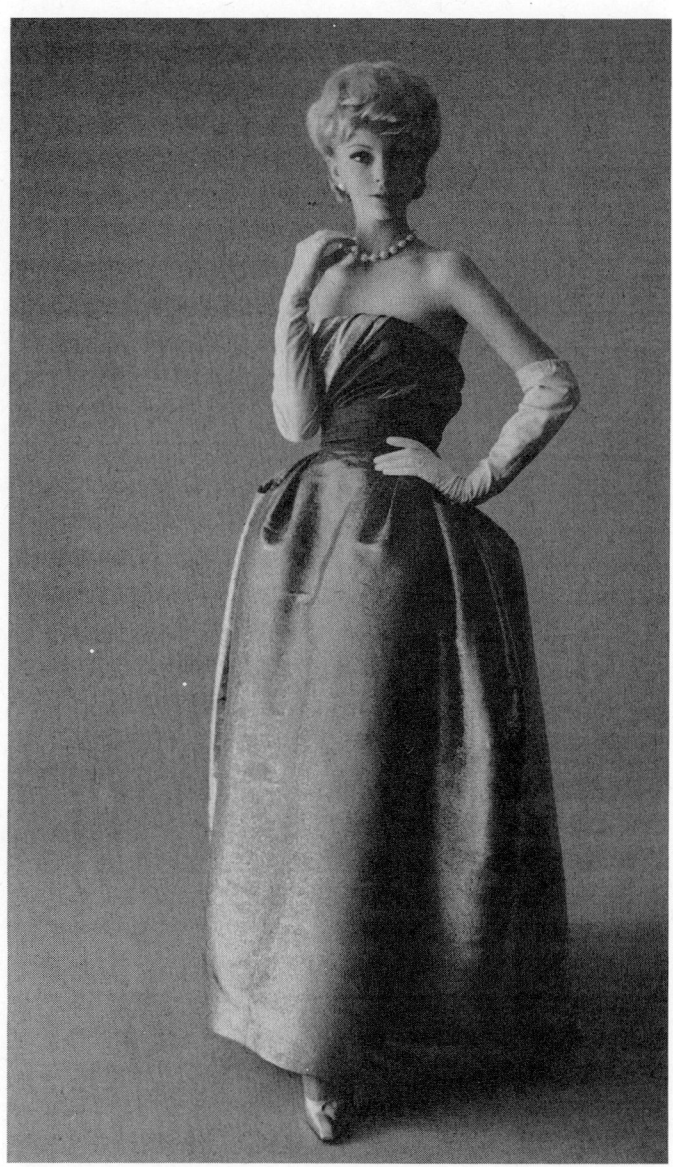

Figure 7. Lamé evening gown by Pierre Balmain, courtesy of L'Officiel. *Photograph by Ph. Pottier.*

134 *The Arts of Costume and Personal Appearance*

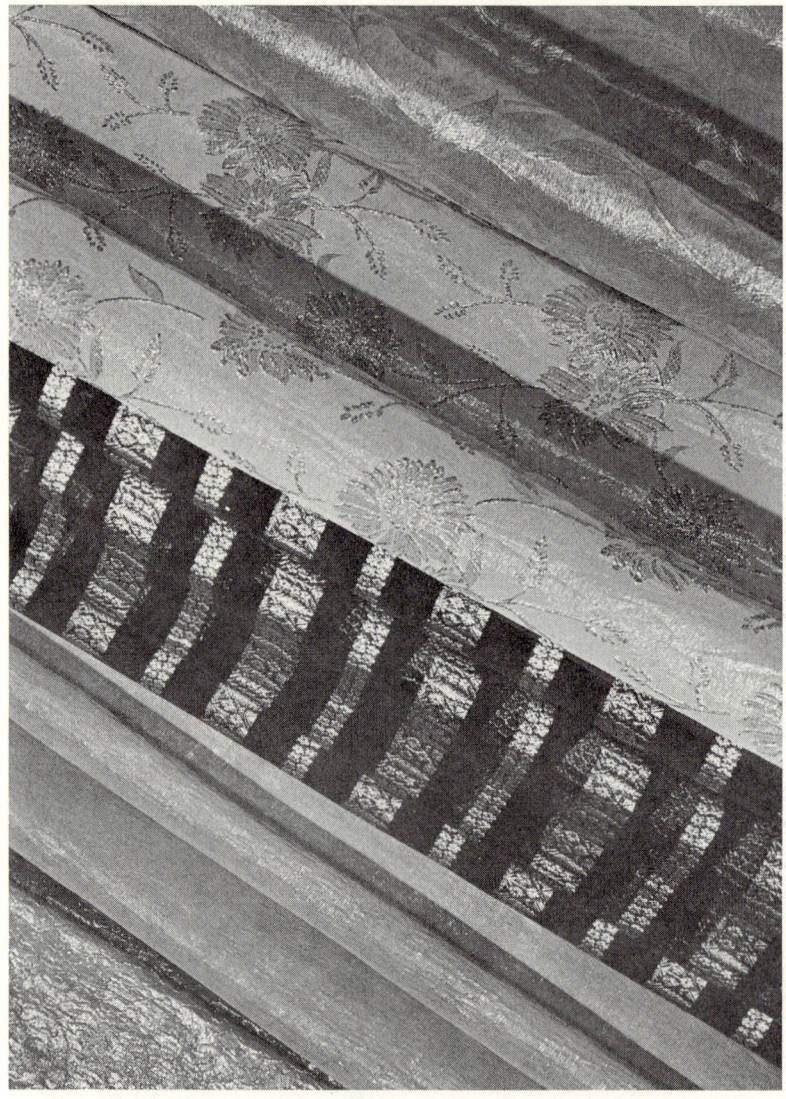

Figure 8. Brocaded lamés of different weights and patterns. The stripe is gold on black silk; the floral pattern, silver metal on a pink silk background; the one to the right of it, light blue and silver. Courtesy of International Silk Association.

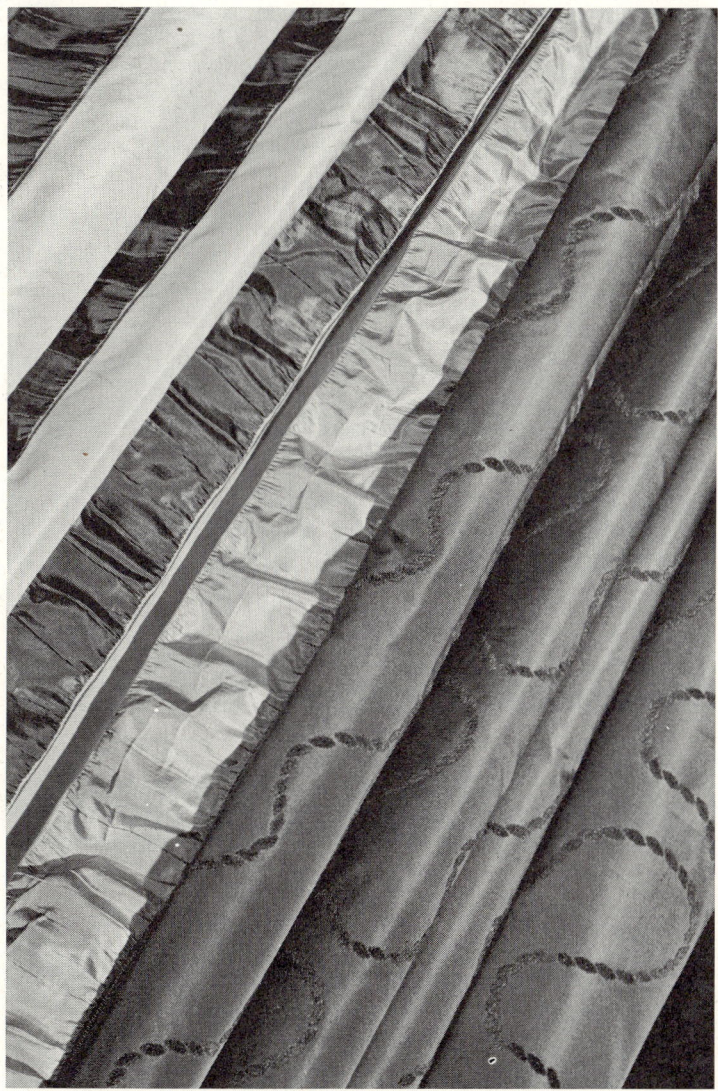

Figure 9. Silk taffetas which have a stand-alone quality. This photograph reveals something of the luster and crispness which characterize the finest quality taffetas. Courtesy of International Silk Association.

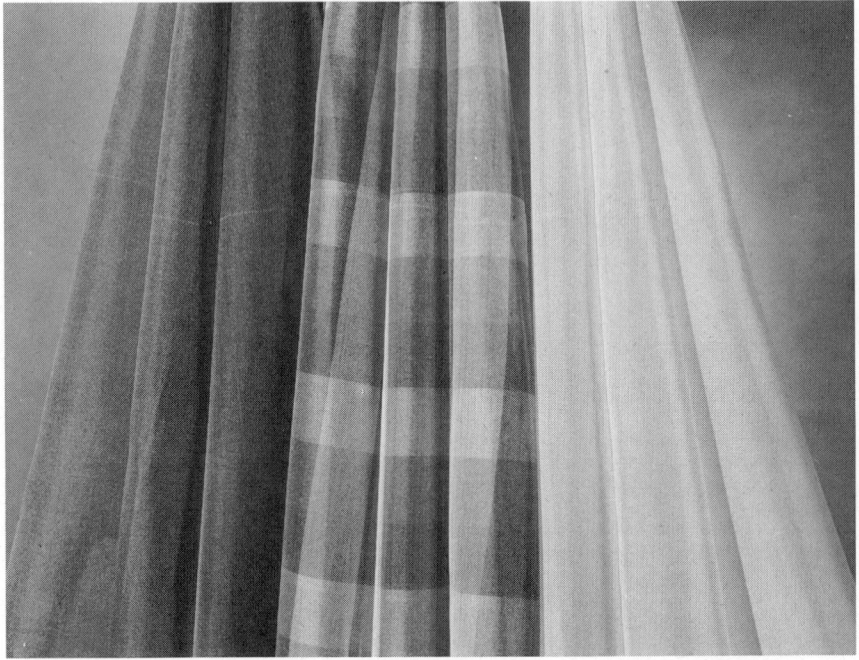

Figure 10. Silk organza. Subtle shadings of one hue tie together the plaid with the plain colors. University of Nebraska photograph.

Fashion at times dictates that fabrics assume the bouffant effect through the use of crinolines or stiff linings.

Bustle effects are accomplished in the same crisp materials mentioned above. When they appear from time to time in modern fashion, they are less exaggerated and more graceful than the shelf-like protuberances of the 1880's. In modern costumes, a bustle effect is suggested by the use of back fullness, as in Dior's evening gown (Figure 13), or by the use of large bows or perky peplums.

THE ART OF COMBINING TEXTURES

Although there are many helpful guides to combining colors, rules for combining textures are hard to convey clearly through words. As one of the plastic elements of design (Chapter Five) texture must be used in such

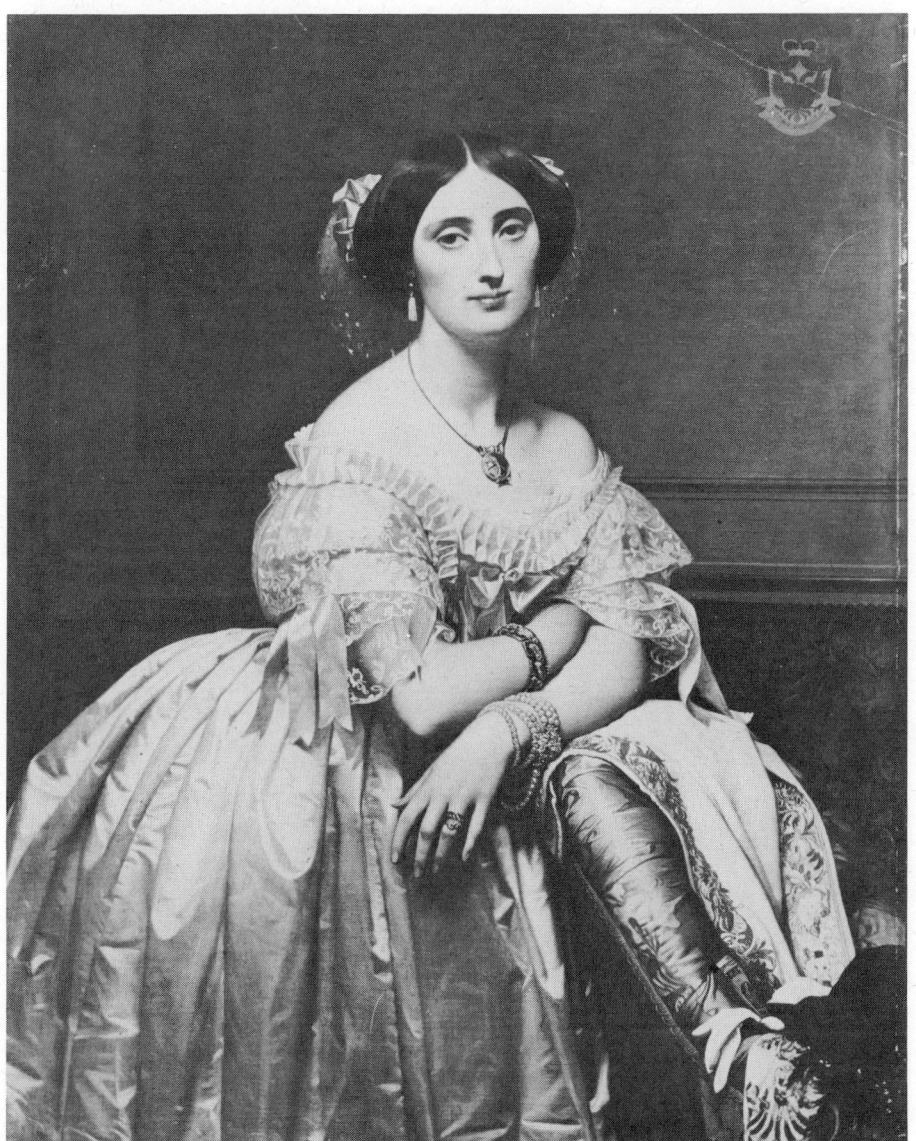

Figure 11. Princess de Brogli. *By Jean Auguste Ingres. From the collection of the Duchess de Brogli, Paris. Courtesy of M. Walter Pach and Harper and Brothers. A charming 1860 version of the* robe de style *worn by a grand lady, and composed of textures used similarly in formal costume today—satin, embroidery, fragile laces, ribbons, and pearls.*

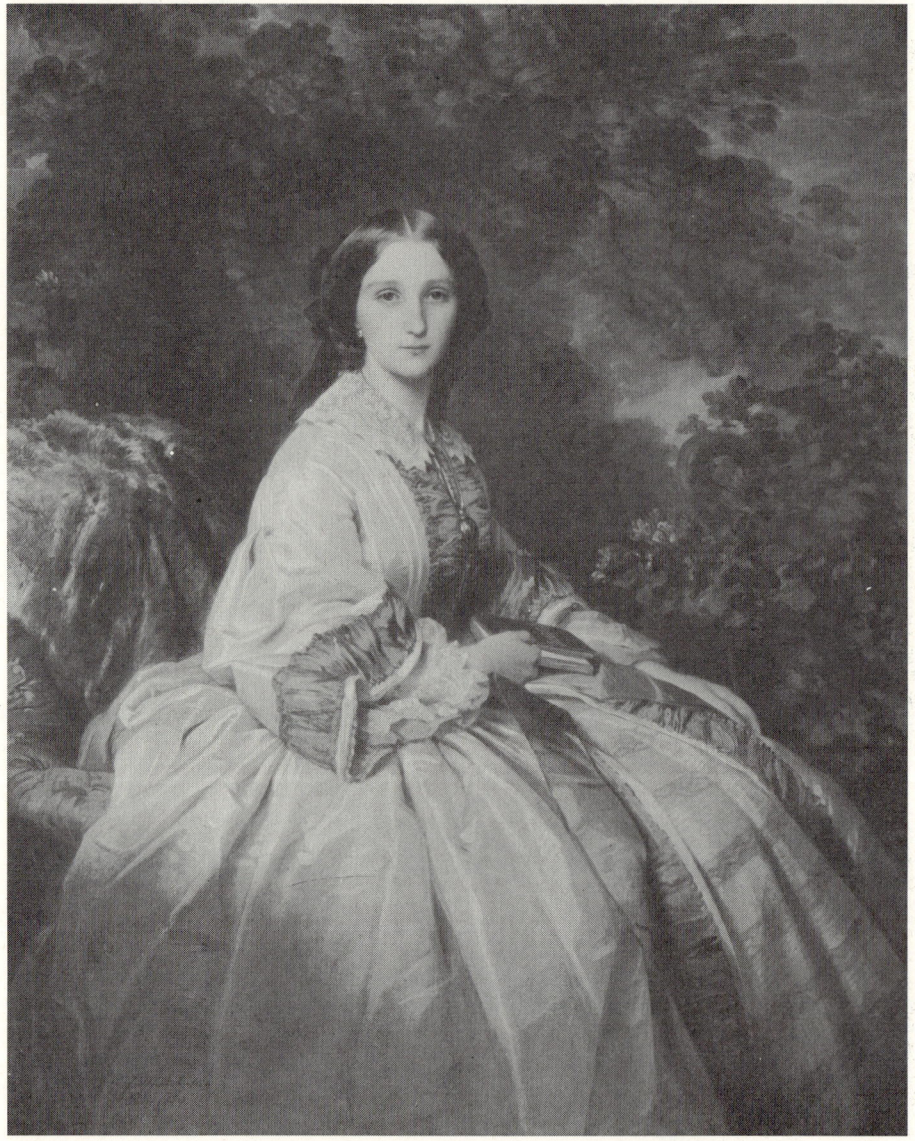

Figure 12. Countess Maria Ivonava Lamsdorff. *By* Francois Xavier Winterhalter. *Collection of Miss Adelaide Milton de Groot. Courtesy of the* Metropolitan Museum of Art. *Soft taffeta, ruchings, tucks, and laces form an enchanting costume which seems right for a demure and dignified young aristocrat.*

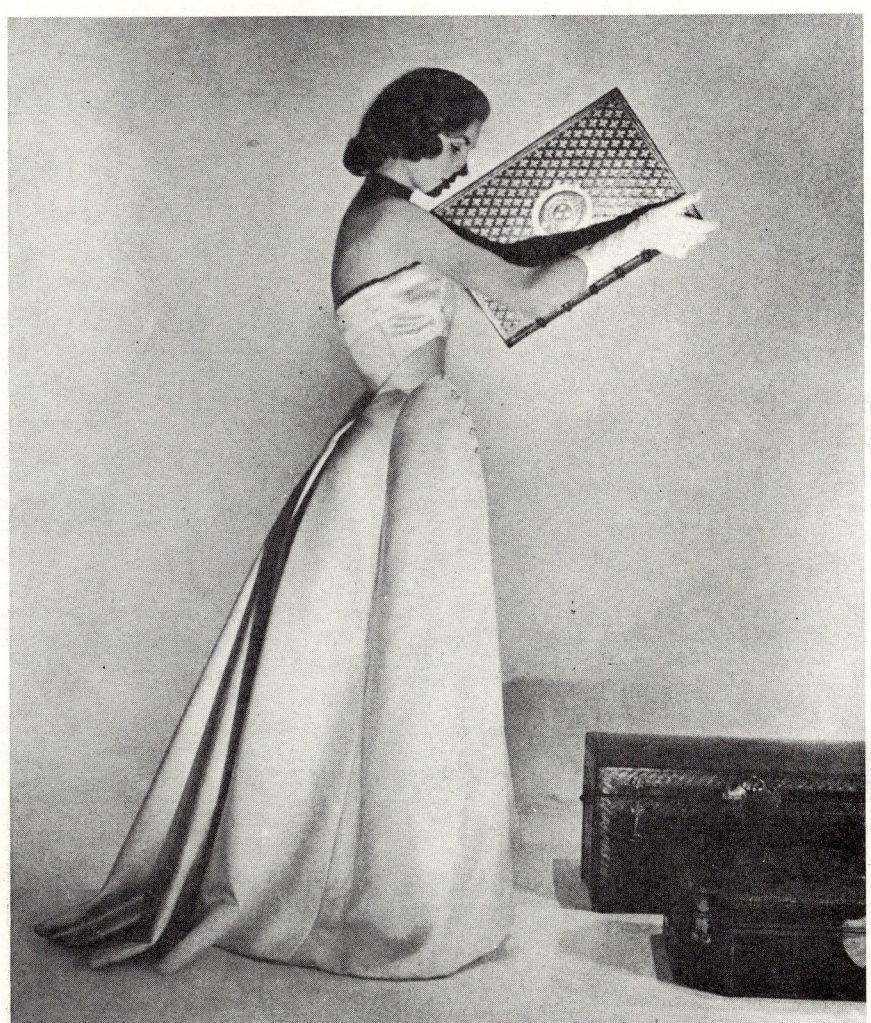

Figure 13. Dior's magnificent backward flight of heavy pink satin. A stiffened arched band curves downward over the rib cage, diminishing the waist before it flows out in the skirt. Photo by Louise Dahl-Wolfe. Courtesy of Harper's Bazaar.

a way as to contribute to the total effect of the design. Harmony of texture is as important to a fine design as harmony of color. Variety may be introduced by a judicious combination of textures, but always within the framework of a central idea. Texture can introduce a change of pace in the design as the spaces and shapes within the composition are developed. The great secret of good texture combinations seems to lie in two factors:

Unity of idea with accompanying variety—similarity with contrasts. Unity means harmony of weight or hand, such as sheer with sheer, heavy with heavy, rich with rich, smooth with smooth, sheen with sheen. Obviously this means no heavy leathers with soft delicate textures or sheer textures with tweeds. It is necessary to have similarity with a little of the unexpected, but always a consistency of idea.

Association of ideas—textures that seem to belong together because associated in one's mind with certain recollections. We delight in the consistency of textures used together (Figure 14). The soft luster of taffeta, textured by soft pleats and shirring, the polished coiffure of the young woman, the delicate lace of her chemise, the sheen of ribbons, the glint of Sèvres porcelain, the richness of velvet and fringe, and the gilt of the mirror's frame seem right to one's sense of the appropriate.

APPRECIATION OF TEXURES OF PAST TIMES

One very important means of gaining appreciation of textures is through acquaintance with the fabrics of the great periods of costume history. We are impressed with their beauty of design, color, and texture, and with the variety of weaves. They can and do still provide inspiration for the fabric creations of today. Perhaps our only important addition to fabric knowledge is in speed and efficiency of manufacture and care, rather than in intrinsic beauty. Knowing the significance of the sumptuous, patterned damasks and velvet brocades of Renaissance Florence and Venice helps us to understand something of the era which produced them.

We have an opportunity to study these precious fabrics and costumes through the glass of museum cases in the United States and Europe and in the portraits of such masters as Botticelli, Memling, Van der Weyden, and Ghirlandaio. For the student of textiles it is fortunate that it was the fashion among artists to show every detail of texture and design in fabrics, so that it is possible for modern textile designers to reproduce them per-

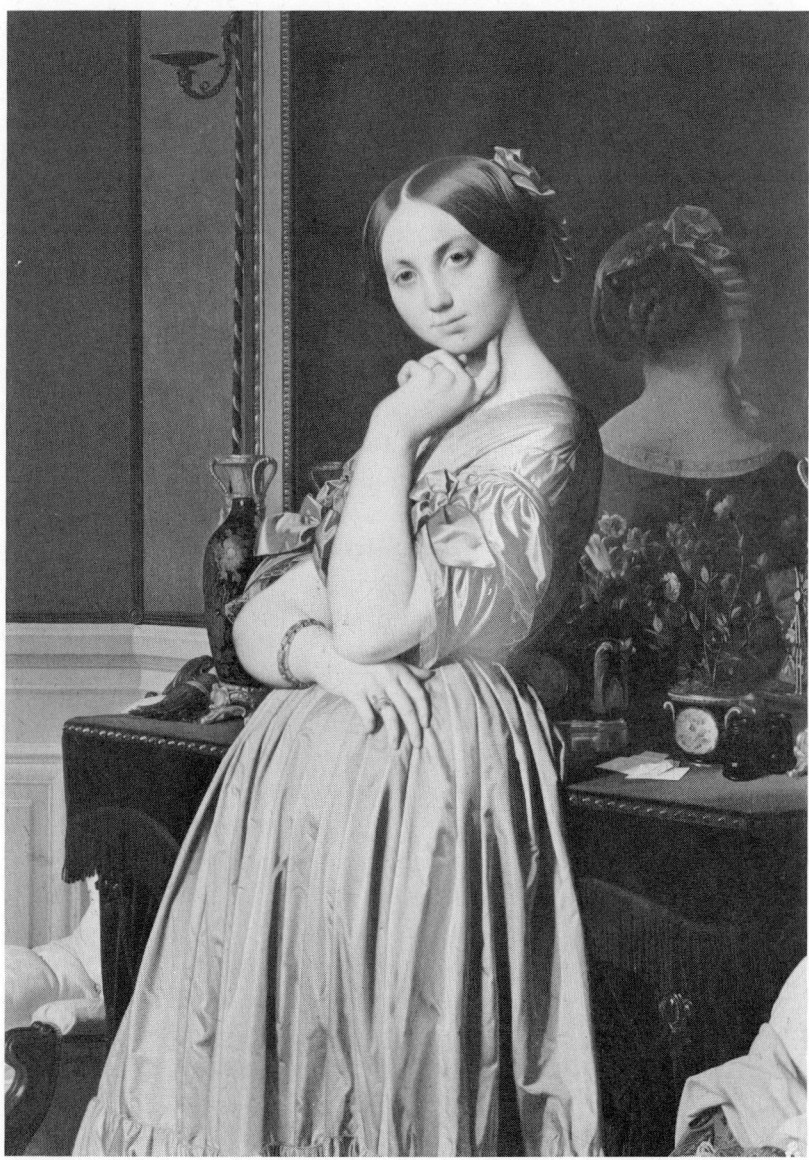

Figure 14. Comtesse d'Haussonville. *By* Jean Auguste Ingres. *Courtesy of* Frick Collection. *Portrait of a demure young woman in a setting of rich and elegant textures which are right together.*

fectly or to use them as inspiration for modern adaptations. We may be amazed to see the richness of pearls stitched on cloth of gold, and gauzes almost finer and more sheer than anything of today. We may be impressed by seeing rich woolens, perhaps from Flanders, hanging in thick, organ-pipe folds, as shown in Gothic tapestries (Figure 11 Chapter Five) or in portraits by Massys and Jan Van Eyck. We return again and again to enjoy the elegance of brocaded satins, pastel taffetas, delicately brocaded and embroidered velvet, and cobweb laces which were created by skillful French fingers in the time of the French Louis, as seen in Le Brun's *Portrait of Marie Antoinette* (Figure 8 Chapter Five).

Our Western world is grateful to have been introduced to the beauty and intricacy of Kashmir shawl weaving, and to the delicate designs of Indian and Persian cotton prints, whose importation upset governments and overturned industry in seventeenth and eighteenth century Europe. The latter became the inspiration for the lovely French toiles and English chintzes, the quaint calico patterns, and the delicate embroidered mulls of the following century (Figure 15). The rich silks and delicate laces of the mid-nineteenth century are charmingly recorded by such meticulous artists as David, Ingres, and Winterhalter (Figures 11 and 12).

The Metropolitan Museum of Art in New York City houses a distinguished collection of dresses dating from the beginning of the reign of Queen Victoria. Many of them are from the hands of famous French and American designers of the nineteenth and twentieth centuries. From time to time, various ones are on display, and the collection is available at all times to designers, who have the privilege of studying and sketching them. The ascendancy of France as the world's fashion leader may be partly due to the availability of fine collections of costumes and textiles in the European museums. American museums and designers are learning the value of this kind of study, as evidenced in the outstanding exhibit of costumes from the House of Worth displayed by the Brooklyn Museum in the spring of 1962.

It is good for us to realize even in a small way something of the toil and devotion, the skill and genius, which have gone into these creations, which are the basis of our modern textiles. It is worthwhile for us to see how closely bound is their history with that of modern European and American culture. Out of this experience should come a new respect and fondness for fabrics and with it an almost intuitive sense of how to use them suitably.

A Glossary of Costume Textures will be found in Appendix C for the convenience of the reader who may not be familiar with a wide variety of

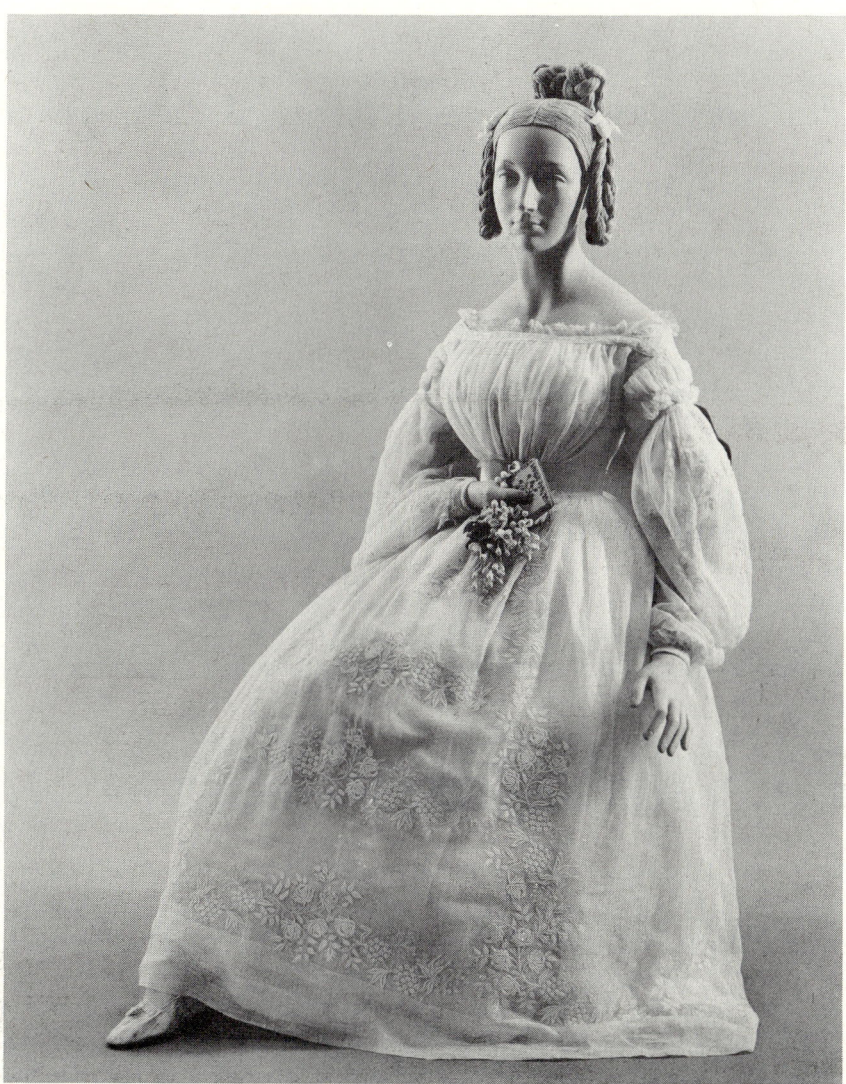

Figure 15. Wedding dress of embroidered India muslin of exquisitely delicate texture. French, about 1837. Courtesy of Metropolitan Museum of Art.

fabrics. The aim is to tell how the fabric may best be used, rather than to give a technical definition.

For further study of fabrics and suggestions for their use in costume, the following references will be helpful.

American Fabrics, *Encyclopedia of Textiles,* Prentice-Hall, Inc., Englewood Cliffs, N. J., 1960.
American Fabrics (a quarterly magazine), Doric Publishing Company, New York.
American Home Economics Association, *Textile Handbook,* Washington, D. C., 1960.
Donald M. Anderson, *Elements of Design,* Holt, Rinehart and Winston, New York, 1961.
Grace G. Denny, *Fabrics,* J. B. Lippincott Company, Philadelphia, 1962.
Fairchild's *Dictionary of Textiles,* Fairchild Publications, New York, 1959.
Maitland Graves, *The Art of Color and Design,* McGraw-Hill Book Company, New York, 1951.
Dorothy S. Lyle, *Focus on Fabrics,* National Institute of Drycleaning, Silver Springs, Md., 1959.

Eight

Dark and Light

THAT quality in nature which we speak of as light and shade, in works of art we term *dark-light*. The Japanese have a word for the use of dark and light in compositions; they call it *notan*. It is fitting that we should borrow this art term from a people who so thoroughly appreciate this form of art expression. Light and shade in nature is usually accidental, though often productive of beauty. *Notan* conveys a fuller meaning, in that dark and light masses are used creatively to achieve a harmony of tone relations. In costume design we should think of *notan* or dark-light as a kind of pattern made when the structural parts and their background spaces are composed of different tones or values contrasting harmoniously.

The sculptor plays with dark-light when he models relief and depression from a solid form. The architect strives for a pattern of dark-light in the structure of his doorways and windows. The painter strives to create an interesting pattern of dark-light in the shapes and spacing of his picture. He makes his various tones melt together into a harmony (Figure 1).

Dark-light is the quality we enjoy in fine etchings, lithographs, woodcuts, and mezzotints when beautiful shapes of varying darks and lights are fused with their contrasting backgrounds. It is fundamental to fine compositions in painting (Figure 2), to photography when it is artistically done, to the pattern in woven and printed fabrics, and to the design in fine laces (Figure 3). Good costume often depends for its effectiveness on dark and light con-

146 *The Arts of Costume and Personal Appearance*

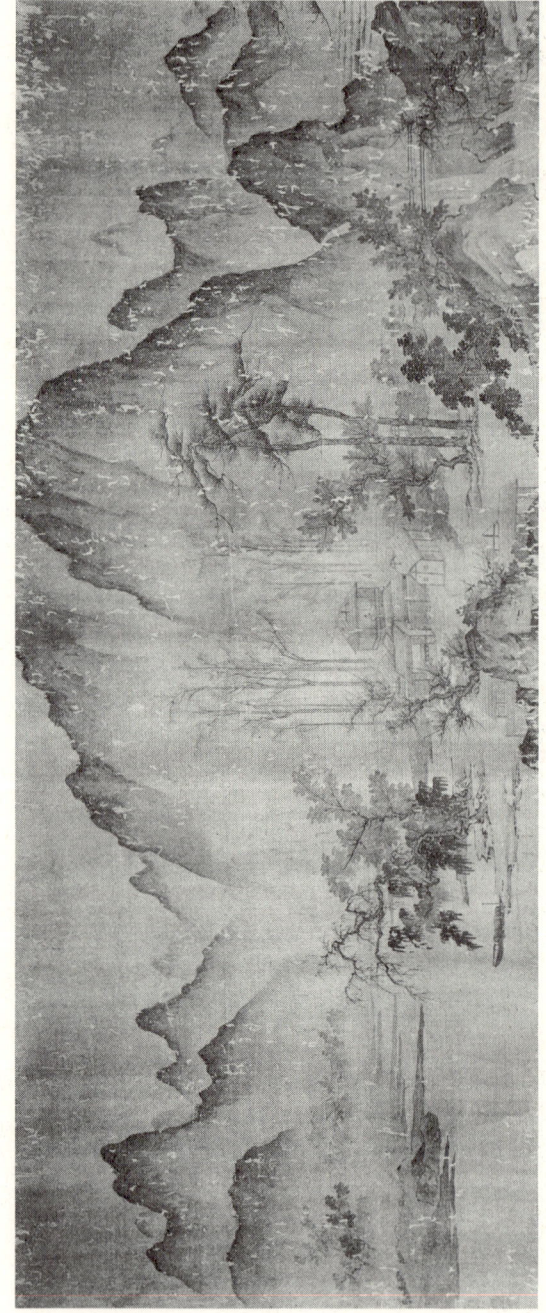

Figure 1. Landscape, Late Autumn. By Wen Tung. Sung Dynasty. Courtesy of Metropolitan Museum of Art. Painted nearly a thousand years ago, this landscape illustrates a great mastery of blending dark tones into light ones, creating an effect of delicacy and femininity.

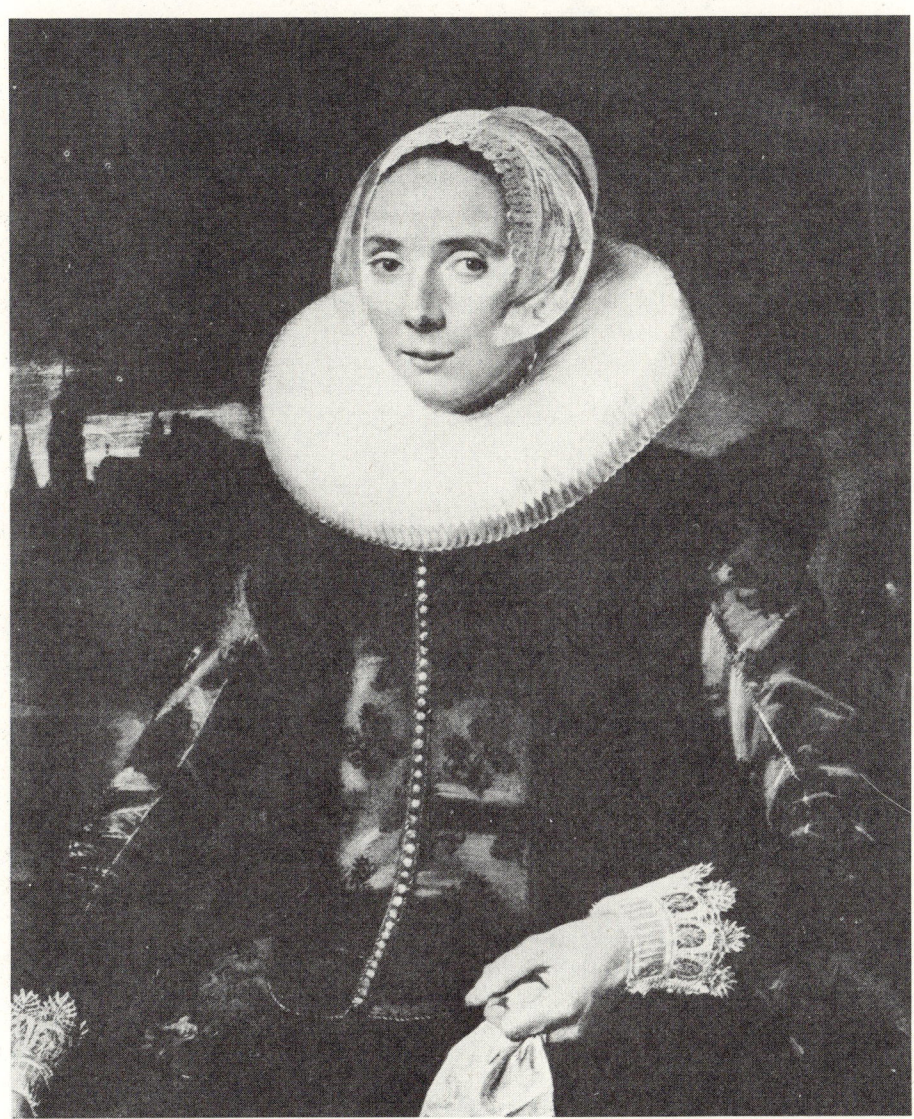

Figure 2. Portrait of a Lady. *By Frans Hals.* Courtesy of Connoisseur. *The artist has centered attention on the face by the white, gauze-like fabric of cap and ruff. He has carried interest throughout by buttons, rich sheen of brocade, and lace cuffs, much as we find them in good costume today.*

148 *The Arts of Costume and Personal Appearance*

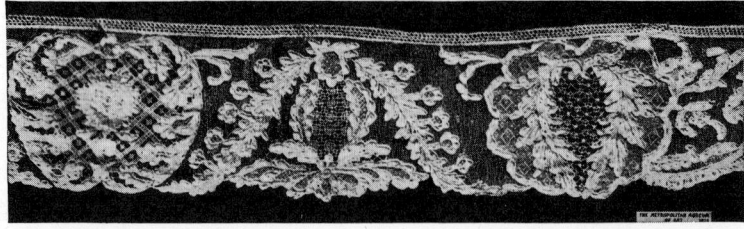

Figure 3. Strip of French needlepoint lace, eighteenth century. Courtesy of Metropolitan Museum of Art. A lovely pattern of pomegranates is effectively brought out against its darker toned background.

trast between the parts of the garment or on the contrast of accessories used with the garments which compose an ensemble. In the final analysis, dark-light in costume serves as a foil for the wearer.

In the hands of a master, dark-light is a kind of visual music, emotionally stirring, much as a great musical composition is to those who have the knowledge to understand it. How does the artist or designer produce these movingly beautiful effects of dark and light? He has an understanding of tone quality or *value*. Value is a term of modern coinage that refers to degrees of darkness and lightness. We can see differences of dark-light if we crumple a piece of colored velvet in the hand and toss it on a table under a bright light. Scattered over its surface will be a great many tones or values of the color ranging from light to dark. Where the most light is reflected, will be seen the lightest values; and in the deepest parts of the folds, where the least light is reflected, will be seen the darkest values.

Degrees of value ranging from light to dark are measurable, and for practical purposes may be reduced to a scale. The Munsell Color System uses such a scale in nine values between absolute white and absolute black. The different steps or tones in the Munsell Neutral Value Scale are shown in Table 1 with their appropriate designations.

The secret of good dark-light in the hands of the artist or designer lies in controlling his variations in value to suit his purpose. "We may use value," according to Maitland Graves, "without considering color, as in a lithograph or etching, but we cannot use color without considering values."[1] At the outset, the artist chooses a dominant tone or value, called a *value key*, to pervade his scheme. If a high value key is chosen for the pervading note, the

---

[1] Maitland Graves, *The Art of Color and Design,* McGraw-Hill Book Company, New York, 1951, p. 277.

dominant tone or value will be somewhere between white, high light, and light on the value scale. If an intermediate value key is desired as the dominant note, it is chosen from the range of low light, medium, or high dark of the value scale. If a low key is wanted, the dominant value will be chosen from the range of dark, low dark, and black of the scale.

It is important to control the choice of the particular degree of value contrast wanted, since it is at the point where the tones meet in contrast that the eye of the beholder is especially drawn.

Quite as important as the dominant note or the kind of contrast we select is the arrangement or placing of our dark-light values in a pattern. The designer, whether by intention or by feeling, makes use of some or all of the design principles. The following illustrations may serve to clarify this point.

DARK AGAINST LIGHT, LIGHT AGAINST DARK

The designer sees to it that he has distinguished shapes in his dark-light pattern. He also manages his background spaces well, for he wants these areas to be pleasing in order to be effective in contrast with his dominant shapes. One way to do this—a way most applicable to costume—is to use a leading mass or shape of dark or light; then other darks or lights of related shape, but smaller size, are grouped around, lending support and seeming to belong to it. This principle is illustrated in Titian's distinguished portrait *Man with the Glove* (Figure 4). The face, a very light shape, leads into the shirt front with its frilled collar; and the interesting shapes of hands and glove are silhouetted in a strongly contrasted pattern against the dark background space. This is quite in the manner of one of today's methods of drawing attention to a center of interest.

An example of this principle chosen from contemporary costume might be a white wool tweed suit strongly peppered with black. The suit has a short jacket with three-quarter length sleeves and black buttons; it is worn with a black overblouse of linen. Black kid gloves slightly wrinkled around the wrist, black opera pumps with a soft luster, a black brimmed hat of rough straw, and white beads and earrings complete the dark-light value scheme.

Another example could be an exotic pajama outfit of chocolate brown shantung (low value) with box-like Chinese jacket opening over a violet-blue jersey bodice in medium tone. As accessories there are Chinese strapped

150   *The Arts of Costume and Personal Appearance*

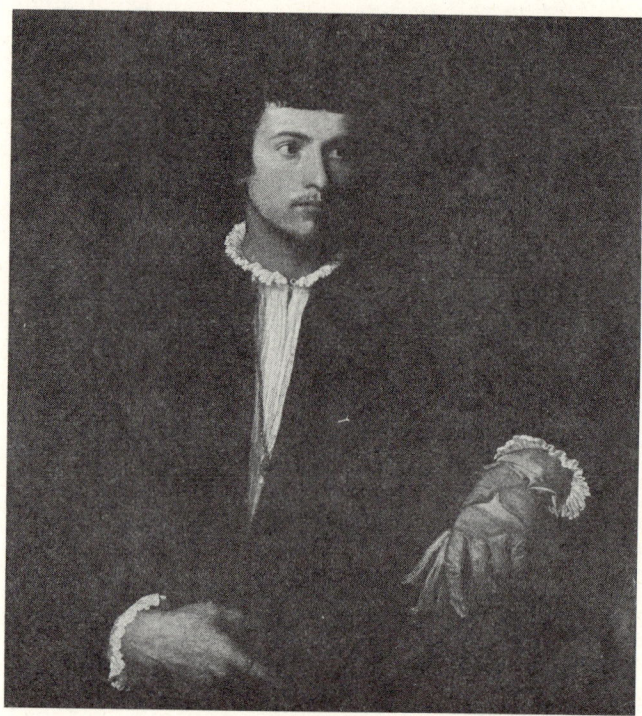

Figure 4. Man with the Glove. *By Titian. National Museum, Florence.* Of aristocratic bearing and very much alive seems this young prince in deep black, sharply relieved by his frilled and pleated linen chemise, forming a pattern of light values.

sandals, a large metal bracelet, and a huge coolie cartwheel hat of grayish beige shantung. Here a pattern of light in bodice and accessories is carried into the dark of the suit. This idea could quite as well be reversed, with the bodice of a dark pattern carried into a lighter background.

The designer manages a balanced contrast of his darks and lights as seen in the Japanese print by Toyokuni (Figure 5). The eye is attracted first to the deep black of the beautifully draped obi, which contrasts strikingly with its background. Bands of deeper black then lead the eye from the obi up over the shoulders, enhancing the lines of the robe's delicately patterned facings and the white folds of the kimona worn underneath and visible at opening edges. Several embroidered motifs, significantly placed, help to complete this dramatic picture in which black is contrasted strongly with higher values in a finely adjusted balance.

DARK AND LIGHT 151

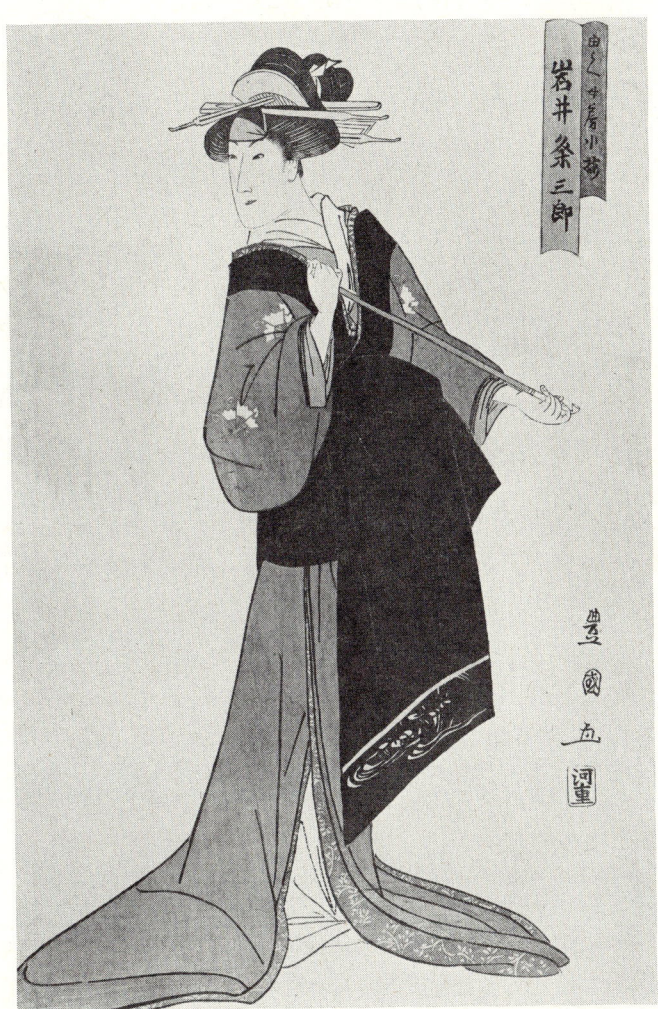

Figure 5. Japanese print. By Toyokuni, 1886. Crown Copyright, Victoria and Albert Museum. *An actor in a dramatic role in which strong contrasts best express his mood, creating a masculine quality.*

In contemporary costume, this balanced contrast is noted in a striking ski outfit composed of a white lamb's wool coat and long white flannel trousers of stretch wool tapering down to interestingly laced black cowhide ski boots. A black wool sweater gayly embroidered in red and white, black mittens embroidered in the same colors, and an old-fashioned white stocking cap ending in a red tassel complete this scheme, in which a dominantly high value key is contrasted strongly with red and black.

The designer may arrange his values in a series of related areas that lead the eye progressively to a culminating point, as in Edward Hopper's painting of a lighthouse (Figure 6). Each area is similar in proportion but larger than the last, until we reach the culminating shape, the lighthouse tower. Here our eye travels from dark mass to lighter mass to dark again; the arrangement of lights and darks produces a logical rhythm.

The designer may arrange a gradation of values to lead from one part of the design to another. Very effective use can be made of two values only; however, one usually desires to use several values in interesting gradations. The painter is a master in his use of small intervals and close gradations of value, whether in tones of grays or in color. A contemporary evening gown by Nina Ricci employs a warp-printed silk taffeta with a large, conventionalized floral design in many shades of warm gray; the design almost completely covers the white background of the silk. The white filling yarns woven through the print frost the grays and the white with a silvery sheen. With it are worn a matching stole and sixteen-button white gloves; long earrings of pearl and silver are the only jewelry.

A Dior evening gown of silk damask, with a dainty and feminine floral design, shows a graceful rhythm and upward movement (Figure 7). The matching stole is velvet lined. In this gown, a low key of close values is achieved by differences in textures and by the way the light is reflected in the satin background of the damask pattern.

Whatever method is chosen by the designer, he knows that a sense of wholeness or unity must seem to carry through the design; every shape and area must be in just the right tone so that one would not desire anything changed. To satisfy himself that the values are right, he frequently tests his work by studying it through half-closed eyes. This habit must become second nature to the student who wishes to acquire proficiency in selection. It helps her to distinguish the essential pattern and to perceive shapes that jump out in a spotty fashion, destroying unity and rhythm, because they seem not to lie on the same surface.

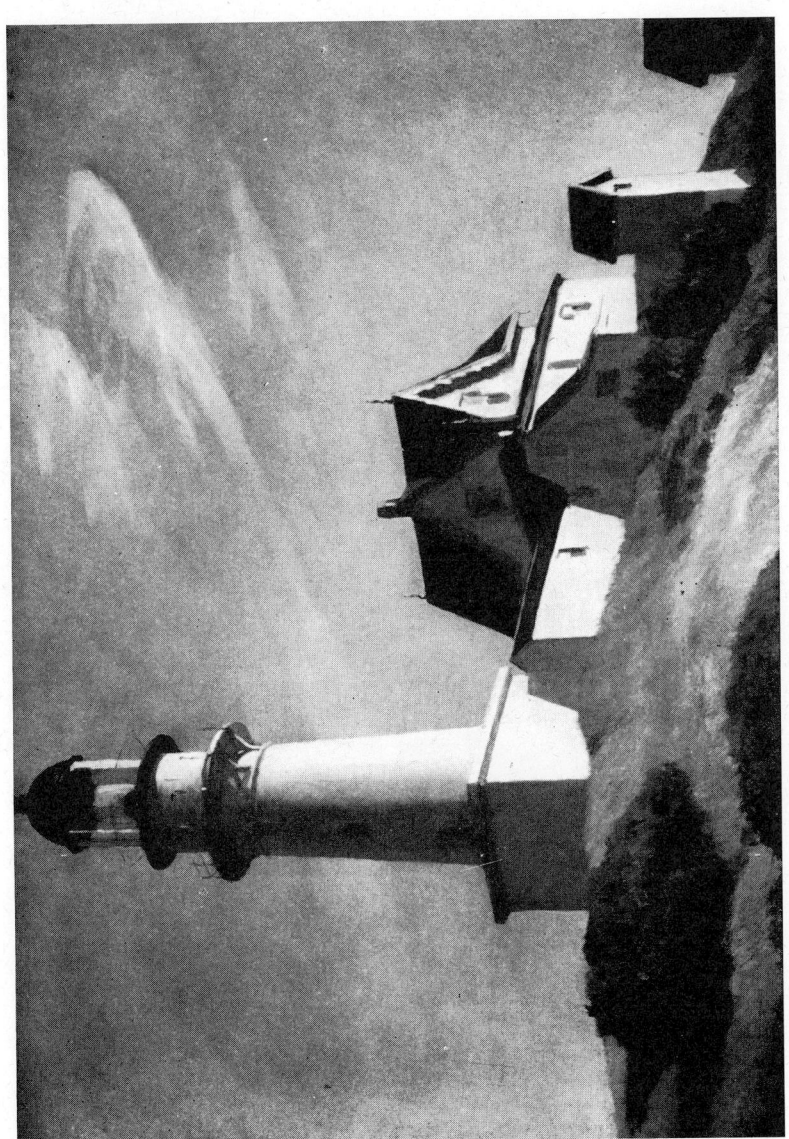

Figure 6. Light House at Two Lights. By Edward Hopper. Courtesy of Mrs. Samuel Tucker. The darks and lights in this delightful painting make a pattern of contrasts leading the eye in succession from light to dark to light again, with its most interesting shape in the tower itself.

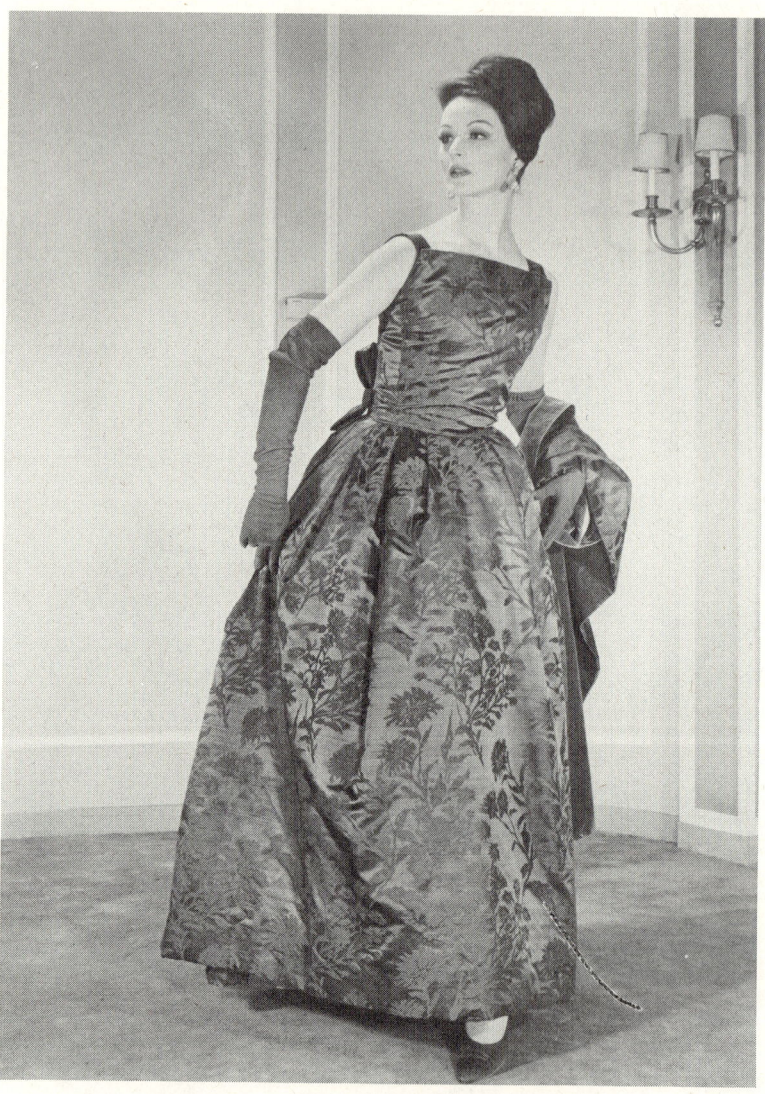

Figure 7. Silk damask evening gown by Christian Dior. Courtesy of Muriel Morris of Christian Dior, New York. Close values in a low key, in which the contrast is obtained by difference in light reflectance in the damask pattern.

EXPRESSIVENESS THROUGH VALUE CONTRASTS

Aside from those qualities which make for good arrangement, it will be seen that a dark-light pattern may be used to convey certain emotional qualities—the kind of expression to which we refer as *empathy*. An understanding of this property of dark-light is important, because it enables us purposefully to control the ideas or moods which we wish to express in any particular costume. When our purpose is vague or indefinite, our results are apt to have little point; but when we know what we are trying to accomplish, our efforts have wider scope and effectiveness.

The purpose controls choice; we must know what values we wish as our dominant notes and what quality of contrast will fit the occasion, express the temperament, or create the illusion desired. In order to help us realize the many possibilities of value schemes to express mood and intention, we present several variations of the dark-light scheme seen in the peasant costume (Figure 8). The original costume has the larger areas in intermediate key with contrasts from white to black in smaller areas of the costume. Several possible variations of this scheme are shown in Figures 8a to 8d. These may be analyzed in a more exact way by referring to the *Plans for Value Contrasts* shown in Tables 2 and 3. These tables are based on the value scale shown in Table 1. They suggest many possibilities for both analyzing and planning good dark-light schemes.

Dark-light patterns may be in strong contrasts, moderate contrasts, and close values; the dominant key may be high, medium, or low. When the values are but three or four steps apart in the scale, they may be considered as close values; six to eight steps between extremes represent strong contrasts. The effects produced in costume by these different combinations of values may be described as follows:

> Table 2 illustrates value contrasts where the dominant background is in low key with a lighter pattern. When the extremes of value are close, as when a dark background has imposed upon it a pattern in high darks, the effect is apt to be quiet, dignified, and, in certain textures, ponderous. Close values in low keys also tend to reduce size (Figure 8a). When dark values are used with notes of strong contrast, the effect is more striking and impressive, for example, black with accents of stark white or high light (Figure 8b). In this scheme one feels an effect of great

TABLE 1 THE MUNSELL NEUTRAL VALUE SCALE
(Permission of Munsell Color Company)

NAME	MUNSELL NOTATION	PER CENT REFLECTANCE	REFLECTED PERCENTAGE OF THE INCIDENT LIGHT
White	N9/	74	80–90
High Light	N8/	56	70–80
Light	N7/	45	60–70
Low Light	N6/	30	50–60
Medium	N5/	19	40–50
High Dark	N4/	13	30–40
Dark	N3/	7	20–30
Low Dark	N2/	4	10–20
Black	N1/	2	0–10

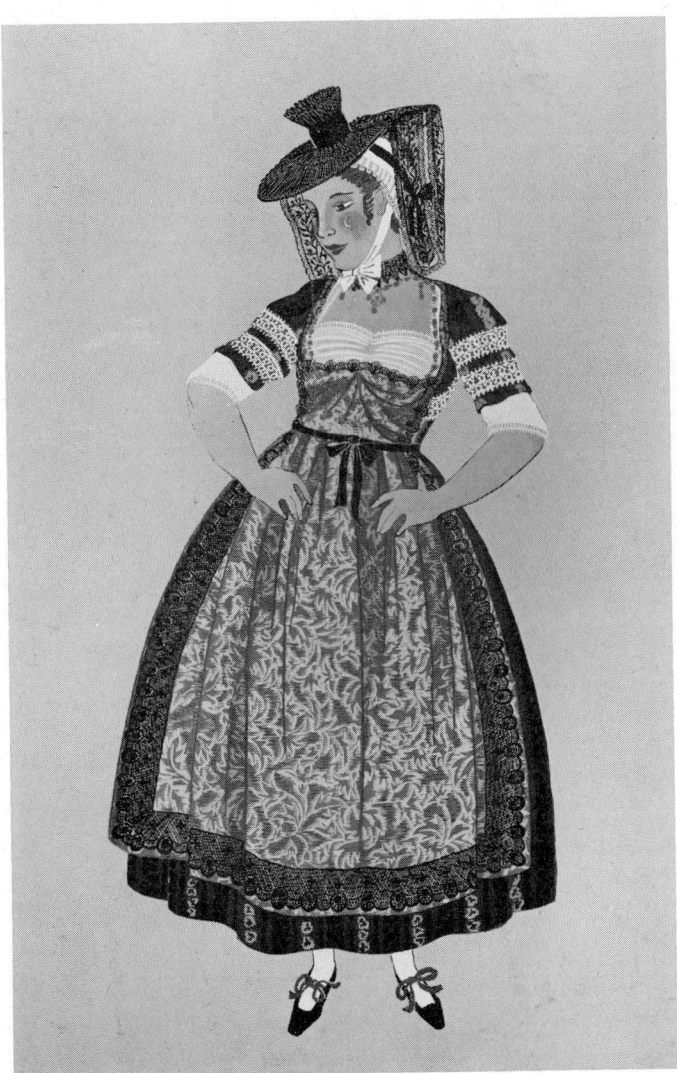

Figure 8. French peasant costume, La Bourgogne. A woman of Bressane; nineteenth century; from Les Costumes Régionaux de France *by Gardilanne and Moffat. Original in the Metropolitan Museum of Art. Courtesy of the Metropolitan Museum of Art.*

158 *The Arts of Costume and Personal Appearance*

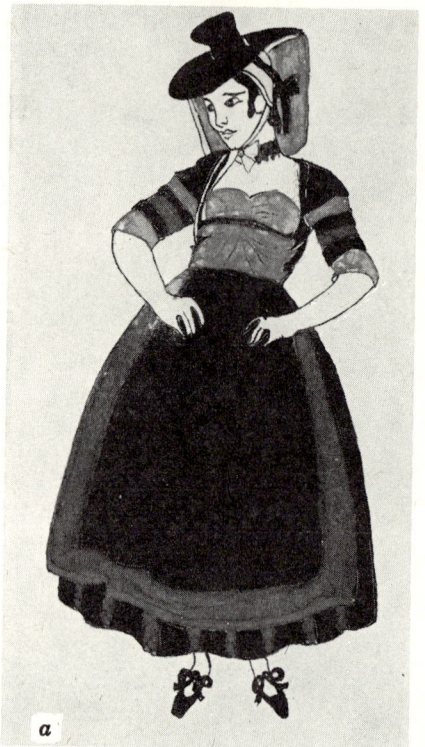
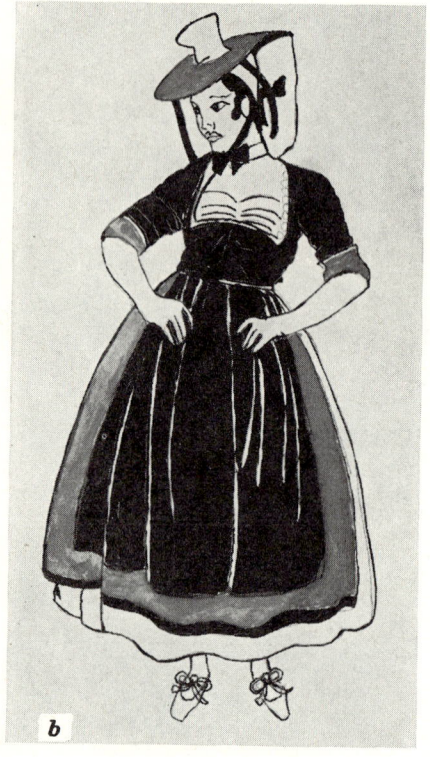

Figure 8, a–d. Value schemes adapted from the French peasant costume shown in Figure 8. a. Dark value dominant, with close interval. b. Dark value dominant, with

strength or force. Low key schemes based on values dark or low dark with accents of light or low light, giving moderate contrast, are less striking and severe, and may prove more wearable.

Tables 2 and 3 suggest combinations for value contrasts in an intermediate key. Here the dominant key is between high dark and low light of the value scale. For example, if medium value is dominant, accented by either a lighter or a darker but close value, the effect is subdued and receding when seen against the usual background of city streets or interiors. It is suited to street apparel for individuals who have sufficient contrast in their own coloring to rise above its retiring, effacing quality. This value key camouflages figure faults and is usually the

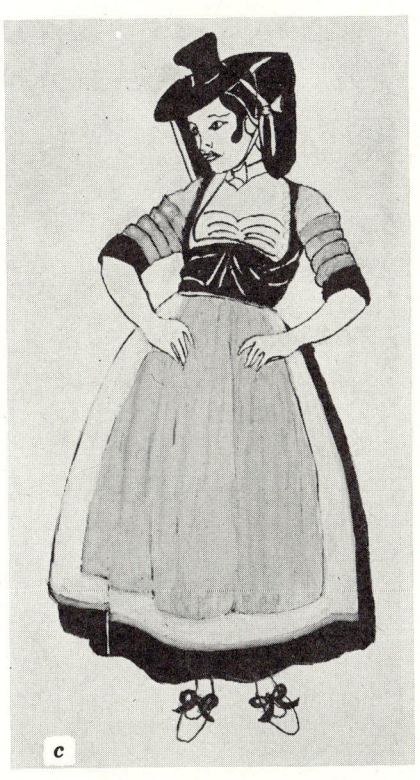 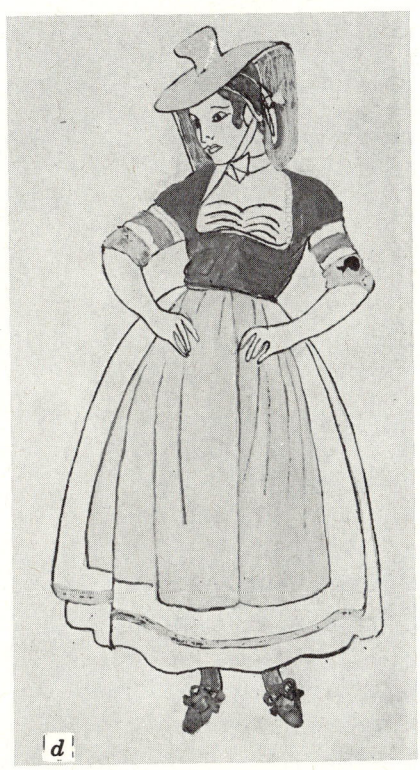

strong contrast. c. *Light value dominant, with strong contrast.* d. *Light value dominant, with close interval.*

expression of the conservative temperament. On the other hand, a dominant value in intermediate key contrasted forcefully with white and black results in a strong, rich, masculine quality important in dress of forceful, compelling personalities. This scheme is suited particularly to spectator sports and evening attire (Figure 8c).

Table 3 shows value contrasts in high key in which the dominant range of value is from light to white, with dark pattern superimposed on lighter ground. When the pervading value is in close intervals, there is achieved a refined feminine quality of great importance in the dress of women of delicate feminine tendencies (Figure 8d and Figure 12 Chapter Seven). On the other hand, when a high key has strongly accented notes of black and white, the result is too harsh and overpowering for

160   *The Arts of Costume and Personal Appearance*

TABLE 2 PLANS FOR VALUE CONTRASTS *
(Light Pattern on Dark Background)

Value Scale	CLOSE VALUE					MODERATE CONTRAST				STRONG CONTRAST OF VALUES					
	4					5				6			7		8
9	•	•	•	•	•9	•	•	•	•9	•	•	•9	•	•9	•9
8	•	•	•	•8	•8	•	•	•8	•8	•	•8	•8	•8	•	•
7	•	•	•7	•7	•	•	•7	•7	•	•7	•7	•	•	7.5 •	•7
6	•	•6	•6	•	6.3 •	•6	•6	•	•	•6—	•	•	6.5 •	•	•
5	•5	•5	•	5.3 •	•5	•5	•	•	5.6 •	•	•	•5	•	•	•
4	•4	•	4.3 •	•4	•	•	•	4.6 •	•4	•	•4	•	•	4.5 •	•
3	•	3.3 •	•3	•	•	•	3.6 •	•3	•	•3	•	•3	3.5 •	•	3.7 •
2	2.3 •	•2	•	•	•	2.6 •	•2	•	•	•	•2	•	•	•2	•
1	•1	•	•	•	•	•1	•	•	•	•1	•	•	•1	•	•1

Each column suggests a possible value scheme in close, moderate, or strong contrast, depending upon the value limits indicated. The bold-face numerals suggest the keynote for a darker background on which to impose a lighter pattern.

* Adapted from Maitland Graves' *Art of Color and Design*. Courtesy of the author and McGraw-Hill Book Co.

most women. The exception is the very forceful personality with decided contrasts in her own coloring.

In contemporary costume the use of dark and light is illustrated in the evening ensemble worn by Miss Rosalind Russell (Figure 9). The stylized flowers of the warp-printed taffeta gown, light values in gloves and beads, and medium value in the slippers suggest a scheme of intermediate key. The contrast introduced by the dominant dark tone of the jacket and repeated in the darkness of Miss Russell's hair produces a more forceful and dramatic scheme, well suited to her compelling personality.

The allover print (Figure 10) shows the use of a scheme that is predominantly in low key, with grays from high dark to medium, contrasting with a white background. This contrast is related to the coloring of the model and is not too severe for her rather large features.

Another costume (Figure 11) shows a use of close values, a dominant light scheme with motifs in high light and light, worn by a model with medium value contrasts and finer features.

TABLE 3   PLANS FOR VALUE CONTRASTS *
(Dark Pattern against Lighter Background)

Value Scale	CLOSE VALUE (4 Value Steps between Extremes)					MODERATE CONTRAST (5)				STRONG CONTRAST OF VALUES (6)			(7)		(8)
9	•	•	•	•	•9	•	•	•	•9	•	•	•9	•	•9	•9
8	•	•	•	•8	•	•	•	•8	•	•	•8	•	•8	•	•
7	•	•	•7	•	7.7	•	•7	•	7.4	•7	•	•7	•	•	•
6	•	•6	•	6.7	•6	•6	•	6.4	•	•	•6	•	•	6.5	6.3
5	•5	•	5.7	•5	•5	•	5.4	•	•5+	•5	•	•	5.5	•	•
4	•	4.7	•4	•4	•	4.4	•	•4+	•4	•	•	•4+	•	•	•
3	3.7	•3	•3	•	•	•	•3+	•3	•	•	•3+	•3	3.5	•	•3
2	•2	•2	•	•	•	•2+	•2	•	•	•2+	•2	•	2.5	•2	•
1	•1	•	•	•	•	•1	•	•	•	•1	•	•	•1	•1	•1

Each column suggests a possible value scheme in close, moderate, or strong contrast, depending upon the value limits indicated. The bold-face numerals suggest the keynote for the lighter background on which to impose a darker pattern.

* Adapted from Maitland Graves' *Art of Color and Design*. Courtesy of the author and McGraw-Hill Book Co.

DARK-LIGHT IN PRINTS OR ALLOVER PATTERN

No better opportunity is afforded for conveying mood and expressing personal taste than through the selection of pattern in fabric, whether in the form of prints, other surface patterns, or woven designs. Many women are afraid to wear prints. Instinctively they feel the prints set up a competition with their faces and figures. They are indeed right, unless they know how to select the proper ones. It is true that few women have the strength of personality or are sure enough of themselves to wear large, bold prints. It is not a matter of size, but of their psychological make-up and the manner in which the prints are handled. Prints fill a need in the costume of American women; they add vivacity to the social scene, express temperament, and aid in camouflaging figures. It must be remembered, however, that prints always look best when only one is used in a costume. What special guides can be used to cultivate one's sense of quality in regard to choosing printed materials?

162   The Arts of Costume and Personal Appearance

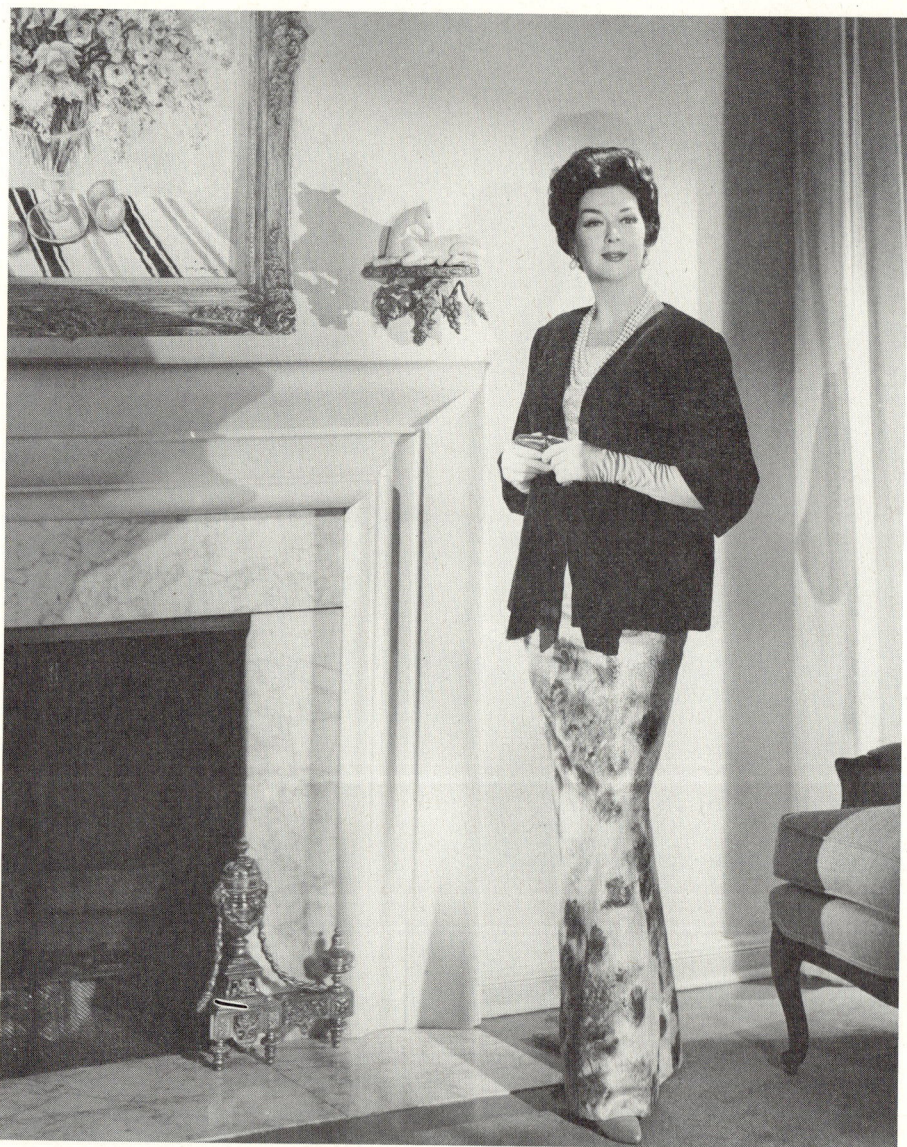

Figure 9. Miss Rosalind Russell. Photograph by John Engstead, Beverly Hills. Courtesy of Columbia Pictures Corporation and Miss Russell. An evening ensemble showing contrasts of dark and light and of texture.

DARK AND LIGHT 163

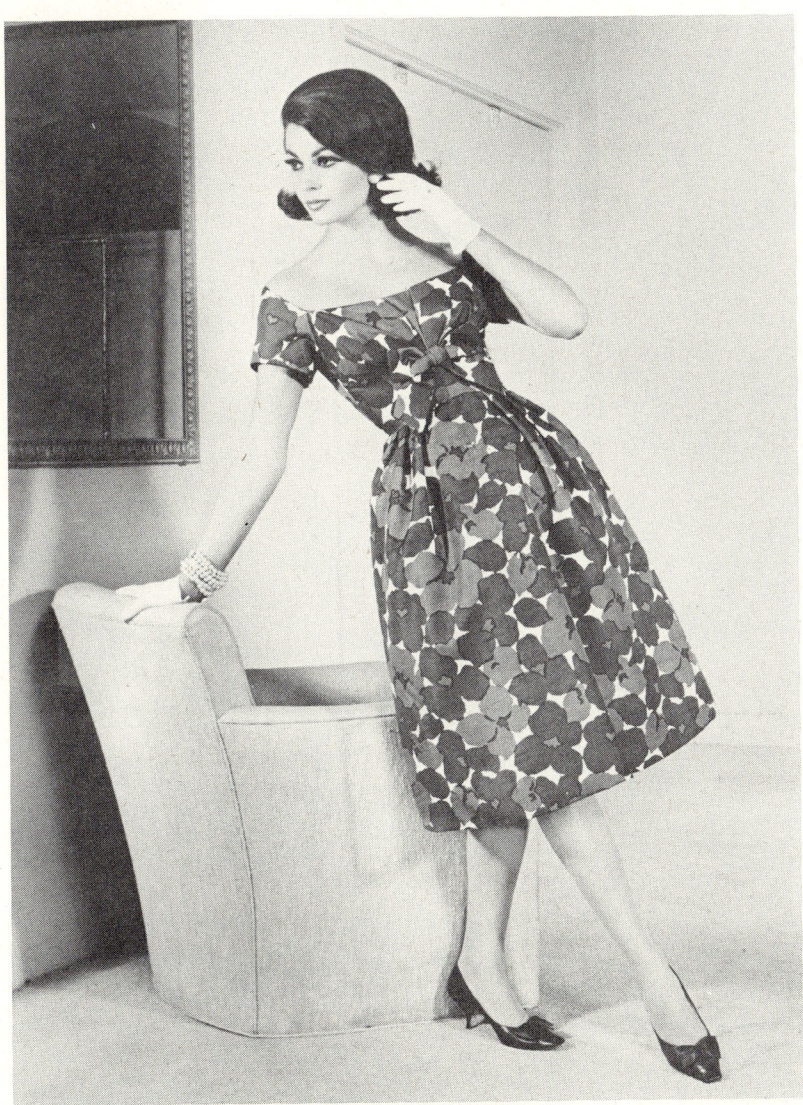

Figure 10. A Jane Derby dress in gray and white silk print. Courtesy of the New York Couture Group. A stylized floral print in predominantly low value key with stong contrasts of dark and light.

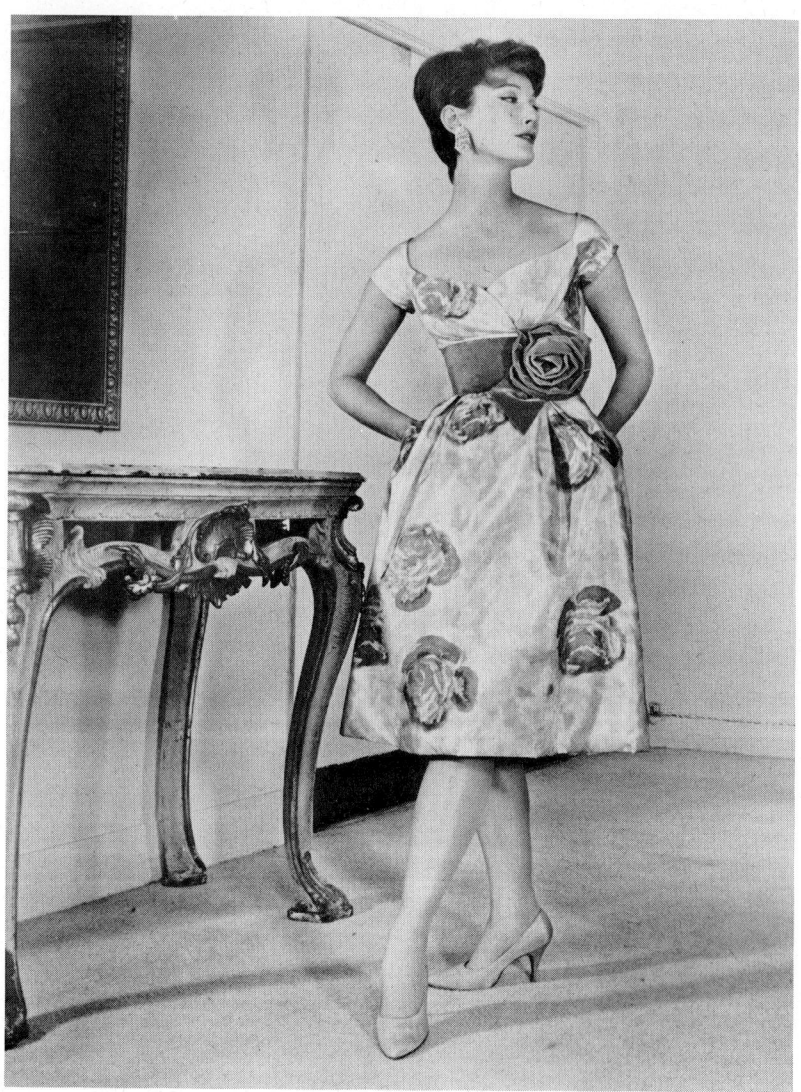

Figure 11. A warp-printed silk by Jane Derby. Courtesy of the New York Couture Group. A value scheme of close values, predominantly light.

Criteria for Judging Prints

The shapes or motifs which make up the design should be interesting in contour and arranged in a pleasing rhythmic pattern. Usually it is better if the rhythm moves in all directions to give a feeling of balance and stability. The movement may be horizontal, vertical, or diagonal; this needs to be taken into consideration when designing costume, as well as in choosing a costume for an individual wearer.

When more than one motif makes up a pattern, these should be harmonious in shape and size; there should be unity with variety.

The spaces which form the background areas must have interest in themselves, so that the pattern as a whole will be pleasing.

Pictorial or strictly realistic treatment of animal and plant forms and scenic landscape effects are never suitable for wearing apparel. Good prints may have their motifs based on nature, but the designer will have added to nature something of his own. This may be something amusing, gay, smart, or exotic; but it must always be something creative.

The design as a whole when viewed from a distance through half-closed eyes should give a satisfying impression that the lights and darks lie on the same surface so that no part appears to jump out or claim too much attention. In other words, a fabric is two-dimensional and should appear so.

A fabric is continuous, and this fact should be borne in mind in designing prints for costume; the print should not appear as an isolated motif. The fabric will be cut and sewn, and the print should lend itself to this kind of treatment. The illustration (Figure 12) shows an imaginative print in which the design is derived from a floral motif but is not a photographic representation of a specific flower. The pattern covers the background so that it forms interesting shapes and spaces. The fabric is chiffon in soft tones of pink, mauve, and white on a violet-blue background.

The scale and contrast of dark-light or color need to be evaluated in relationship to the person by whom they are worn. Prints may emphasize the size of the wearer as do texture and color.

Allover patterns may be poor or commonplace for several reasons:

The motifs have no interest or significance.
The motifs are unrelated.
The arrangement of the pattern does not give a sense of movement or rhythm.

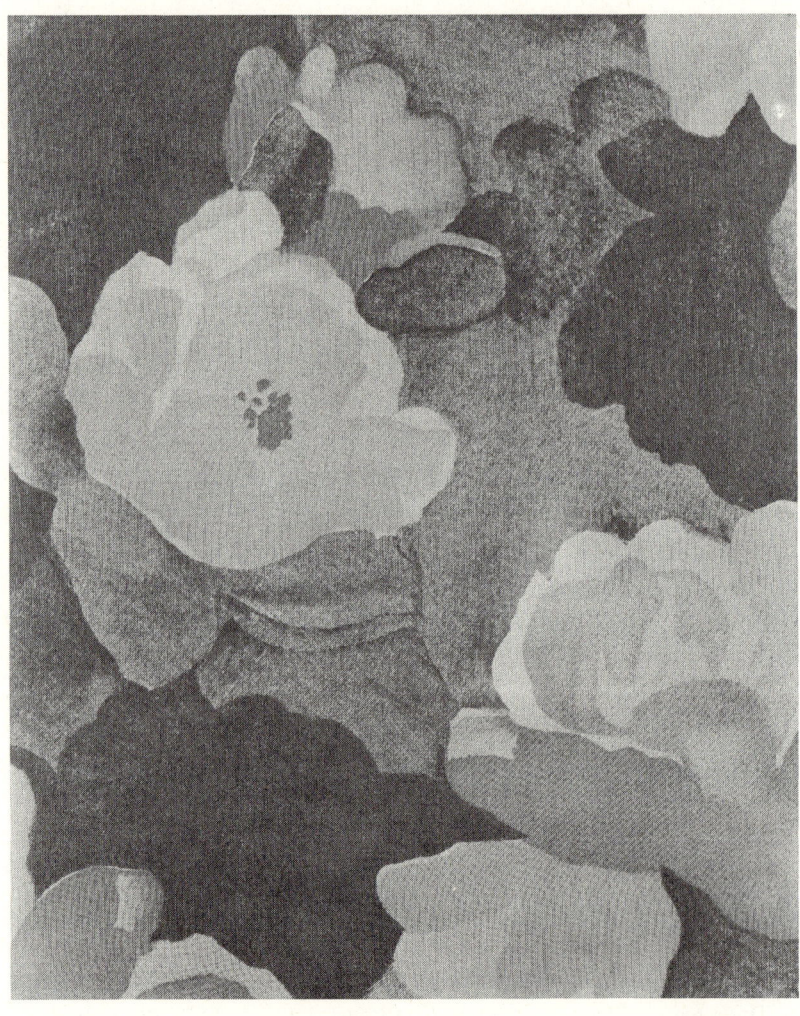

Figure 12. A stylized floral print on chiffon, with lovely subtle gradations of hue and value. Suitable for a draped silhouette or straight-hanging fullness.

The darks and lights are spotty and stand out, calling attention unpleasantly to certain parts. The values are unrelated; darks do not carry into lights and vice versa.

Characteristics of Different Types of Prints

Prints may be classified according to many different features:

Large scale as distinguished from small scale motifs.
Widely spaced motifs as compared with compactly spaced motifs.
Strong contrast in value as distinguished from close values.
Strong or intense colors as distinguished from soft and grayed hues.
Motifs purely abstract or geometric as compared with those based on nature forms.
Prints of formal or conservative character as compared with those which may be considered informal, free, or exotic.

Some allover patterns give the impression of force, vigor, and the dramatic and should be used by sophisticated women (Figure 18). Others seem dainty, refined, and ladylike, as though they were intended for delicate, feminine women (Figures 13 and 15). Some suggest the dignified and mature. Others give the impression they belong to youth and are gay and amusing.

Some seem very impersonal and conventional and suggest the conservatism needed when one is engaged in business and professional pursuits (Figures 16 and 20). Some are highly stylized, formal, or traditional in their treatment. One print might have been inspired by an Italian Renaissance brocade (Figure 14). Others are freer and more imaginative, suggesting but not copying forms in nature (Figures 13, 15, 17, and 22). Still others are so exotic that they are suitable only to express personal moods and gala social occasions (Figures 12, 17, and 19).

The texture of the fabric on which the print is used will also change the effect of the print; a large and rather bold design in chiffon, draped with much soft fullness over a slip of a neutral hue, will produce a different impression from the same print on a taffeta. A hand-blocked print on a soft wool challis will be quite unlike the same composition on a shiny satin. Contrast the imported silk shantungs (Figures 21 and 22). One is a warp print in subtle shades of greens, golds, and yellow-greens; the other, patently a copy of the first, is a direct print in much bolder hues and lacks the artistry of the true warp print.

168 The Arts of Costume and Personal Appearance

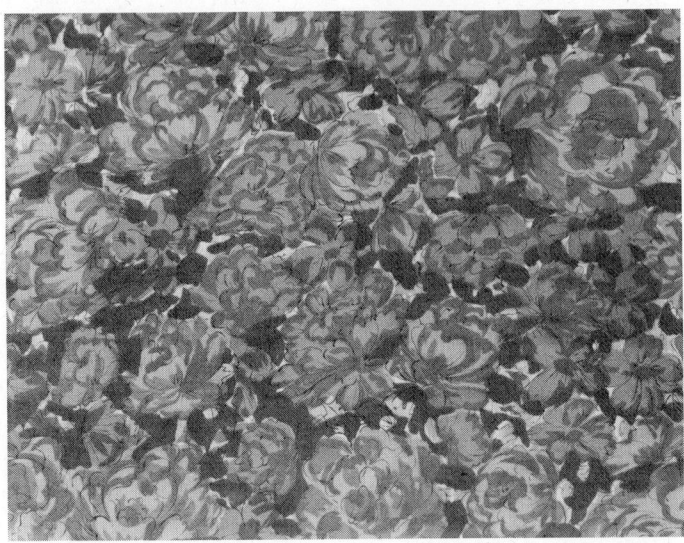

Figure 13. A print in close values in a modern treatment of a floral design, compactly spaced. The design lends itself to many types of color harmony.

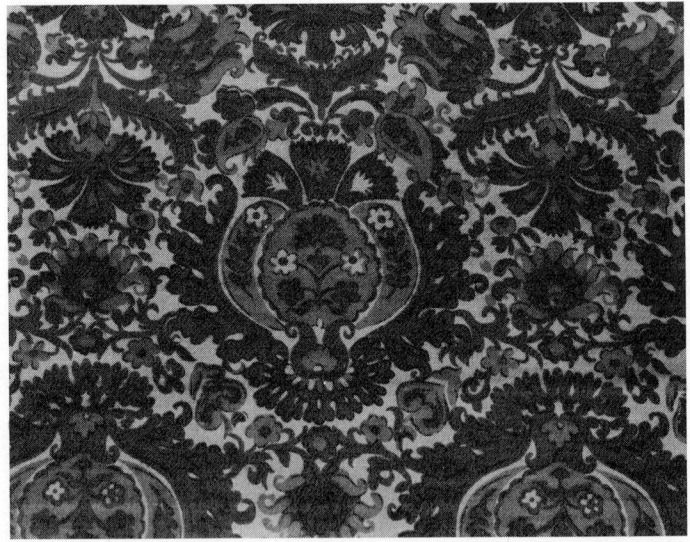

Figure 14. A traditional design in formal style reminiscent of an Italian Renaissance brocade.

DARK AND LIGHT 169

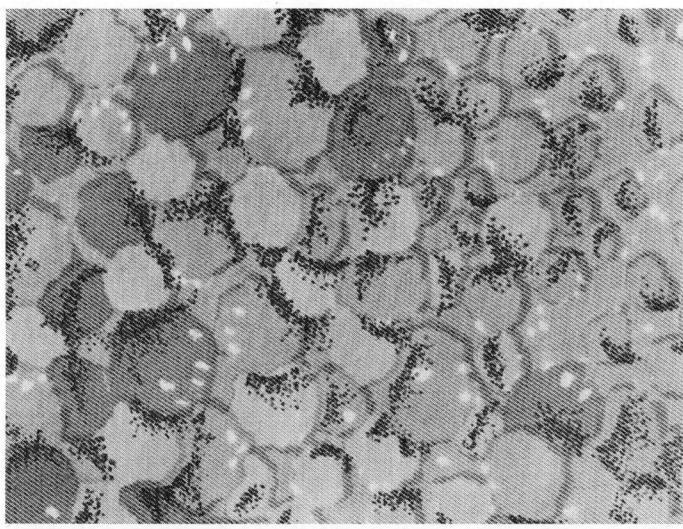

Figure 15. A print in subtle shades of blue and blue-violet in close values on silk surah. Many such prints are used on fine cottons or silk-textured nylons and polyesters for spring and summer wear.

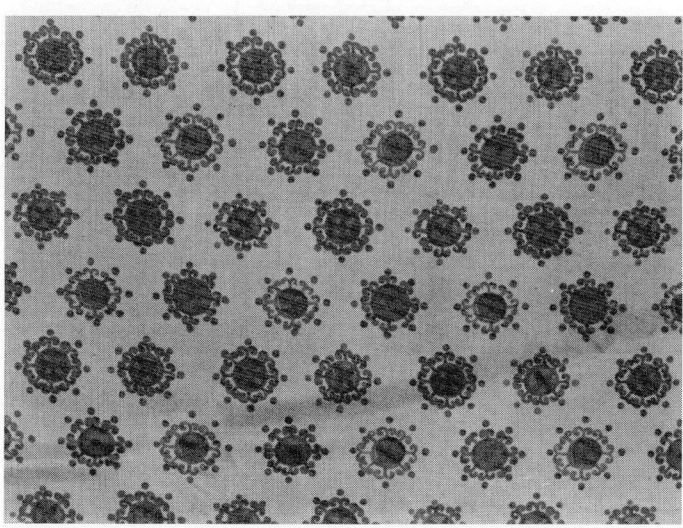

Figure 16. A conventional design with more imagination in its styling than the usual polka-dots. It is impersonal enough to lend itself to wear by women of different types and figures.

170   The Arts of Costume and Personal Appearance

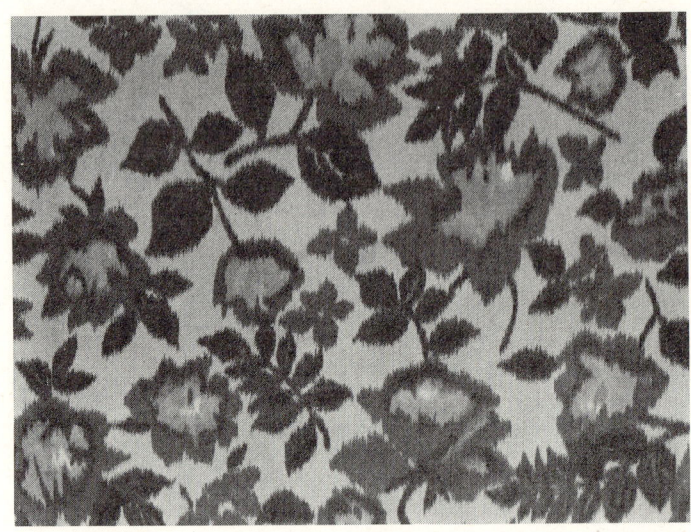

Figure 17. A warp-printed taffeta with rather strong contrasts in low-light to dark key. Suited to dressy wear for a person of the Yang type. (See Chapter Four)

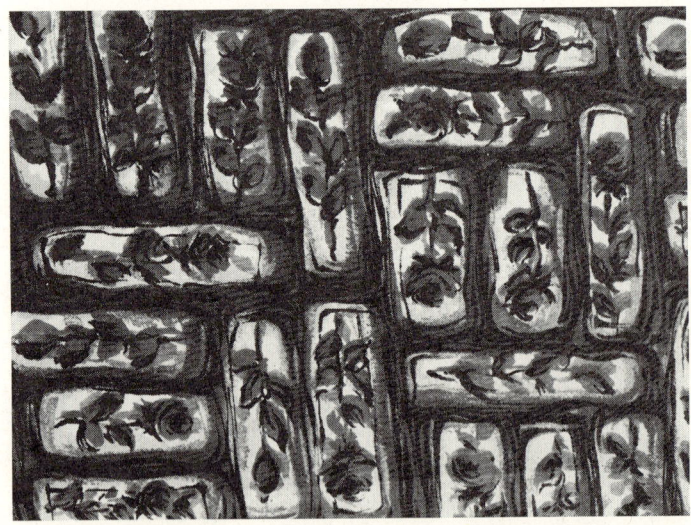

Figure 18. An imaginative design, modern in feeling, with strong contrasts of dark and light.

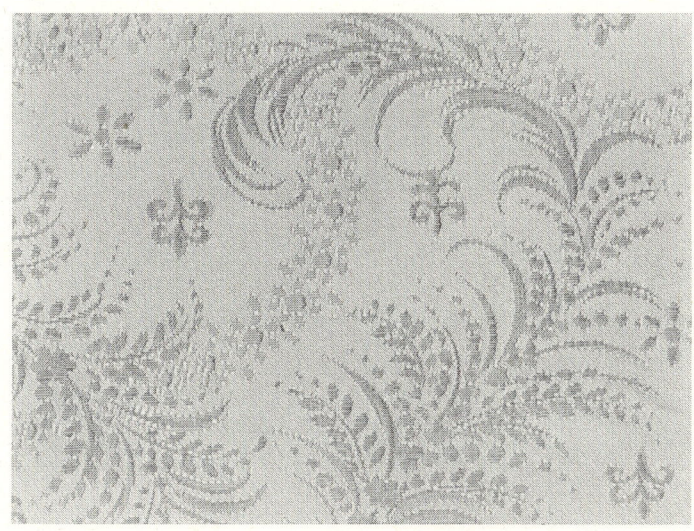

Figure 19. This is a white brocade (not a print) in which the variations in value are due to the reflection of light from the weave of the fabric. An elegant, dainty, and feminine fabric suitable for a robe de style or a bridal gown.

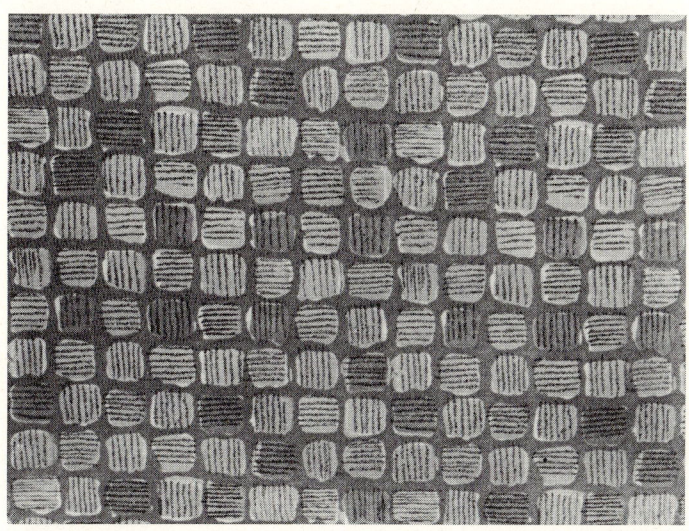

Figure 20. A conservative pattern in close values, so inconspicuous as to seem almost a textured fabric rather than a print. Suitable for street wear for any type of wearer.

172   *The Arts of Costume and Personal Appearance*

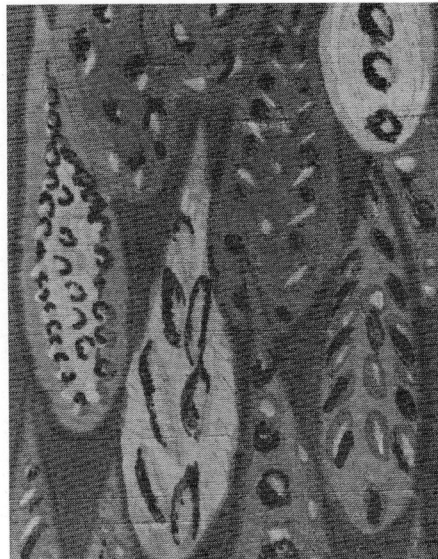 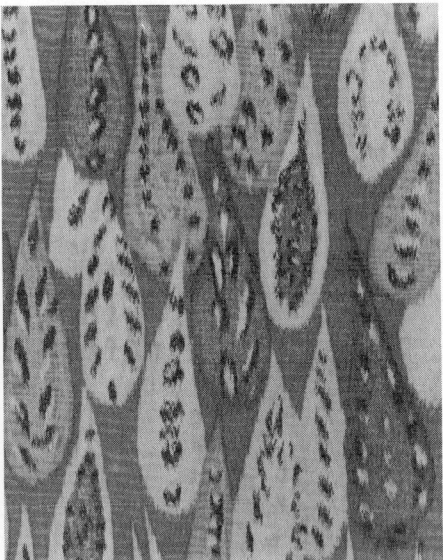

Figure 21. This fabric is patently an imitation of the warp print in Figure 22. It is interesting and wearable, but lacks the fine sublety of the latter.

Figure 22. A warp-printed silk shantung in close values in rich and unusual tones of gold and green.

Exercises

1. A well-known teacher of design gave his students the following guide for composing good dark-light pattern: See that you have (a) one large leading shape or form, (b) one or more long narrow shapes, and (c) several small shapes. Study some examples of fine old paintings and modern works, noting to what degree this rule is demonstrated.
2. Make a collection of clippings of fine examples of dark-light in costume.
3. Select one design of simple but interesting shapes and make a careful tracing. Transfer this design to several sheets of water-color paper. According to the suggestions in Table 2 and 3, make different value schemes: high key, low key, close value, strong contrast.
4. From a fashion magazine select one large-sized example which has good possibilities for making an original scheme in several values. Trace and transfer it carefully to a sheet of construction paper in a nice color. Using tempera paint, make an original scheme of values, letting lights into darks and darks into lights.
5. Make a collection of prints of good design to illustrate the following points:
    Wide spacing—compact spacing
    Large scale—small scale
    Strong contrast—close values

Abstract or geometric patterns—patterns based on nature forms
Conservative, conventional or formal patterns—informal, free, exotic patterns
Mount these swatches and label appropriately; mention the occasion for which they seem suitable.
6. Illustrate by actual swatches the kind of surface pattern you would consider to be most suitable for afternoon, evening, and street wear when worn by:
   The demure young debutante
   The sophisticated woman of thirty
   The short, stout woman
   The small, slight, mature woman
   The tall, too slender, young girl
   The gay young miss
7. Find examples of prints which you consider outstanding and analyze them to show how they meet the criteria of good design.

Nine

Fundamentals of Color

ONE who responds sensitively to color, who thrills keenly to nature's endlessly varied effects or to the skillful use of color in daily environment, knows something of life's rich experiences. And one who develops a growing understanding of its use has opened up to himself intriguing new vistas of enjoyment and satisfaction.

Color is claiming an increasingly important place in modern living. Currently color application to every facet of interior design is of great interest to a wide segment of the population. It is of major concern in all aspects of marketing, store exteriors and interiors, advertising, and packaging, because of its influence upon buying habits. In women's clothing, color has always ranked with line and fabric as a necessary consideration, but carefully studied color has invaded the field of men's apparel to an extent not seen for many decades.

On every hand we are confronted with the need for making color decisions; in no realm is this appreciation of color more a revelation of a woman's taste than in the selection of her clothing. Some people are afraid to use color because they do not understand how; then again, there are some who use it without sensitivity.

It is unfortunate that so many are unaware of the joys that come from a knowledge of color. They scarcely realize the varied palette of the modern world—ours for the taking. There are no sumptuary laws to restrict its use, as in early times, when the use of color was controlled by economics or social position. When we know how, we are free to use those hues which have thrilled people in all ages and lands. We may appropriate the earthy tones and lapis lazulis of old Egypt or the rich glowing jewel tones of the aristocrats of the Renaissance, whose costumes were stitched with sparkling gems. We may choose the refined and smoky tones of rose and green, fawn and blue-violet of the late eighteenth century; the joyous pomegranate reds, heavenly blue-greens, and topaz of Chinese embroideries; or the strong magentas, rich, dark sunset oranges, and brilliant greenish yellows of Mexican folk arts. Many other types of color, mirroring the life and tempo of their time, can be employed to express mood and idea by those who know how.

People ordinarily go through different stages in developing color appreciation. The child learns to recognize pure primitive hues and to identify them, knowing red from green or blue. Beyond this elementary stage, one's advance depends upon interest, ability, and environment. A second stage comes when one learns to copy nature or to imitate schemes he sees or remembers. He begins to appreciate differences of value and intensity in arrangements that please him. The varied hues of flowers and sky take on new meaning. Gradually he comes to see that there is nothing haphazard about fine arrangements; each element in a fine harmony conforms to the principles of color use.

Discernment and the creative application of color principles become the third step in development. New beauties are disclosed. The ceramic glazes of hand crafted pottery, Finnish rugs, Japanese prints, Chinese textiles, and contemporary painting reveal undreamed-of beauties in their infinite gradations. One discovers new joy in the ownership and the study of some beautiful color print or bit of fabric, and feels power in working out new schemes.

Here and there is one whose sense of color is instinctive, but most people reach a high level of taste through study, careful observation, and experimentation. To understand and to use color beautifully, one must have an integrated fund of knowledge and must be familiar with its vocabulary and the contributions of the artist, physicist, physiologist, psychologist, and chemist.

THE PSYCHOLOGIST'S CONTRIBUTION

Color is dynamic. It not only appeals to the intellect, but influences our emotions. The old expressions, "seeing red" and "feeling blue," are indications of definite attitudes toward color. Certain hues are connected with the various seasons of the year, holidays, and national and religious symbolism.

The association of specific colors with particular civilizations is hardly accidental. They are expressions of the life and psychology of their people and time. Thus the light, mirthful, feminine hues of French eighteenth century costumes and interiors seem to express to us the gaiety and the frivolity of that brilliant and pleasure-mad era; the pure reds, vivid jades, and elephant-pinks of seventeenth century Indian painting give us an impression of the rich, unrestrained imagination of a people living in a warm climate.

Different cultures attach differing connotations to the same color as a result of a host of interrelated environmental circumstances, so that colors have not meant the same thing to all peoples during all times. Nevertheless, the manner in which color is used expresses the philosophies of any culture at a given stage of its development. Custom is of great importance in maintaining the meaning of color, and custom prevails over long periods of time with greater force than fashion. In a somewhat similar manner, individuals have color preferences, some of them apparently innate; others develop from an experience in all probability forgotten. Thus individual color preferences are personal expressions, but are shaped within the framework of one's culture. There is some evidence that certain colors have greater appeal than others; some appeal more to men, others to women, and still others to children. The intermediates seem to be preferred by only a limited group who have a more highly developed aesthetic discrimination. However, color preference may be habitual because of culture.

Some rather common color associations of the western world:

YELLOW. Warm, sunny, bright, cheerful, friendly, optimistic, feminine.

RED. Courageous, vigorous, virile, fiery, stimulating, exciting, exhilarating, restless, rich, hospitable, warm, aggressive, overpowering, dangerous.

ORANGE. Combines the sunniness of yellow with the warmth of red; lively, joyous, stirring, cheering, warm; very intense orange may be irritating.

GREEN. Combines the qualities of blue and yellow; quiet, calm, restful, soothing, soft, friendly, cheerful, refreshing, cool; one of the least strident of standard colors.

BLUE. The coolest of colors; serene, tranquil, reserved, serious; in excess, cold, melancholy, depressing.

PURPLE. Rich, aloof, royal, dignified, dramatic, enigmatic; combines the extreme warmth and coldness of red and blue and is melancholy and exciting, sad and warm at the same time.

WARM COLORS. Stimulating, aggressive, exciting, cheerful, buoyant, lively, active, intimate, advancing.

COOL COLORS. Restful, soothing, quiet, aloof, reserved, somber, withdrawn, receding.

LIGHTER COLORS. Feminine, friendly, youthful, gay.

DARKER COLORS. Masculine, old, reserved, sophisticated.

WHITE. Pure, light, cool.

BLACK. Villainous, dead, sophisticated, warm.

As increasing amounts of cool color are added to the warm colors, they become less emphatic and take on some of the character of the cool color; cool colors to which warmth is added shift toward the expression of some of the qualities of the warm colors. Changes in lightness and darkness alter the character of a color.

A fundamental property of color from the standpoint of psychology is its degree of warmth or coolness. The association of warmth and coolness with certain colors is strengthened by some of the findings of both the physicist and the physiologist. The warm end of the spectrum is actually warm. Warm colors accelerate pulse, temperature, and appetite. The red-orange-yellow range of color is regarded as warm; the green-blue-purple range, cool. According to some psychological investigations, emotional character seems to be tied up with warm-cool color preferences. Those who prefer warm colors are extroverted, accept new ideas readily, adjust easily to social situations, are friendly, interested in others, and think quickly. Those who prefer cool colors are introverted, detached, reserved with others, adjust slowly, and express themselves with difficulty.

It is important, then, that those who would use color to express mood and temperament, whether on stage or in costume for daily life, understand the psychology of colors. In general, this entails understanding the red-orange-yellow range of colors as insistent, forceful, advancing, restless, stimulating, radiating warmth and vitality, and helping to create illusions of increased size. By contrast, the cool range, green-blue-violet, will be understood as receding, aloof, tranquil, passive, and creating by suggestion a sense of distance and smaller size. The power of color to express personal temperament, convey feeling, and create illusion is a valuable tool in assembling costume to make the most of individual beauty.

THE PHYSICIST'S CONTRIBUTION

The physicist has contributed much to our scientific understanding of the nature of color. He is concerned with the source or stimulus that the eye perceives as color. This stimulus is part of the enormous radiant spectrum (Figure 1). Only a small portion of it may be seen, and this is the portion called light. White light, which contains all colors, emanates from the sun and reaches the earth as energy or light waves; when dispersed or broken down, it appears to the eye as color. Sir Isaac Newton first separated white light into the sequence of colors which he called the spectrum. The rainbow is nature's way of breaking down these light waves; passing light through a glass prism or a spectroscope produces the same result. The light emerging from the other side is no longer white, but many colors, ranging from red to orange to yellow to green to blue to violet with infinite gradations between, and always in the same order. The fixed order of the colors seen in the spectrum is explained by their differences in rate of energy as they radiate from the sun and is expressed by the physicist as wave length. The light rays are slowed down and spread as they pass through the prism; the differences in their wave lengths cause them to be deflected to varying degrees.

Light waves are measured in terms of the millimicron (1 mμ = 10^{-7} cm.) of the Ångström unit (1 A.U. = 10^{-8} cm.). The whole visible spectrum is contained approximately between 760 millimicrons and 390 millimicrons. Expressed in another way, red light has a wave length of 33,000 to an inch, and blue light has a wave length about one-half this size or 66,000 to the inch. This helps us to see that reds are produced by long wave lengths of a low frequency, whereas blues and violets are produced by shorter wave lengths of a higher frequency, that is, more vibrations per second. Beyond the red rays are the still longer and invisible wave lengths which are called infrared rays; beyond violet are waves of shorter lengths called ultraviolet. Table 1 gives the frequency of the primary colors found in the spectrum. The range of values is given to accommodate the differences of hue of any one color.

TABLE 1 WAVE LENGTHS OF VARIOUS COLORS

COLOR	mμ RANGE
Red	630–760
Orange	590–630
Yellow	560–590
Green	490–560
Blue	450–490
Violet	380–450

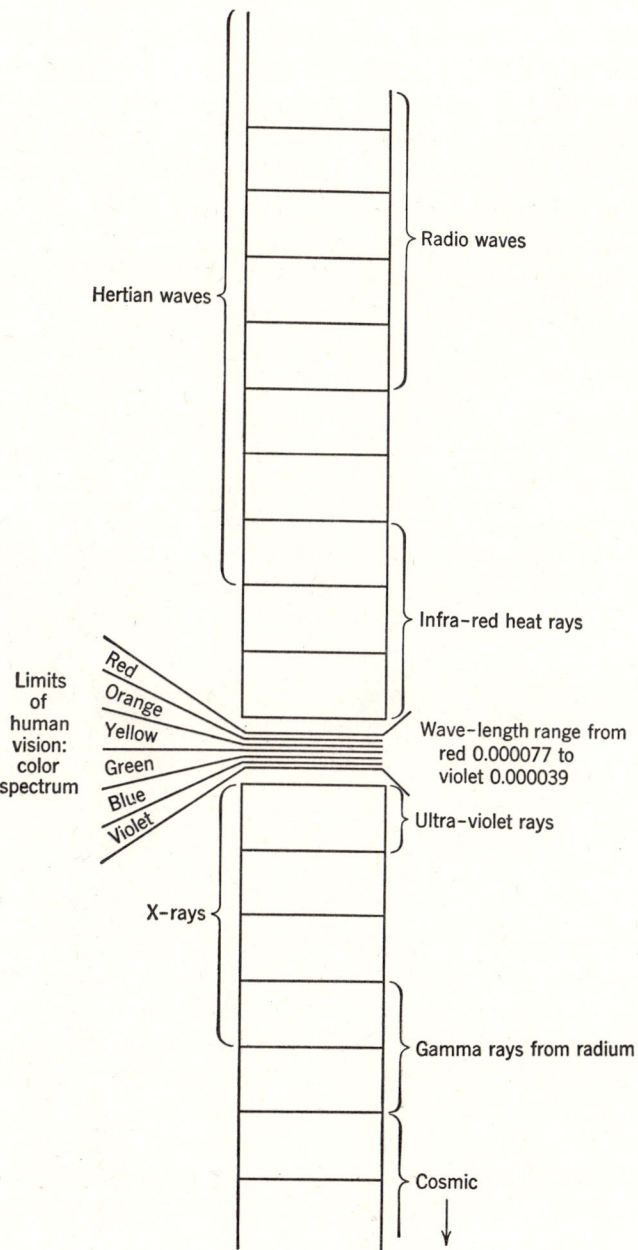

Figure 1. The complete electromagnetic wave spectrum.

When white light, which contains all colors, strikes the surface of an object, certain wave lengths are absorbed and others reflected. Those which are reflected produce the sensation of color. Different substances have the power to reflect different colors; they absorb all the colors in light except one, and throw that off as visible color. A red fabric is red because it absorbs all the colors in light except red and reflects from the fabric that one. Without light the object would be colorless. Objects that appear white reflect all light waves; those that appear black absorb all light waves.

The chemist is concerned with the chemical or molecular character of pigments and dyes, and the formulation of coloring materials which will produce different colors. The color molecule will absorb certain wave lengths and reflect others. It is necessary to put into a dye molecule all colors except that which is to be reflected. The pure colors of the spectrum consist of one wave length; but nature's colors and the colorants of the chemist are impure and may contain many lengths. Colors which have been changed in value, intensity, or both contain a considerable range. Very few dyes are of a single wave length, and for that reason many of the theories of light cannot be repeated in actual practice. The dominant wave length determines the color seen.

The impure colors have a different appearance under various kinds of illumination; two hues which seem alike under one illuminant will not match when viewed under another, a phenomenon called *metamerism*. Each kind of light source has its own spectrum. Even the sun exhibits light of varying quality. Bright sunlight at noon, morning light, evening light, north light, and that of a cloudy day produce a diversity of effects. The spectrum of the incandescent bulb has a different energy distribution from that of the sun. It contains a preponderance of red and yellow and a scarcity of blue and violet. Therefore, under ordinary artificial light the dominant hue of most colors shifts toward the longer wave lengths. This means that each color shifts a step toward the warmer end of the spectrum: reds tend to become orange-reds; greens, to become yellowish greens; blues under the yellow incandescent lamp tend to be neutralized and become dull or grayed. One lavender taffeta evening gown, very beautiful by day, was gray and colorless at night. Standard fluorescent lights contain a greater amount of blue and tend to de-emphasize the warm elements in a colored object. Other fluorescent and incandescent lights have been designed to yield a softer light, more nearly that of natural daylight.

In shadow or low illumination, colors tend to shift a step to the shorter wave lengths or to the cool side of the circle. We often observe this in nature: green grass in sunlight becomes blue-green in shadow. A red-purple flower in sunlight will be bluish purple in shadow. Thus the cool colors are at their best under the natural illumination of sun and shadow. Under artificial illumination, unless vivid, they tend to be unattractive, because they are to some extent neutralized.

THE PHYSIOLOGIST'S CONTRIBUTION

Light reflected from the surface of an object and entering the human eye produces the sensation of color. Both the eye and light are requisite to the perception of color. Reflected light rays enter the eye and are focused on the retina as an image. The image is transmitted through the optic nerve to the brain for completion of the sensation of sight. The retina contains the photosensitive part of the eye, receptor cells called the rods and cones. All the complex nervous system of the rods and cones is connected to the brain through the optic nerve. The rods are assumed to be primarily brightness sensitive, and perceive only achromatic or neutral colors, white, gray, and black. They respond to very small amounts of radiant energy and account for night vision. The cones are assumed to be primarily color sensitive and more complicated. They perceive chromatic color and permit the distinctions between red and green and between blue and yellow in normal vision. Most color blindness is the inability to distinguish differences of red-green. The cones are almost entirely responsible for daylight vision and are held to be operative only at moderately high light intensities. So complex is the sight system that it is not completely understood.

The physiologist's well-known fatigue experiment shows that the nerve endings of the human eye are quickly exhausted by exposure to any one color. Place a disk of bright red on a sheet of white paper and gaze at it intently for about thirty seconds. Remove the disk and transfer the gaze to the white paper. An afterimage, its complement blue-green, will appear in place of the red. The term complement means that color which lies directly opposite on the color wheel (Figure 5). The red sensitivity of the eye is decreased, and the blue and green receptors of the eye predominate. It is now rather generally assumed that color vision contains three mechanisms capable of independent activity that are sensitive to the red, green, and blue wave lengths. Repeat the experiment with any other bright color, and its *chromatic afterimage* will appear on the white paper. A list of complements will be found in Table 6.

By staring at an object against a gray background under ordinary light and then transferring the gaze to a point on the gray ground, a dark afterimage will result. This is called a *negative afterimage* and results from the depression of the light adaptive factor. Less frequently, *positive afterimages* are experienced by viewing objects in intense illumination; a light afterimage results. One explanation is that the excitation of the lightness receptors continues.

The implications to be drawn from these phenomena are that complementary colors, or colors which have nothing in common with each other, used in their purest form give extreme contrast and are likely to offend one's sense of beauty by reason of the shock of their difference. However, complementary colors do tend to produce a balanced stimulation of the nerve endings of the retina, a fact of primary importance in producing color schemes that are satisfying. Warm colors, therefore, need the relief supplied by accents of cool colors, and cool schemes need accents of warm colors. But in costume we must use true opposites or contrast with care and discrimination.

COLOR SYSTEMS

The colors of the spectrum in their ordered succession form the basis of our color systems. If a cross section of the variegated color strip of the rainbow or the band of colors seen through the spectroscope is arranged with the ends together in a circle, a color wheel is formed which is the basis of all color systems (Figure 2).

Several color systems are in use today. The Brewster or Prang theory of color was developed from the work of Isaac Newton and was demonstrated in the nineteenth century by David Brewster. It declares red, yellow, and blue to be the three primaries from which all colors are derived. This system is used extensively by those dealing in pigments.

The Young-Helmholtz theory claims that the three primaries are red, green, and blue. These scientists and their followers proved the red-yellow-blue pigment theory to be inaccurate when working with light. James Maxwell, approximately a contemporary of Helmholtz, devised a triangular diagram for the analysis of light which he adapted to a rotating disk in one

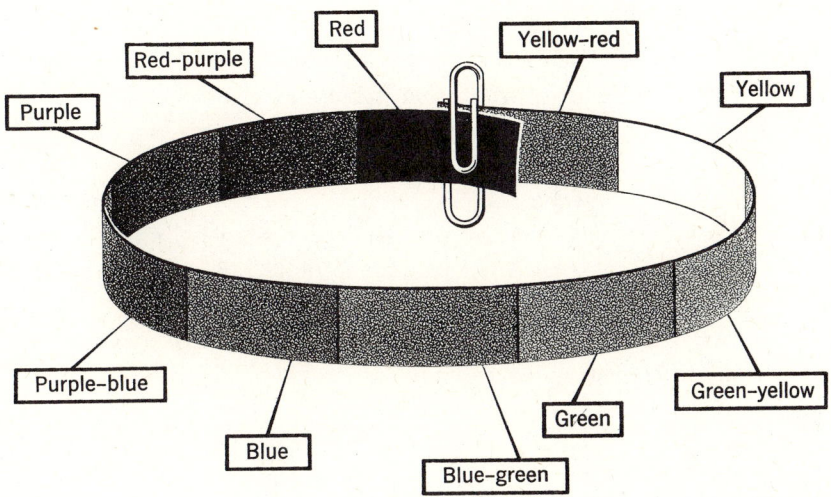

Figure 2. The colors of the spectrum, spaced evenly by Munsell and arranged with ends lapping into a circle. Adapted from diagram courtesy of Munsell Color Company.

of the first attempts to analyze color mixtures. F. E. Ives first produced a practical instrument for color measurement. The Young-Helmholtz system is frequently used in tristimulus psychophysical color matching equipment and stage lighting.

The primaries of the Ostwald circle are four in number and suggest the corners of a diamond; but when expanded to include the secondary colors, it becomes spherical. The Ostwald system is shown as a color solid, rather than a sphere as in Munsell, and is composed of complementary triangles joined at their base through a vertical value scale; each independent color array forms a triangle. Six basic color sensations are recognized. Four are chromatic, yellow, blue, green, and red, the primaries; two achromatic, black and white. The secondaries are yellow-green, blue-green, purple, and orange. The system recognizes the whiteness, the blackness, and the grayness, or the chromaticity of each color. Intensity scales extend from each step of the value scale and form a triangular pattern, which terminates at the apex marked by the color in its most saturated form. There are eight steps of gray between black and white. The system is sometimes referred to as psychological, as it corresponds to visual color sensations.

The Munsell System

One of the greatest contributions of the Munsell system is that it brought standardization out of existing confusion in the names of colors. The artist's pigments, based on the accidents of their chemical and physical nature, and the picturesque but inaccurate names used by the layman or promoted by commercial interests have been reduced to designations that are measurable standards. Any color described by the Munsell system is immediately comprehensible, and the color need not be seen to be recognized. The worth of such a system is recognized by any person who uses color.

The Munsell system introduces the student to the three dimensions which measure color differences: hue, value, and chroma or intensity. These differences can best be understood by thinking of them in terms of a color sphere. The hues of the light spectrum, unevenly divided and merging one into another by indistinguishable degrees, Munsell spaces evenly into a band with sections of equal dimensions (Figure 2). The colors of the band now become segments of the color sphere and are placed in sequence around a neutral axis (Figure 3). At any given level of the axis, all the hues are the same degree of value, growing increasingly lighter to white at the top, and increasingly darker to black at the bottom. As the hues change from the neutral gray of the axis, outward, their strength or chroma increases to the full strength or saturation of each individual color.

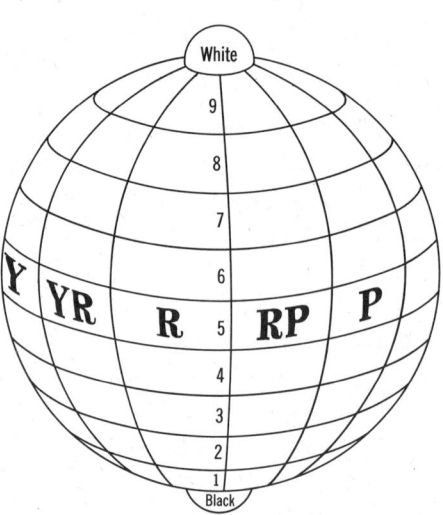

Figure 3. Diagram of the color sphere. The hues are in sequence around the neutral axis. The axis and all hues surrounding it are of the same value at any given level, increasingly lighter to white at the top, and darker to black at the bottom. From neutral gray at central axis the hues increase in color strength as the distance outward from the center is increased. Courtesy of Munsell Color Company.

Hue

Hue is the name by which one color may be distinguished from another. Green is the name of a hue which distinguishes it from another known as red. There is a name for any hue in the color sphere regardless of its value, intensity, or gradation. One of the most helpful of the Munsell charts is the 100-hue circle or color clock on which names of hues are designated with scientific precision (Figure 4).

On the 100-hue Munsell circle red, yellow, green, blue, and purple are designated as the five principal colors. Yellow-red, green-yellow, blue-green, and purple-blue then become intermediate hues, because they are halfway between the principal colors. "These ten hues are called major hues and have been chosen not because they are ten in number—although the decimal system is very convenient—but because they represent mutually equidistant hue-points to the eye."[1] The Munsell system is concerned with light and the sensation produced within the eye, while the Prang system deals with pigments. It was early found that the Prang primaries when rotated rapidly on a spinning disk produce a warm rather than a neutral gray. Therefore the orange of the Prang system has been eliminated, and a true neutral results from the five Munsell primaries. If the orange of the Prang system is omitted, "red and yellow do not usurp too great a portion of the circumference."[2] A perfect balance of warm and cool hues is obtained, and the true complements come directly opposite each other on this color circle (Figure 4).

The Munsell system further distinguishes hues by their warmth or coolness. In terms of the physicist's spectrum, the red end of the spectrum with longer wavelengths gives the sensation of warmth, while short waves at the violet end cause the sensation of coolness. Midway between these extremes is green. As green is neither warm nor cool itself, it can be used as a balancing point to determine warmth or coolness. The hues to the left of green on the color wheel are the warm colors, because they contain yellow and red: green-yellow (GY), yellow (Y), yellow-red (YR), red (R). Colors to the right of green on the color band are the cool colors: blue-green (BG), blue (B), purple-blue (PB), and purple (P).

Carrying this idea still further, it is important to note that all colors may be considered to have a warm or cool aspect depending on the amount of red, yellow, blue, or purple which they contain (Figure 4). Thus:

---

[1] Albert H. Munsell, *Color Notation*, Munsell Color Company, Inc., Baltimore, 1936, p. 67.
[2] Albert H. Munsell, *Color Notation*, Munsell Color Company, Inc., Baltimore, 1905, p. 50.

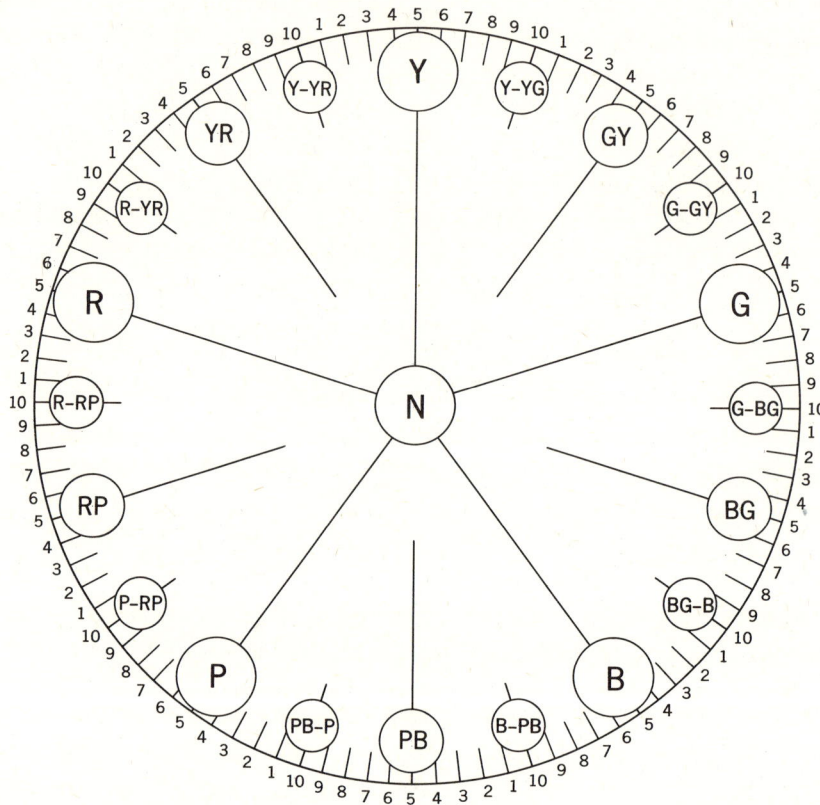

Figure 4. 100-hue circle. Courtesy of Munsell Color Company. This chart shows 5 principal hues, 5 intermediate hues, 10 second intermediate hues, and 80 special intermediate hues at constant value, arranged in clockwise sequence around the circumference of the color sphere. The principal hues are notated with one initial letter, the intermediate hues with two initial letters, and the second intermediate hues are notated with three initial letters. The one occurring twice (at the beginning and end of the notation) is that of the adjoining principal hues. Since more than three initials would be clumsy, the special intermediate hues are notated by numerals—according to their position in relation to the major hues. In clockwise sequence each of the ten major hues has the position of 5 on the circuit, the numerals 1, 2, 3, 4 and 6, 7, 8, 9 indicating the graduated steps of the special intermediate hues.

Green may contain yellow and be warmer, or contain blue and have a cool aspect, apple green compared with turquoise.

Blue when pure and saturated is cool, even cold; but if blue contains a small amount of green, it has a warm aspect. Blue which contains a small amount of purple is cooler in aspect: peacock or cobalt blue compared with violet or ultramarine blue.

Purple becomes warmer when mixed with red and cooler when mixed with blue: amethyst compared with heliotrope.

Red when mixed with yellow is very warm, even hot; but when mixed with purple, it has a cooler aspect: pimento compared with cerise.

Yellow when mixed with any amount of red becomes warmer; when mixed with even small amounts of green, it becomes cooler: gold compared with lime or chartreuse.

A knowledge of the Munsell system will enable one to use color charts and scales in evaluating any materials encountered in professional work with color. Lists of color terminology and of popular color names have been included in Appendices A and B.

Value

Value, the second dimension of color, is the variation of the light strength in a color. The value scale becomes the vertical axis of the circle of hues (Figure 5). Theoretical black is at the lower end, representing total absence of light, and white at the top, representing pure light. The eye can readily distinguish between these extremes a nine-step gray scale, regularly graded from visible black to white. The degree of lightness or darkness of any color is determined by comparing it with the neutral value scale; refer to Table 1, Chapter Eight.

Home value level is the step or level on the value scale at which any hue reaches its maximum intensity or point of greatest saturation. By referring to Table 2, one will see that hues reach their greatest strength at different levels

TABLE 2 HOME VALUE LEVELS

HUE	STEP OF THE VALUE SCALE
Yellow	eight
Green	five
Red	four
Blue	four
Purple	three

on the value scale. In combining green and red in their natural order of value, the green, no matter whether it has been made lighter, a *tint,* or darker, a *shade,* will remain lighter in value than the red combined with it.

Ogden Rood, whose work preceded that of Munsell, demonstrated the principle of a natural order of values which Munsell has called the "home value level." Rood states that colors in nature have a "natural order" and that any "two contiguous colors should have their luminosities arranged to correspond to nature." He reminds us that the "relation of green-yellow to green is shown beautifully by the foliage under sunlight, while the interval of cyan-blue to blue to ultramarine-blue is displayed on the grandest scale in the sky."[3] Later colorists, following Rood's example, use color in the following relationship of values:

Yellow, the lightest value in the scheme
Yellow-red, darker than yellow
Red, darker than yellow-red
Red-purple, darker than red
Purple, darker than red-purple

And on the other side of the circle:

Yellow, the lightest value in the scheme
Green-yellow, darker than yellow
Green, darker than green-yellow
Blue-green, darker than green
Blue, darker than blue-green
Purple-blue, darker than blue
Purple, darker than purple-blue

No other principle of color harmony is so fundamental to the understanding of good usage as the law of Rood; it is extremely important, since most color schemes hold to this relationship.

Dissonance is another aspect of color based upon value. It is the term given to the occurrence or use of hues in reversal of their natural order of value. An example would be a composition in which the major area was yellow-red with small accents of yellow in a darker value than the yellow-red. The English colorist, Carpenter, basing his investigations on Rood's natural order,

---

[3] Ogden Rood, *Modern Chromatics,* D. Appleton-Century Co., New York, 1903, p. 274.

found another principle demonstrated repeatedly in nature and art and called it *discord*. "Discords," says Carpenter, "are at once the most dangerous and the most delicately beautiful of color effects. In large masses unendurable, but in small quantities they add much to brilliance, help greatly in vibration. [Carpenter found] . . . no explanation of this reversal of the order . . . until an analogy presented itself in the case of music, wherein the use of discords is perfectly well understood—indeed, music without them would seem imperfect. This analogy between music and color . . . [is noted where a minor note is introduced into a major theme, and vice versa] . . . both requiring a discord to complete the chord." [4]

Tables 3 and 4 have been adapted from Carpenter to help in composing schemes with some element of dissonance. The prevalent use of dissonance in the contemporary use of color makes it important that one learn how to handle it successfully. It must never be allowed to dominate; the more important its position, the less one can afford to use. Look for the unexpected; in the mastery of some dissonant element, one gets a thrill of conquest.

TABLE 3 DISSONANCE ON THE YELLOW-RED-VIOLET SIDE OF THE CIRCLE

DOMINANT COLOR	LIGHTER VALUE DISSONANT	DARKER VALUE DISSONANT
Yellow	Yellow-red	
Yellow-red	Red	Yellow
Red	Red-purple	Yellow-red
Red-purple	Purple	Red
Purple		Red-purple

TABLE 4 DISSONANCE ON THE YELLOW-GREEN-BLUE SIDE OF THE CIRCLE

DOMINANT COLOR	LIGHTER VALUE DISSONANT	DARKER VALUE DISSONANT
Yellow	Green-yellow	
Green-yellow	Green	Yellow
Green	Blue-green	Green-yellow
Blue-green	Blue	Green
Blue	Purple-blue	Green-blue
Purple-blue	Purple	Blue
Purple		Purple-blue

[4] J. Barrett Carpenter, *Colour*, Charles Scribner's Sons, 1932, pp. 25, 27, 30.

Chroma or Intensity

Chroma, the third dimension of color, is the distinction between a strong color and a weak one. Chroma is the degree of *saturation* or purity of a color, or its color strength, intensity, or *luminosity*. Chroma may be illustrated by the difference in strength between a pale pink and a vermilion red, a grayish blue and a vivid blue. The more saturated or intense the color, the narrower is the range of wave lengths predominating; in colors less pure or less saturated, there is a mixture of wave lengths. Strong or saturated colors are designated as brilliant or intense; those of weak intensity or chroma are spoken of as grayed, dull, or neutralized hues or tones. A scale of intensity for any hue runs through gradations from neutral gray to the specific point of saturation for that color. Each of the colors at its greatest distance from the pole is at its most intense; by gradual steps inward it is reduced in intensity until neutral gray is reached (Figure 5).

Each color does not reach its full saturation at the same step on the intensity scale. The greater the natural chroma of the color, the greater number of steps it will be removed from gray at its full saturation. Table 5 gives the number of steps or degrees from neutral gray at which the principal hues reach their full chroma.

It will be seen that the strength of blue-green is actually one-half the strength of its opposite, standard red. This table explains the carrying power of the warm colors, red and yellow, in comparison to the cool colors, blue, green, and purple. Because colors do not reach full intensity at an equal number of steps from gray nor at the same home level of value, an array of the values and intensities for any particular color is irregular and does not conform to a spherical outline.

When the home level of value of a color is changed by making it lighter or darker, the intensity of the hue is reduced. Adding the complement or gray

TABLE 5 CHROMA STRENGTH OF COLORS
AT THEIR HOME LEVEL OF VALUE

COLOR	STEPS FROM NEUTRAL GRAY
Red	ten
Yellow	nine
Green	seven
Blue	six
Purple	six
Blue-green	five

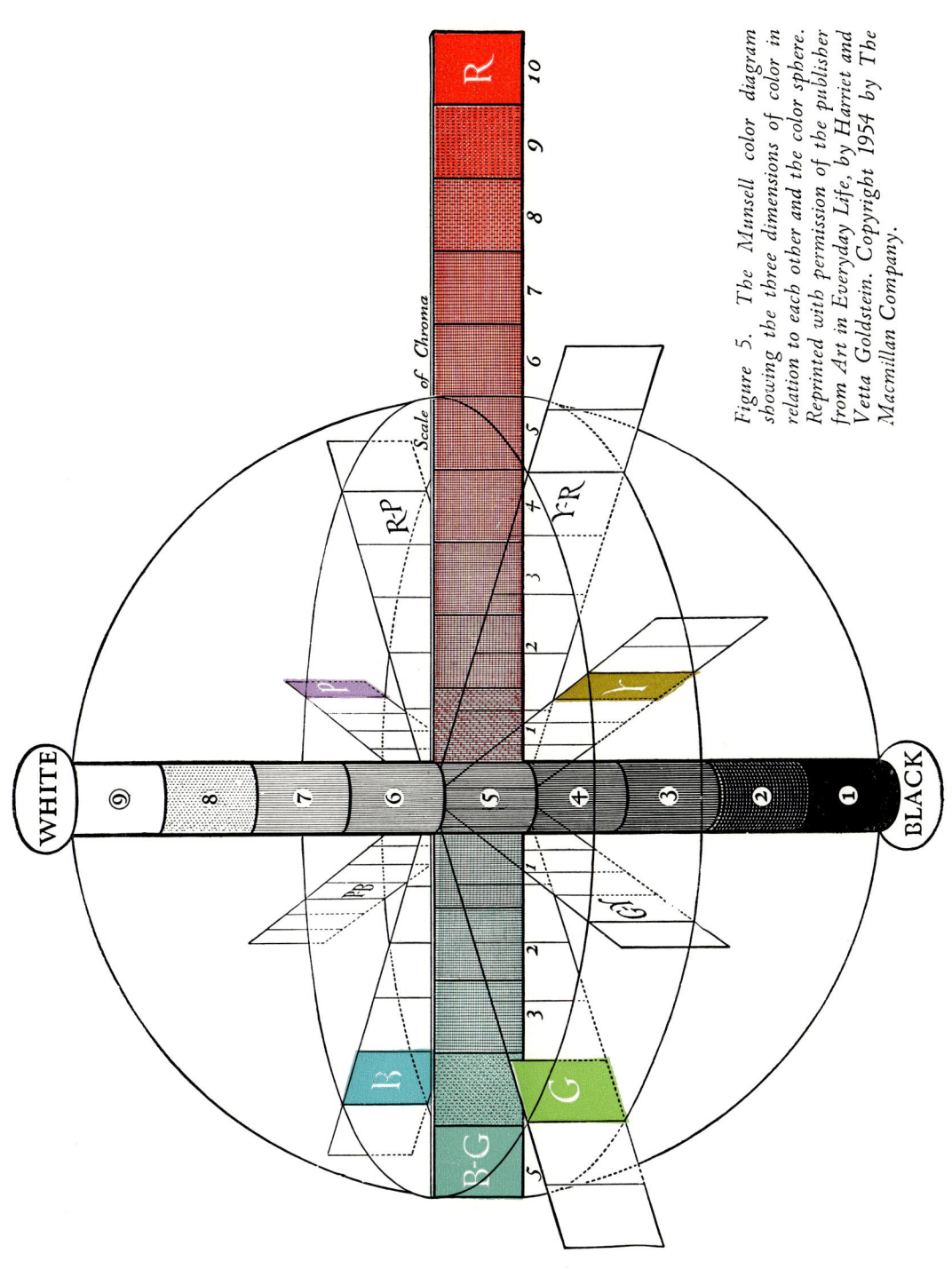

Figure 5. The Munsell color diagram showing the three dimensions of color in relation to each other and the color sphere. Reprinted with permission of the publisher from *Art in Everyday Life*, by Harriet and Vetta Goldstein. Copyright 1954 by The Macmillan Company.

to a hue produces the same result, and texture will affect apparent intensity. Bright colors increase size, advance, attract attention, and excite; dull colors decrease size, recede, and soothe or depress.

HOW COLORS INFLUENCE EACH OTHER

The chromatic afterimage was discussed earlier in the chapter. Table 6 gives a list of the complementary colors.

When complementary colors are placed in juxtaposition, their dissimilarity is accentuated. Red placed next to blue-green makes both the red and the blue-green more intense or saturated; and if the colors are very bright, they produce a shock to the eye. This phenomenon is known as *simultaneous contrast*. Juxtaposing black and white makes the black more black and the white more white. A combination of dark gray and light gray has the same effect.

When any combination of analogous colors is used together, one sees not only the original colors, but also their neighbors beyond. Analogous or related colors contain a common hue, as green in the combination of green-yellow and blue-green. Thus in a scheme of blue and purple-blue one gets the impression of greenish blue on one side and purple on the other, and an effect of rhythm is set up which may be very exciting.

Monochromatic hues, a combination of tints and shades of one color, react differently to juxtaposition; they appear more dull and less saturated. For this reason a combination of shades or tints of one hue will tend to lack sparkle and interest unless these intensities and values are varied skillfully and there is the right amount of each.

White, because of its luminosity, will combine best with the cool colors, such as green-blue, violet, and purple. Black will give the most pleasing results in combination with luminous colors, such as vivid reds, yellows, and

TABLE 6 COMPLEMENTARY COLORS

COLOR	COMPLEMENT
Yellow	Blue-purple
Yellow-red	Blue
Red	Blue-green
Red-purple	Green
Purple	Green-yellow

green-yellows. As gray is neutral, it will harmonize with both luminous and somber colors. This principle has applications in the selection of hues for blondes and brunettes.

Color is seldom used in isolation; it is more commonly used in relation to other hues that alter impressions. The textures on which colors are used create varying effects; and the kind, strength, and source of light also alter the appearance of color.

These references will help in your study of color.

Faber Birren, *Color, Form and Space,* Reinhold Publishing Corporation, New York, 1961.
Faber Birren, *Creative Color,* Reinhold Publishing Corporation, New York, 1961.
Faber Birren, *The Story of Color,* University Books, New York, 1958.
Committee of Colorimetry Optical Society of America, *The Science of Color,* Thomas Y. Crowell Company, New York, 1953.
Ralph M. Evans, *An Introduction to Color,* John Wiley & Sons, Inc., New York, 1948.
Johannes Itten, *The Art of Color,* Reinhold Publishing Corporation, New York, 1961.
Egbert Jacobson, *Basic Color,* Paul Theobald, Chicago, 1948.
Dean B. Judd, *Color in Business, Science, and Industry,* John Wiley & Sons, Inc., New York, 1952.
Aloys Maerz and M. Ray Paul, *A Dictionary of Color,* McGraw-Hill Book Company, Inc., New York, 1950.
A. H. Munsell, *A Color Notation,* Munsell Color Company, Inc., Baltimore, 1954.
The Munsell Book of Color, Pocket Edition, Munsell Color Company, Inc., Baltimore, 1960.
H. D. Murray, editor, *Colour in Theory and Practice,* Chapman & Hall, Ltd., London, 1952.

Exercises

1. Study an exhibit of modern paintings, and note the effect of intense illumination produced by using hues of longer wave lengths to create sunlight effects. Note, too, how these hues are shifted to shorter wave lengths to produce shadow.
2. Study colored dress fabrics under both sunlight and artificial light to note changes in hue.

3. Using a set of 100 colored papers, classify the hues according to their values, arranging them in order from the lightest to the darkest.
4. Select from colored papers or fabric swatches one hue in as many intensities as possible, grading them from brightest to dullest.
5. Study the *Atlas of the Munsell System* or any series of scales of value and intensity available to you. Using colored papers or fabric swatches,

   Select two warm hues, each of them medium value and medium intensity. Mount together and tabulate after checking with charts.

   Select two cool colors, medium value and medium intensity. Mount them together and label.

   Select two warm colors, each of them light in value and grayed to approximately one-fourth intensity. Mount together and label.

   Select two cool colors, each of them dark and of strong intensity. Mount together and label.
6. Study some fine examples of color chosen from Renaissance and eighteenth century painting to note the frequency with which the artist uses colors in their natural order of values.
7. Study similarly the work of modern French painters to discover their use of dissonance.

Ten

The Art of Combining Colors

We have been discussing the underlying science of color, but many other factors are involved if we are to put colors together beautifully. Because of the thrilling emotional effect which color has upon most of us, our intuition regarding it is apt to be unreliable. For example, if one has a fondness for a certain blue, she may not be able to dissociate her attachment for this color from the fact that it is inappropriate under certain circumstances. In other words, she gets so much satisfaction from seeing her favorite color that she cannot bring herself to consider a problem objectively when this blue is concerned.

Many people have certain color prejudices, but actually there is no color which is not beautiful if used properly. In order to use color well under varied circumstances, it will be necessary to study it intellectually and objectively. We must study examples of the finest use of color, and try many experiments to cultivate sensitivity in order to understand how to control individual color choices. If we do this, we cannot be satisfied with the stereotyped or banal in currently popular combinations. By objective study we shall come to appreciate aesthetically many colors we thought ugly, and shall find how immeasurably we have broadened our appreciation and personal satisfaction.

COLOR HARMONIES

Colors are harmonious if used in such a way that their relationship enhances the beauty of each one. Selecting hues from specified places on the color wheel will not guarantee perfection, but color chords may assist, as do musical scales and theory. The truly fine composition develops when the artistic instinct is allowed to emerge.

Related Hues

Color harmonies that are related may be one hue, or adjacent hues on the color wheel. When only one hue is used in its varying values and intensities, it is referred to as a *monochromatic* scheme. "Mono" means one; "chroma," the hue or color. If two or three neighboring hues are used, they are harmonious because they have one hue in common. These color schemes are called *analogous* or small interval.

No effect of color can surpass the beauty of movement created by merging and blending colors into one another. This may be illustrated by blending hues between magenta and violet, yellow-green and turquoise, or scarlet and purple; colors are chosen that embrace a small arc of the 100-hue circle, but their intensities and values are varied. It must be made clear, however, that the smaller the interval between hues, the greater the need for variety of tones or values in these hues. When closely related hues varied in value and intensity are used, their next neighbors, even though not physically present, are also seen by illusion, setting up a stimulating vibration. Refined and beautiful harmony results when hues range from green-blue to olive green, from tones of olive green to emerald, and from dark gold to cinnamon brown, as in the French peasant costume reproduced from a museum example by Gardelanne and Moffat (Figure 8 Chapter Eight). In this illustration is seen a reddish brown and black striped cotton frock, gold brocaded apron edged with black lace, white guimpe, and starched white cap tied under the chin. Over the cap is a black hat with fluted brim, diminutive fluted crown, and streamers of the same beautiful black lace on either side. This is a color scheme in gradation of small intervals strongly contrasted with white and black. The diagrams (Figure 1) show a method which can be used for figuring out the hues one may wish to combine in a similar scheme of small intervals. Such a device aids us in arriving at the hues desired. In Chapter Eight,

196 *The Arts of Costume and Personal Appearance*

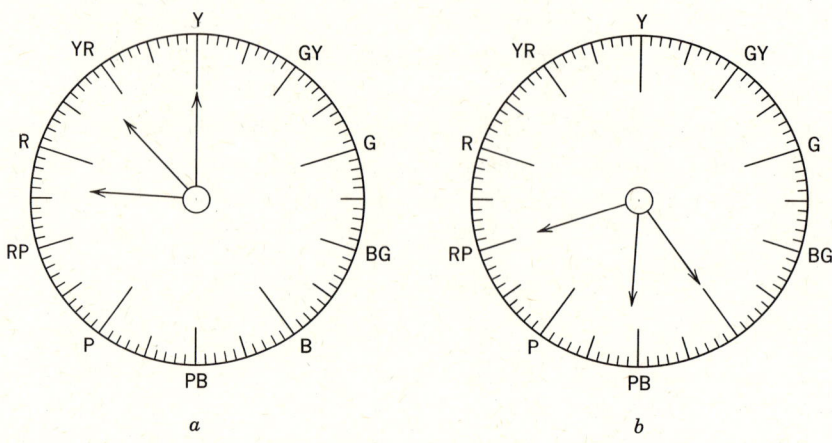

Figure 1. Small intervals charted. a. *A girl with blonde hair wears a rose wool suit with neutral yellow-beige suède gloves and a mink scarf.* b. *A dinner gown of bright purple-blue is worn with a lamé jacket of high value magenta brocaded in silver; sapphire jewelry and sapphire velvet pouch bag.*

Tables 2 and 3 suggest value combinations based on the dominant value desired. Ruskin said that the preciousness of color depends more on gradation than on any other of its qualities, since gradation is to color what curvature is to lines. Many interesting combinations of color in costume are developed around the idea of small interval of hues and close gradation of values and intensities.

Contrasting Hues

On the other hand, much fine color is produced by a skillful use of moderately wide or wide intervals on the color circle (Figures 2 and 3). Our zone of color may comprise the entire circle if we lower the value and reduce the intensity of the hue. This explains the rich and glowing colors in Oriental rugs or in paintings by Renaissance masters, where hues ranging around the entire circle are used together in grayed intensities and in a wide variation of values.

The simplest use of contrast in color harmony is that based on *complements* —hues that lie directly across from each other on the color wheel. The need of the human eye for a balanced stimulation of warm and cool colors must be an essential consideration always. Thus may be combined a medium blue-green with a dash of vermilion, or a grayed blue and a bit of orange.

THE ART OF COMBINING COLORS 197

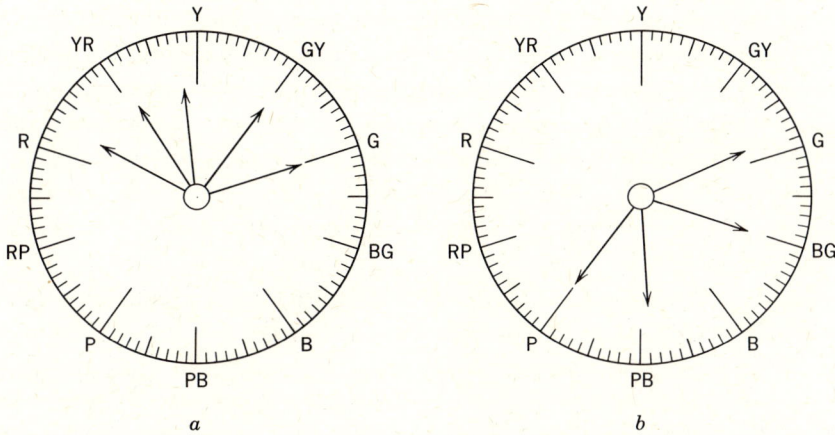

Figure 2. Moderate intervals charted. a. *A girl with orange-red hair wears a spring ensemble consisting of a dress of mustard-colored silk printed in darker reddish browns and off-white flowers worn under a sheer wool coat of olive green, and a bracelet of bright green.* b. *A silk print by Christian Berard has a blue-green background with fanciful birds in purple, purple-blue, green (slightly yellowish), black, and white.*

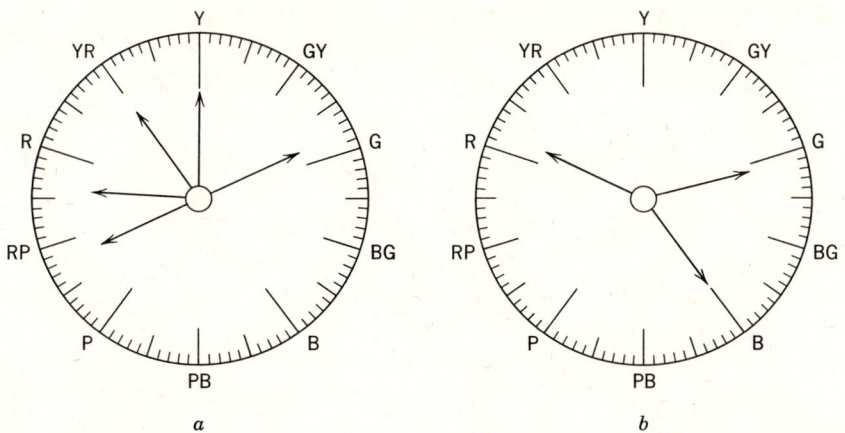

Figure 3. Wide intervals charted. a. *A tweed coat of green, slightly on the yellow side, is cross-barred in a light bluish pink and both colors are very grayed. It is worn by a yellow-haired girl with a suit of green tweed flecked in pink; brown shoes and a felt hat in tones of darker purple-red.* b. *A neat little silk print for a summer street frock has a rust-red background with figures of ultramarine blue, a little green, black, and white.*

For the sake of variety, frequently more than two colors are used. In this case the *split complement* is formed by using one hue and the colors on either side of its complement, purple-blue with yellow-red and green-yellow. Another variation is the *double complement* where two sets of complements are used, such as yellow and purple-blue with green-yellow and purple.

The *triads* are also contrasting harmonies. If a set of colors forms an equilateral triangle on the color wheel, they constitute a triad. An example is the combination of yellow, red-purple, and blue-green.

Persian and Indian paintings of the sixteenth and seventeenth centuries are one of the finest sources for study of distinguished color. In one example, a princess wears a dress in several tones of orange printed in a pattern of pale yellow, green, and white (Figure 4). Her jewels are red and green, and she carries a pale mauve pink or red-violet flower. Here, if it had been possible to reproduce the colors, could be seen hues ranging far around the circle in a fine contrast of pale tones against black hair.

Another type of contrast occurs when a single bright or dominating color is given greater importance by contrast with an extremely neutral color, rather than by using it with other intense hues. Thus warm hues may be contrasted with grayed hues having a warm cast, as in vermilion with beige, peach with ivory and pearls, green with grayed greenish gold and copper, and crimson with warm gray. On the other hand cool hues may be contrasted with neutralized hues having a cool cast, as in cornflower blue with pearl gray, pearls, silver, or rhinestones; emerald green with black or oyster.

Natural Order and Dissonance

When one combines hues in their natural order of value, the yellows or their derivatives are the lightest in value; the reds and greens are darker than the yellows; and the purples and blues are the darkest of all. This principle is illustrated by a very subtle scheme of pastels: a gown of pastel blue-green taffeta, a bracelet of emeralds and diamonds, and a corsage of small pink and pale yellow rosebuds and forget-me-nots with green foliage. The yellows and reds are seen to be the lightest, with green and blue-green in their natural order, darker.

Colors used in the reverse of their natural order of values, dissonance, may result in beautiful effects, provided very small areas of the reverse order are used: turquoise or a darker green-blue with small amounts of olive green; red-purple or purple-brown with accents of blue-violet in lighter value; or chocolate with light green.

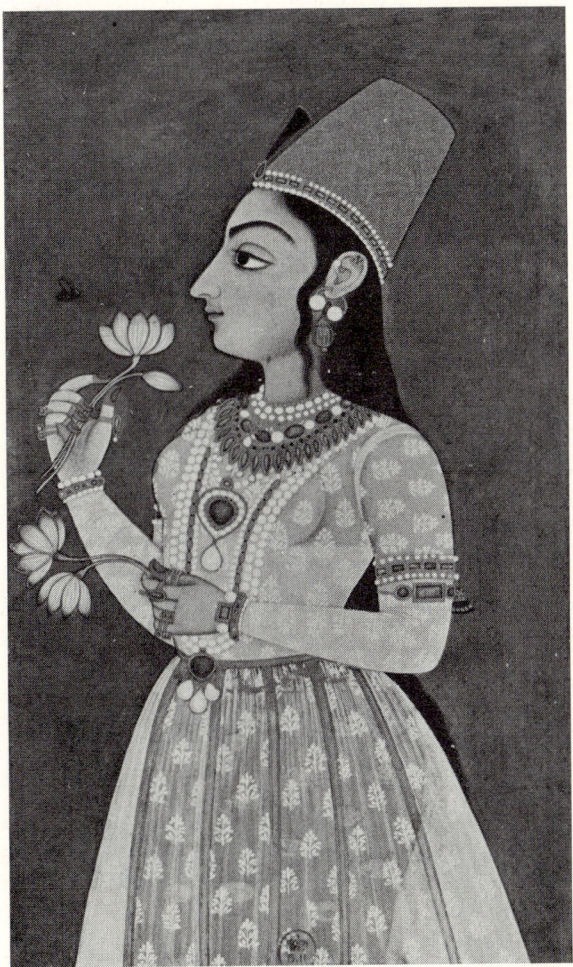

Figure 4. Indian Girl Holding a Flower. *Hindu painting of the seventeenth century. Tones of orange and mustard are used to emphasize dusky skin and black hair against a dark grayed purple-blue background.* Bibliothéque Nationale.

In nature one sees examples of this reversal of the natural order. The bloom of a purple plum is not a lighter purple, but a pale violet-blue. The highlights on an orange are not lighter orange, but pale rose. The lovely fuchsias of our semitropical states combine petals of a kind of salmon-pink (red-orange) with a pale bluish pink (dissonant), or bright scarlet with pale lavender (dissonant). A fragment of sixteenth century Persian brocaded fabric with predominating areas of red-violet in medium value is given sparkle with small bits of pale violet-blue (dissonant). One eighteenth century taffeta with background of medium light turquoise blue is brocaded in floral pattern of reddish browns and deep olive greens (dissonants). Another has a floral pattern in tones of dark blue-green and red-purple (dissonants) on a background of light blue satin.

In the modern school of painting, the works of Cézanne, Van Gogh, Gauguin, and others constantly show us the use of dissonance. It may be a pale blue-green shape against deeper gold and black, or rich coppery hues with accents of pale lavender. The alert student of color will do well to study Cézanne's revolutionary use of color, such as his often-used strong yellow to yellow-green with tones of pale violet-blue and bluish-pink. A student of costume will profit by studying Marie Laurencin's orchestration of delicate hues, as in her *A Lady in Pink,* where pale tints of rose have been used in the hat and darker beige masses in the hair. Although these paintings are done with a much more varied palette than is usually employed in costume, yet modern fashion creators are strongly influenced by them.

Dissonance occurs in printed dress fabrics and in ensembles, but genuine understanding must be had to use it well. It must never be used in excess. In small touches it becomes very important, adding beauty and vibration. As in music, dissonance seems necessary, for too much harmony and too much sweetness pall upon us. The dissonant element thrills the discerning because it is unexpected; however, it may seem discordant to the inexperienced.

LAW OF RELATIONSHIP

Relationship of Hue

The first decision is the selection of a suitable dominant hue that is in harmony with the face, figure, temperament, and occasion. This selection is not necessarily used in the greatest amount, nor is it the most saturated, but it sets the pace. This is the color around which the harmony is built.

If pure standard hues express the mood or tempo desired, they should be combined with others of the same category. In other words, do not try to mix principal colors with the more refined intermediates. They are difficult, if not impossible, to combine successfully.

By the same token, because of relationship of hue, earthy colors—mustards, ochers, terra cottas, browns, sap greens—make agreeable schemes wherein may be combined both cool and warm elements. Acid colors—versions of turquoise, marine blue, periwinkle, magenta—may be used together because of their hue relationship; at the same time they offer warm and cool elements. But earthy and acid colors are difficult to use together until one thoroughly understands dissonance.

Relationship of Value

Value, you recall, is the degree of lightness or darkness of a color. In a color scheme the values should be related but not identical, and one should find some value contrast.

Sharp contrast in value is garish in effect and tends to destroy color. Any dark color placed on a light ground intensifies the dark and makes the light lighter. Therefore it is necessary to reduce the contrast in value in order to secure a pleasing effect. Through half-closed eyes one should be able to detect colors which "jump out" at the eye because they are out of key or unrelated to the scheme.

Relationship of Intensity

Similarly, the intensity or saturation of the dominant hue sets the stage, or limits to some extent the intensities one would use with it. Vivid hues are combined with others that are comparable in tone. On the other hand, when the basic hue is less intense, one uses other less intense tones. But because of the danger of too much dullness, the intensity must be varied as well as the value. Consequently, very subdued colors can be used with small areas of brighter tones, but not too bright, in accessories; for example, yellowish brown may be combined with mustard, and very dull green may be combined with brighter greens in small areas.

Blue grays may be used with soft but brighter blues. The subtle, refined tones of Japanese prints illustrate this principle, and help us to realize the jarring effect of an off-key intensity, because they are so right in their degree of intensity variation.

COLOR HARMONY AND THE LAWS OF DESIGN

The total effect of any color harmony depends on the hue chosen, but more than this on its relation to other tones in the composition. Color tones must complement each other; each must make the other more attractive, more interesting, more enjoyable. In order to achieve this fine quality of relationship, it is necessary to apply the basic design principles.

Color must be and can be balanced by using the warm and the cool colors, the light and the dark, and the bright and the dull. The amounts of color and the contrast can be accomplished by using the law of areas or law of backgrounds, which states that large areas of color should be quiet in effect, whereas small amounts may show strong contrasts. The larger the amount used, the quieter it must be; the smaller, the more striking. It is entirely possible to exercise great care in the selection of colors that balance but forget to arrange them according to their weight—hue, value, and intensity. If the colors used are alike in their power to attract, then ratios such as two to three and three to five will be a good proportion.

In order to lead the eye through the costume, there must be a repetition or crossing of color dimensions. Subtlety of movement is of utmost importance, so as not to jar the senses. But the eye must not move continually; it must be allowed to rest for a time on the prime focal point. Color, well arranged, will help to emphasize the dominant features and subordinate the others.

The problem, then, is to consider first the impression to be made or the feeling to be conveyed, because one idea must dominate. One hue, one value, and one intensity must be chosen to occupy a larger place than the others, but for variety there must be some degree of contrast.

COLOR TO EXPRESS EMOTION AND CONVEY MEANINGS

The above decisions as to qualities of color are also influenced by the emotional effect to be expressed. Here again one has the opportunity to exercise control. What impression is the scheme to convey—vitality, force, joy, gaiety, dignity, maturity, conservatism, or the dramatic? Is the costume intended to make the figure recede or be extended? For what occasion will it be worn?

All these factors must enter into the decision in order to control results. This idea may be illustrated by working out the color harmony for a dinner dress to be worn by a vivid young woman with a gay, sparkling temperament. She has black hair, green eyes, and a rich creamy skin.

A high value key of a fairly bright intensity will suggest the gaiety and festiveness needed for the girl's temperament and the occasion. Chartreuse, a greenish yellow—high light on the value scale and of bright intensity—could make the dress. For the evening wrap move clockwise around the 100-hue circle to find a related, but cooler hue. The choice will be silver brocade in a bright green that is low light of the value scale. This gives a lovely scheme of small interval. For contrast and in keeping with her forceful temperament, use the 100-hue circle again, and passing counterclockwise, decide to introduce a red note. Vermilion, a bright orange-red in medium value, used in small amounts, will supply this needed drama. The vermilion may be used in the slippers, the jewelry, or the evening bag, but one or two notes only.

In this instance color has been employed in the following manner:

High values and bright intensities, to express temperament, appropriateness to the occasion, and to be a complement to personal coloring.
Chartreuse in largest areas—light and medium bright.
Green and silver brocade, second in area—medium light and somewhat brighter.
Vermilion in the least amount and of brightest intensity.

One might wish to select an afternoon ensemble to express stateliness, refinement, and feminine grace. The dominant hue used in the coat and dress might be a bluish purple or plum wool crepe that is dark in value and of moderate to grayed intensity. Perhaps the lining of the coat could be a dissonant—purple-blue of lighter value. The hat of purple-red could be trimmed in lighter tones of red and blue-purple and some small notes of bone. The gloves too might be bone color, and for a note of excitement one might wish to introduce a bit of turquoise jewelry. In this illustration color has been used in the following manner:

Hues dominantly low in value and medium in intensity, to express the dignity and refinement of the wearer.
Close intervals of hue and value to express conservatism and maturity.
Cool colors to relate to the wearer's gray hair and blue eyes.
Hues in combination suited to an afternoon occasion.

Procedure for Combining Colors

First, select the dominant hue. Analyze this color as to its specific hue, value, and intensity. Determine its position on the 100-hue circle (Figure 5

Chapter Nine). One should know the 100-hue circle so thoroughly as to be able immediately to see any hue according to its position on the color circle. It becomes essential to recognize the warm and cool as well as the bright and dull aspects of color.

Second, determine the colors to accompany the dominant. These, too, must be judged according to their warmth or coolness and degree of saturation, as well as to what takes place when they are juxtaposed with the dominant hue.

Third, ascertain the placement of hues according to design principles of balance, proportion, rhythm, and emphasis.

And finally, be aware of the fact that the laws of color harmony are needed as a foundation, but the *true artist* will go beyond all laws to express an impeccable taste all his own.

Exercises

1. Some color names are located in Appendix B. Look through current fashion magazines to find other color names being used and interpret them according to the 100-hue circle.
2. Analyze the fine examples of colors in historic and contemporary textiles and paintings. Use a finder or cup the hands around certain areas to isolate them for study.
3. Plan and execute in water color or tempera paint a series of experiments demonstrating distinctive use of the following types of combinations:
    One-hue schemes
    Earthy hues
    Acid tones
    Warm colors with accents of cool and vice versa
    Important single color enhanced by neutralized hues
    Very neutralized hues with dashes of brighter tones
    Vivid hues together

Eleven

Enhancing Personal Coloring

In the study of personal coloring and the means of enhancing it, we come to another of the high points in the subtle art of costuming. Taste and personal distinction are evidenced in the colors a woman chooses and wears. Surely one who plans to work professionally with the problems of clothes and personal appearance must be able to speak with authority in the matter of colors which enhance individual coloring. For advisement of this nature one needs to call upon all her fundamental knowledge of color and texture, illusion, and costume to express personal temperament or mood.

The more thorough our understanding of what colors do to each other when combined, the more able we shall be to distinguish the subtle nuances of color with which one deals in making color schemes for personal coloring. This knowledge facilitates a more creative approach to cosmetics and to costume color. In order to recognize more clearly assets and liabilities, the first step must be the analysis of the color tones in the skin, eyes, and hair.

ANALYSIS OF PERSONAL COLORING

The best procedure for analysis is to remove all make-up with cleansing cream or mild soap and warm water so that natural coloring may be seen realistically. Then compare yourself with some standard. A class or club group affords an excellent means for studying differences in coloring. In a large group there is certain to be at least one girl who approximates a perfect blonde, a brunette, an auburn-haired girl, and others belonging to the various personal coloring classifications. A comparison of these more or less standard types will help in seeing the wide differences there are in skin, eyes, and hair, and the differences even among those of the same color classification. When groups of girls or women are formed for a critical study, a wide variety of hues as well as of values and intensities is found.

Analysis of Skin Tones

In a very general classification of skin tones, there are but two types, warm and cool skins, corresponding to the warm and cool sides of the color circle. Then there are differences in lightness and darkness of the warm and cool types, and differences in the vividness and the subdued qualities of skin tones are commonly observed.

Those whose skins tend to be very light and cool are called fair to distinguish them from dark, creamy, or ivory skins. A fair skin has a basis of orange-yellow. In the cheeks and lips are overtones of red-violet or violet-red, and there are also blue shadows which occur about the nose and under the eyes. The blue and red-violet overtones which give fair skin its coolness determine to a great extent the hues of rouge and lipstick usually most effective.

The skin tones of the warm types have either a creamy or an ivory cast, ranging from very dark, rich, and swarthy to light creamy or ivory tones. Creamy skin has more orange than yellow, and its overtones are red-orange. This is the skin of a vivid brunette. The red-orange overtones set the pace for rouge and lipstick. Then there are the skins which are basically of a yellow tone, called ivory. They usually have no color in the cheeks, but very red or red-purple lips, and their overtones are greenish. Olive skins range from a very light value, as in the pale, ivory skin of Deborah Kerr, to the dark, bronze skins of women of Latin races (Figure 1).

Other types of warm skins are the rich honey- or amber-colored complexions so often associated with a suntanned blonde; this skin color and blonde hair are particularly effective with brown eyes. This coloring would be classed as yellow-orange, but of a lighter value than that of the dark, vivid brunette.

The skin tones of auburn-haired types are yellow-orange, ranging from light, creamy tones to darker, richer ones. The overtones are usually red-orange. Purple-red overtones in this type cause a florid skin, which presents difficulties in selecting becoming colors.

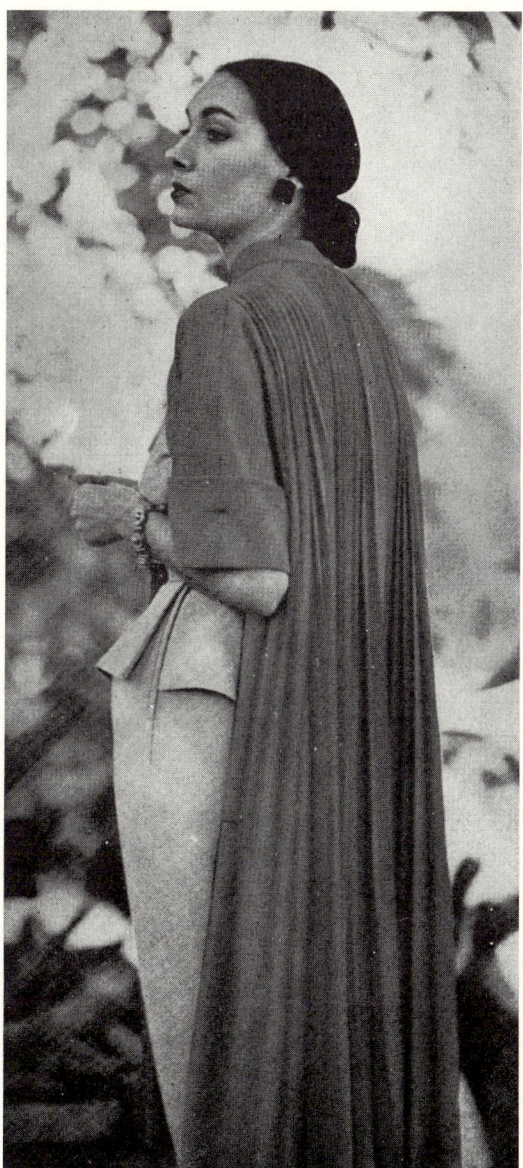

Figure 1. A dramatic costume developed in a strong color contrast of light violet-blue and cherry red, reflecting the striking characteristics of the wearer. Courtesy of American Enka Corporation.

Analysis of Eye Color

The coloring of eyes associated with the cool types are blue, gray, green, and violet; brown, black, and hazel are considered warm eyes. But many people are more interesting as well as more complicated color problems, because they do not conform to these standard combinations. They are, however, usually either predominantly warm or cool.

The eyes are regarded as third in importance when considering becoming costume colors. The areas of skin and hair are large, whereas the eyes occupy a very small area. Their color, therefore, is not seen at any distance. In the best practice the eyes are usually accented in small areas. Eye color repeated in entire costumes often gives no life or interest to the eyes; instead it is apt to drain them of natural brilliance and may be unpleasant against skin tones.

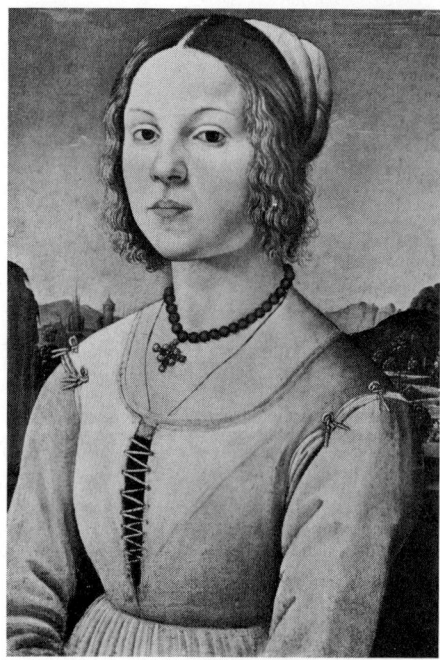

Figure 2. Portrait of a Young Girl. *By Lorenzo di Credi. Kaiser Friedrich Museum. The lovely auburn hair of the young girl has been enhanced by most of the auburn's best colors: the yellow-greens, olives, and bronze-like browns of the Italian landscape. The girl herself is attired in cream white laced over a black chemise; mauve-pink sleeves, tied on; and, not to remain unnoticed, a necklace of clear red.*

Analysis of Hair Color

Blonde hair (YOY) is so much grayed with blue as to be put in the cool classification. The true Irish type of hair is blue-black, and white hair has bluish tones. The pale, neutral blonde hair, often called by the poets flaxen, is a very neutralized light yellow with a greenish cast. These hair tones harmonize with red and blue-violet flesh tones. Ash blonde hair is the very neutralized, darker blonde hair so commonly seen accompanied by pale eyes and a skin of almost the same value. Little contrast is afforded without resort to make-up.

Hair called red is actually a red-orange or a pure orange of bright intensity ranging in value from the golden hair of the vivid blonde through auburn (near medium value) to the darker red-orange of henna cast which Titian immortalized in his beautiful men and women. Lorenzo di Credi painted his lovely *Portrait of a Young Girl* with light auburn hair (Figure 2). Then there is brick-red hair, which is usually accompanied by a transparent pink or florid skin and blue eyes. To tone down this kind of hair great skill is required.

Finally there is brown hair, which is neutralized red-orange in all ranges of value and degree of brightness. In Tables 1 and 2 these color types and their composite combinations are classified to show how they relate to one another.

From the tables it will be seen how varied are the combinations of coloring. Composite coloring can be most interesting and unusual when one knows how to bring it out. When one has mastered basic principles, she will enjoy the freedom of trying to achieve creative effects. It is impossible to set down color rules for composite types because of the myriad variations in individual coloring.

One fact the tables show is that many of us are far from vivid, having rather indefinite coloring, such as the ash blonde. Drab or nondescript coloring is certainly not outstanding, and personal distinction under these circumstances needs to be enhanced with the judicious use of cosmetics.

CHOOSING COSTUME COLORS

It is important to analyze individual coloring of hair, complexion, and eyes to determine individual color ensembles and to experiment under skilled guidance with costume colors which will do flattering things for personal coloring. There is a choice of two methods. Some people may like to remove all make-up and, sitting before a mirror in a strong, north light, see the tricks that color can play when large swatches of colored fabrics are draped about the shoulders. Others may wish to see cosmetics applied before trying on different colors. There is greater value in studying colors without make-up when one is learning to be discriminating. The same fundamental rules used in the making of any color harmony apply here, unity with variety. It will be easier without make-up to see likeness and to decide how much difference will be pleasing. It may be possible in limited instances to increase color choice through slightly different cosmetic tones. However, utmost discretion must be used in this matter.

In choosing colors one should not be influenced by prejudice or attraction

TABLE 1 TYPES OF PERSONAL COLORING

COOL TYPES	SKIN	EYES	HAIR
Vivid blonde	Fair, light neutralized YO or OY; overtones of red-violet in cheeks and lips; faint blue in shadows	Bright, deep blue, gray, violet-blue; less often, green	Vivid Y or YO or "golden" hair in light value; reduced in value it becomes light auburn; reduced in value and intensity it becomes ash blonde
Neutral, flaxen-haired blonde	Pale or very light neutralized YO or OY; hint of red-violet in cheeks and lips	Blue, gray, green, tending to be pale	Light neutralized straw color or flaxen; near same value as skin tones, thus tending to lack value contrast
Irish blonde	Same as vivid blonde, or same tones, darker value	Deep blue, violet, green, gray	Blue-black and with dark lashes and brows, forming a striking contrast with fair skin
WARM TYPES			
Auburn	Fair or a light creamy YO with overtones of RO	Brown; sometimes blue or gray	Bright red-orange in wide range of values from golden to titian, and always the determining factor in choice of color for dress
Vivid brunette	Deep creamy YO with overtones of RO	Brown or black	Brown or blackish brown, neutralized red-orange
Olive brunette	Degrees of OY, ranging from light to dark with overtones of a greenish cast; no color in cheeks	Brown or black; sometimes greenish	Black or subdued RO, dark brown

TABLE 2 COMPOSITE OR INTERMEDIATE TYPES OF PERSONAL COLORING

COOL TYPES	SKIN	EYES	HAIR
Honey-skinned blonde	Honey, amber, or suntanned; YO, darker than fair	Brown, hazel, or green	Light YO or neutral to golden blonde
Ash or drab blonde	Fair to pale or darkish skin with cool overtones	Pale blue or gray	Grayed Y or YO, mouse-colored
WARM TYPES			
Titian	Creamy	Blue, hazel, or brown	Dark red-orange or henna cast
Light-haired brunette	Light creamy	Brown	Golden or neutral blonde with dark lashes and brows
Chestnut	Light creamy	Blue, hazel, or brown	Brown with glint of red, chestnut
Fair-skinned	Fair	Blue or green	Dark brown
GRAY- AND WHITE-HAIRED TYPES			
	Fair	Blue or gray	Mixed gray or gray or white
	Creamy	Brown	
	Sallow	Any color	
	Olive	Brown or hazel	
	Florid	Gray or blue	

to any specific color. Becomingness is the essential factor to consider. This means that the color does pleasant things to the skin, hair, and eyes; that its texture brings out the right characteristics of the person; and that it is suited to the occasion. The color should help to impart clearness and the look of health to the skin; it should not draw or drain from the skin its natural color. The skin tone can be reduced to muddiness by color too light in value, made sallow by bright complements, or may take on an unpleasant florid or red-purple cast when bright green is worn. With the exception of the suntanned skin, a rule to follow is that of keeping the color in a darker value than the skin. Suntanned skins are often agreeably emphasized by cool pastels. Floridness is reduced by any grayed, dark, warm color. Cool skins wear best the darker cool colors and the lighter warm ones. Warm types may wear warm colors in all but the lightest values, and the cool ones when dark and of an intensity related to their own.

Color should bring out the highlights or sheen of the hair and make the eyes more interesting. Blue and gray eyes are particularly sensitive to strong color. They may be washed out by the wrong color or deepened by the right one. For example, an entire ensemble of blue may drain blue eyes of their color, but small accents of the color will emphasize them. Through the use of the right color, gray eyes can be changed to blue, green, or violet.

Only those who are vivid in coloring should wear vivid colors in large areas; the less vivid the individual the less apt she is to transcend strong color. However, persons with little color and value contrast in their personal coloring, the intermediates, need some contrast of hue and value. Large areas of color should blend with skin and hair; small areas, accent other features. Prints worn by intermediates should have a contrast of value. Close intervals of cool colors make for quieter, more subtle combinations; wide intervals produce striking dramatic effects. Intervals of color contrast should be related to contrast in personal coloring.

Texture greatly influences the appearance of color and may be the determining factor in whether or not the hue is flattering. Generally, bright colors are more satisfactory in dull textures than in shiny ones. Very flattering results may be achieved with brighter tones in soft woolens and pile materials. Appropriate textures will not add to size, emphasize thinness, make features appear coarse, or call attention to lines in the face.

Colors for Blondes

There are many types of blondes. Included are the vivid blonde with fair skin and lovely gold hair (Figure 12 Chapter Four, Figure 1 Chapter Thirteen), the more neutral blonde with delicate cameo-like skin and flaxen hair, and the ash or nondescript type with skin, hair, and eyes blended in a monotone grayness which requires a vivacious personality or skill in make-up and costume to overcome.

Few vivid colors are right for all these types of blondes, as they clash with the brilliance of vivid blonde hair, destroy the delicate beauty of neutral blonde skin and hair, eclipse the drabness of ash blonde hair and eyes, and make the skin almost putty colored. An attempt should be made to highlight or emphasize their lightness of skin and hair, make the most of delicate tones of skin, and deepen the color of the eyes for each type. Intermediate hues rather than primaries or principal hues will be more flattering, since they harmonize with the many tones of the complexion. Intermediate hues that belong to blondes have blue in admixture; and if this is understood, blondes will find becoming hues almost anywhere on the color wheel.

Blondes of whatever type will choose as their best colors the green-blues and blue-greens, all the way from soft turquoise to bottle green to midnight blue. The more vivid the individual, the wider will be her range of values. The composite ash blonde will need to keep to the darker values, from middle value and below. Her problem is to gain value contrast and a clear skin, which she can do only with darker values. These dark values then can be given more life through variation in texture and ornament. The complete range of green-blues and blue-greens is right for all blonde types because they both relate to blue overtones and complement skin and hair tones, but their values and intensities must depend on the degree of personal vividness. These basic hues may be made still more enhancing by repeating the lightness of hair in casts of yellow-green or repeating the skin overtones in touches of a bright, darker purple-blue or raspberry, producing a color scheme of wide intervals.

A second group of hues for blondes is in the blue-violet to red-violet color path, which so beautifully enhances cool eyes and violet-red overtones. Again, the value range is varied from light to dark for the vivid blondes and is limited to the grayer intensities for the flaxen-haired blondes and to the darker values for ash blondes. Here there is opportunity for many beautiful effects: large areas of violet-blue or blue-violet may have accents of red-violet, violet-red, or turquoise used in close intervals; medium and darker values may be given added interest by off-whites in pearl, silver, or oyster. The dark red-violets, called wine, seem a bit heavy for the light coloring of most blondes, and are not for their feminine kind of personality.

The familiar eye-fatigue experiment shows that when one looks hard for a moment or so at one color, its complement is called up. Thus if the skin is suntanned or tends at all to be sallow, the stronger intensities and more luminous blues and violets tend to force unpleasant yellows and oranges in the skin. This would mean that only the darker versions of these color paths would be becoming. By the use of green-blues and greens, according to the principle of the fatigue experiment, florid or red-violet tones in the skin would be forced out unpleasantly.

Another color path is that of the cool browns, browns on the red side which have been grayed with blue and purple, rather than orange and yellow reduced to dark values. Browns of this kind are very beautiful with light hair, fair skin, and blue eyes when accented with rose, violet, or blue-violet in a lighter value, a discord. A vivid blonde looks well in cinnamon, cocoa, and maple sugar brown, particularly when they are combined with darker values; but she chooses beiges only when her hair is near the auburn tones. Beige is exactly the thing the mousy or drab blonde should not choose; it affords no contrast, and contrast is greatly needed.

Many reds are most effective for a blonde with a good complexion and light flaxen hair. Cardinal (a bright red with a bit of blue) and vermilion (a light red with a bit of orange) seem right in beautiful textures. Velasquez used this kind of red as the background for the little Spanish Infanta, Margaretta, who had flaxen hair and a pale skin. Red of this quality seems correct today for a blonde with a vivid personality. But there are other becoming reds for blondes: the rose called *bois de rose,* coral if medium strong, and such pastels as delicate peach and shell pink, which blend with skin tones but need accenting with darker values in order to avoid a sugary look.

The soft yellow-greens in chartreuse, almond, and olive are lovely with definite red-violet overtones and vivid gold hair; but they are hardly wearable for the one who lacks value contrast and definiteness of coloring.

The importance of texture must not be forgotten, as a less flattering color may be made more wearable in a texture that is becoming. Lustrous blacks, such as satin, velvet, and silver fox, are beautiful for the vivid blonde and the neutral or flaxen-haired blonde with strong enough contrast; whereas the more ashen blonde needs medium values of warm-cool and cool-warm colors in muted tones, but black only in dull textures. Also flattering are the soft brown of baum marten, the refinement of tourmalines, and the crush pastels such as grayed blues, pinks, or aqua used with darker accents.

To sum up, then, all blondes will look best in grayed intensities to enhance the brightness of their own coloring. Values should be dark enough to highlight their lightness. Cool, intermediate colors, both cool-warm and warm-cool ones, relate to and complement their coloring. Chalk white, black relieved with pale accents, and warm pastels are lovely; and certain vivid light reds and lustrous black may be chosen when the personality is vivid.

Colors for Auburn-Haired Types

One who is possessed of the gorgeous coloring that accompanies auburn hair should surely understand how to make the most of it. As has already been said, auburn hair coloring ranges all the way from red-gold to a dark titian and includes the brick-red (more red than orange) so often seen with a bluish-white or a florid skin. The ideal skin of the auburn-haired is creamy and is found combined with brown, green, or hazel eyes; the composite versions of this type may have blue, often pale blue, eyes (Figure 11 Chapter Four).

As pure, vivid colors are wrong for blondes, so for this type vivid colors tend to compete with brightness and to nullify the beautiful personal tones. The desired effect may be obtained by using darker values to enhance lightness, but lighter hues will accentuate the darkness and richness of titian hair. The warm skin tones and eye colors also help to determine the hues chosen. The intermediate hues, if chosen in the right values and intensities, may range far around the circle. Browns, when used in contrasting tones always darker or lighter than the hair, are particularly harmonious with auburn coloring. Popular color names include beige, buff, golden brown, japonica, safari brown, and Rembrandt brown. The latter is the dark, rich yellow-brown of the old master and is especially fine in rich textures.

A second color path is that of the yellows and yellow-greens from soft chartreuse through olive to a bronze-green so lovely with rust and old-gold jewelry. Greenish-gold velvet with cream about the face or accents of darker green and pearls set in gold would be beautiful for a typical auburn and almost as good for a vivid blonde. And this same beautiful scheme carried out in greenish-gold soft woolen or jersey, with the green notes changed to brown, is right for all those with coloring which ranges from gold to titian.

Another color path is that of the green-blues. These complement the hair and skin tones without forcing the hair to seem truly red as does green, except in dark values. This range of colors can be used in rare and beautiful schemes of close intervals of hue but in a wide range of values.

Purple-blue, too contrasting in large areas, is lovely in small accents with red-gold hair; it supplies all the primaries, red, yellow, and blue, in a complete harmony. Some authorities would have auburns use reds and purples, but this surely depends on skin tones, personality, and the particular reds and purples used.

For the auburn with clear, light skin there is nothing quite so beautiful as delicate, warm pastels—cream with gold jewelry, pale green-yellow and yellow-green with darker accents, or delicate shell pink, as seen in de Credi's *Portrait of a Young Girl* (Figure 2). Contrary to earlier teaching, there is a tint of delicate pink, between peach and coral, that is right for most auburns. Darker-skinned auburns may take their cue from this to select darker values of these same hues, remembering always to choose them in a grayer intensity than their hair.

The brick-haired individual has a less simple problem, because there is much blue in her white skin and a very strong orange in her hair. This person should be careful not to force these colors but to tone them down with a close interval of cooler hues. Cream white, blue-gray, beige-browns with strong contrast of darker brown, cool browns with accents of lighter violet-blues, or light violet-blues with accents of darker purple-blue will be interesting as schemes. They must, of course, be related to hair and skin to tone down high color.

The auburn types, by way of summary, will choose their colors from the grayed, warm and cool-warm colors, with accents of cool colors. Suggestions include the earthy tones, cream white, black, and any value from light to dark which contrasts with the hair. Cold blue and the purple ranges, almost prohibitive in large areas, should be selected with care.

Colors for the Vivid Brunette

No type of coloring is quite so easy to suit in the matter of becoming colors as the vivid brunette. Strong value contrast, made by dark brown hair, eyes, and brows against rich creamy skin, makes possible the wearing of vivid, almost unrestrained color. The choice of colors is limited only by what they do in forcing sallowness or a hard, unpleasant, orange cast into the skin. The range of value is wide. Dark values may be worn and sometimes relieved by accents of light; light values are likewise flattering if the complexion tones are not made unpleasantly darker by the still lighter pastels. Black is good for this type when the skin is clear; white will emphasize the rich, healthy tones of a dark, swarthy skin; and warm gray may serve as a foil for the dark hair.

The dominant, barbaric hues of Old Mexico and South American Indian cultures or the exciting colors associated with the Russian Ballet suggest color ensembles for a vivid brunette. Chinese and geranium reds, bright pinks, cerise, emerald green, topaz yellow, and strong green-yellows, which drain color from the faces of more subtle or neutral types of coloring, should enter into the apparel of this vivid type. These vivid colors, so well suited to sport and evening clothes, should include from the cooler side of the circle deep purples and brilliant ultramarine blues. No other type wears them quite so well. These same lavish colorings in subdued versions, reduced almost to earthy tones, are correct for daytime wear in soft woolens and jerseys. Vivid prints on strongly contrasting backgrounds and such unusual and exotic furs as leopard and ocelot are for this type.

Colors for Composite Brunettes

Composite brunette colorings are found very commonly in America. One type has dark hair, fair or creamy skin, and brown or hazel eyes (Figures 12 and 13 Chapter Thirteen). Many composite brunettes combine the advantage of dark, contrasting hair and brows with cool skin and eyes. This combination enables them to use almost any hue around the circle, providing the value is darker than the skin and the intensity is not so bright that color is washed from cool eyes. The warm colors, less strong than those given the vivid brunette, and the bright, cool colors, in darker values including Wedgwood blue and peacock, are becoming. The off-whites are also good, and the warm pastels that range from orchid around the warm side of the circle are wearable if dark enough not to force the skin to look darker.

Colors for Dark-Skinned Blondes

Those who come under this classification have light yellow to yellow-gold hair, sometimes quite neutral. They are called blondes for this reason, but they could quite as well come under the brunette classification, because their eyes are brown (sometimes hazel) and their skin is creamy, honey-colored, or amber. The skin determines the color characteristics of this type.

According to the laws of unity the best colors are warm, because they are related to hair, skin, and eyes. However, the bright, warm colors, correct for vivid brunettes, are so intense they destroy the richness of honey-colored skin. Bright, cool colors will force an unpleasant orange into the complexion. Color paths of golden browns and red-browns from dark to light will accent brown eyes and blend with honey-colored skin and light hair. Beiges and tans, however, are so near the coloring of dark-skinned blondes that they are made drab and uninteresting. Other color paths are in the darker greens, blue-greens, and earthy tones; turquoise, bright green, and white are enhancing by night.

Colors for Light-Haired Brunettes

The light-skinned, light-haired brunette or blonde with brown eyes is another unusual type; and in this instance costume colors are influenced by the brown or hazel eyes. The French peasant costume (Figure 8 Chapter Eight) suggests the browns, from yellow to red-brown, for this type. For this kind of coloring, light and dark values in either warm or cool brown produce beautiful effects. Dark yellow-browns with gold and cream, red-browns with rose, or chocolate browns with violet-blues or soft turquoise may be used. The beauty of cream white with cool pastels of turquoise, green, and pale violet-blue may be accented with gold jewelry. Soft rich furs such as beaver, seal, nutria, mink, and kolinsky are becoming.

Colors for Olive-Skinned Brunettes

The dark brown or black hair and very deep, ivory skin which has a definite greenish cast is associated with women of Latin background (Figure 1). The most distinguished of the olive types is the person with pale ivory skin against dark hair. Also included in this classification are the many olive types with lighter hair and hazel eyes and those with suntanned olive skin, which has a rich bronze cast.

Our best conception of hues for dark olive skins is obtained from old Egyptian murals. Elizabeth Burris-Meyer has beautifully assembled some colors which include dull tones of yellow-greens, mustard, yellow, ocher, copper, and rust-reds, with here and there a note of lapis lazuli or turquoise found in a typical Egyptian palette.[1] These colors are called earthy and relate to dark olive and bronze coloring without making it sallow or giving it a ruddy glow. Black can be very interesting against young, fresh, glowing skins, but it makes older ones look dull. However, when combined with the earthy tones of gold, copper, and ocher, it is rich and striking. Dark bright blues, wines, and bottle greens are also right. Bright green, turquoise, and white for evening complement this dusky kind of beauty, and set it apart with an individual distinction. Rouge will widen the color repertoire of the olive type, but in using it women in this group become more nearly vivid brunettes and lose some of their uniqueness.

Olive-skinned brunettes thus are at their best in grayer hues and particularly the earthy tones of yellow-green. The values will be dependent upon the darkness of the skin. These persons may use the red hues around as far as red-purple if it is grayed. Of the cool colors, they have all the greens, blue-greens, and pure, bright blues. In this way full importance is given to the bronze or the dark, rich, greenish tones in skin and eyes. Light-haired olive-skinned brunettes may wear a wider range of values in the same color paths.

---

[1] Elizabeth Burris-Meyer, *Historical Color Guide,* Wm. Helbrun, Baltimore, 1938, p. 2.

Colors for Irish Blondes

One of the most fortunate of all color types is the Irish blonde of cool coloring with dark and light contrast. Added to fair skin, red-violet overtones, and cool eyes is the advantage of blue-black hair that provides contrast, which the blonde so often needs. The Irish type has the whole range of acid colors, from blue-greens around the cool side of the circle to red-violet, in all values darker than the skin. They may wear chalk white and unrelieved black, the sharp contrast of black and white, all the grays, silver lamé, the gray and black lustrous furs, and precious stones which repeat their cool qualities. Beiges which are unrelated to their coloring and the reds which have a base of orange or yellow are less wearable; yellow-green is unflattering, unless accented with something very becoming. But reds with a tinge of blue, such as crimson and American beauty, are most effective. The very best colors, however, will come from the wide cool range mentioned above, and they often are chosen to enhance eye coloring. Pastels of the mauve, orchid, and periwinkle versions, not too grayed, are excellent for evening; an example from the past is an arresting 1880 gown in light purple-blue with tiny ruffles in American beauty at the edge of the skirt.

Colors for Gray- and White-Haired Types

All those who have lost part of their original coloring in hair, and usually skin as well, come under this classification. These women may draw on a great variety of colors if they understand their original coloring and the tones in their changed coloring. Indeed, those who have clear complexions and fine eyes can make themselves most distinctive if they have courage and taste.

There are those whose hair is still mixed with dark. Sometimes these women use a rinse that tides them over until the hair is entirely gray or white. There are others whose skin has changed and is florid, sallow, or a darkish orange against the mixed coolness of the hair. These women will not look their best in the colors they originally wore, but there will be some colors from their original classification that will suit them when neutralized and darkened. There is the stage when one must avoid those colors which emphasize the yellow, green, or brown tones in the hair. Thus browns, beiges, yellows, and yellow-greens, most prints because of their patterns, and strong complements are barred. Dark values, grayed colors in the cool range from blue-green around the cool side of the circle to wines are usually good. Cool, muted colors and pastel pinks and blues are right if kept darker than the skin. Discreet use of carefully chosen make-up in the color path which tones in best with the skin is very helpful. The faintest tinge of eye shadow often does lovely things, but again it must be used with discretion.

When hair has turned entirely gray, the problem is simpler in that one has the opportunity to complement its gray tones in costume colors which take the skin tones into account. Certain dark greens and taupe-browns are lovely with brown eyes; cool eyes afford opportunity for use of a wide range of cool colors, limited only by the brightness and freshness of the skin.

The white-haired woman, especially if she is fair, affords a magnificent canvas for artistic achievement in color ensembling. She may choose from the whole range of blue and purple tones, from black, chalk white, coral, blue-green, ultramarine, and from the lovely pastel pinks, mauves, and violets, but not the yellow-greens. Her natural coloring may be accented with rouge and lipstick of the most delicate, light, cool hues. Perhaps a hyacinth rinse, if necessary, and eye shadow of lavender blue may be used. In this way the white-haired lady is able to eclipse all the young things in her striking beauty.

Exercises

1. Study the blondes in a class group. Have them stand in a row in order of the darkness or fairness of their skins. Compare the color of their hair by having them stand with their backs to the class so that a larger area of hair is visible for study. Note the difference in sheen, in value, and in range of hue from yellow to yellow-orange. Study brunettes, auburns, and intermediates in a similar way.
2. Make a collection of fabric swatches to illustrate the colors that are becoming to standard types.
3. Experiment with colors for yourself and make a chart to show the values and intensities of each becoming color.

Twelve

Creating Illusions

The contemporary woman's striving for the semblance of a perfect figure corresponds to the creative artist's admiration for personal distinction and aesthetic refinement. This is where art steps into the picture, for it is good design that helps us to enhance the good and conceal the less desirable.

MEANS OF IMPROVING FIGURES

Diet and exercise are foremost considerations in the development of a figure of more nearly ideal size and proportions. These two factors are interrelated in arriving at and maintaining a beautiful body.

A fine posture is paramount to physical attractiveness; without it the most perfect proportions will be ineffective. The stoutest and the thinnest will gain enormously in distinction from a good carriage. As never before, contemporary standards of feminine beauty demand a head held high, an elevated chest, a slender waistline, and hips tucked under (Figure 2b Chapter Three).

Foundation garments if well-fitted contribute to the smooth, well-groomed appearance of the average woman irrespective of age. There are two schools of thought relative to the wearing of foundation garments. One disapproves on the ground that they restrict and weaken the muscles of the torso. On the other hand a properly fitted foundation need be neither restricting nor uncomfortable. Foundation garments, whether brassière and girdle or one-piece, should be tried on to determine whether or not they fit correctly, as garments are designed for a wide variety of figure types. If necessary, have a foundation altered by an expert fitter. A heavier figure requires a sturdier garment than does the slender one which may achieve a smooth line through a light weight, spandex two-way stretch. Good-quality, sturdy garments are expensive. The person who conscientiously loses weight will have more money for the purchase of much more interesting clothing.

Foundation garments should never fit so tightly that they displace flesh; a garment which is too tight will roll and produce bulges which defeat its purpose. Characteristics of a well-fitted garment are that it will support the bosom, control the hips and abdomen, and come down over the heaviest part of the thighs. An advantage of a pantie girdle is that it may be worn quite long and yet not impede movement of the legs. Hosiery of the correct length is important in the comfort of a girdle. A garment should be equally comfortable whether one is sitting or standing (Figure 1). Other articles of lingerie also contribute to the semblance of a good figure. Costume slips, too, should be tried on. A good slip molds smoothly over the bust, under the arms, about the waist, and down to the hips. The outer skirt silhouette may determine whether or not a slip which hangs straight from the hips or flares outward from this point is purchased.

Finally, optical illusion may be used to minimize figure irregularities through skillful handling of line, texture, and color. It may be employed while trimming or rounding the figure and improving posture to make a person appear at her best; it should not be

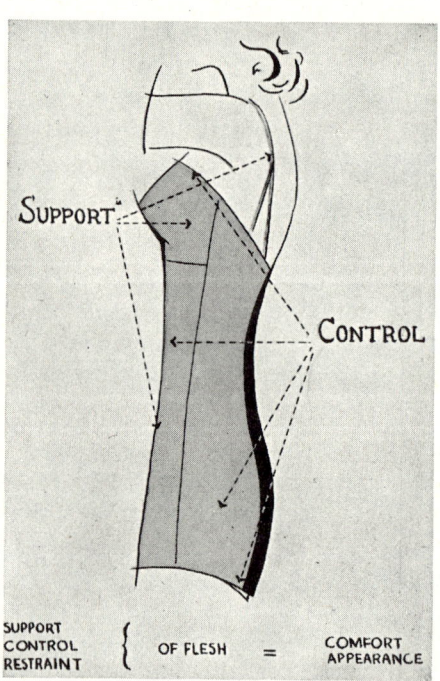

Figure 1. Today's foundation garment showing how correctly fitted garments can improve figures. Courtesy of Women's Wear Daily.

used as an escape from discipline. Optical illusion is of extreme importance in camouflaging the problems of irregularities beyond correction. It is at this point that art assists enormously in creating a more beautiful appearance.

TECHNIQUES OF OPTICAL ILLUSION

To create optical illusion an understanding of the use of line movement, the psychology of color, and the effect of various textures in expanding and reducing size is essential. Then it is possible to create the appearance of a more pleasingly proportioned figure by covering irregularities, by breaking up overly large, plain expanses into smaller areas, and by shifting attention to other points more favorable.

It is not enough to know good design. We must be sensitive to the effect of:

Line direction: whether vertical, horizontal, or diagonal.
Nature of the spacing: whether broken up into long narrow verticals, wide horizontals, or diagonals.
Proportion and scale: whether large, unbroken areas or small, broken spaces.
Silhouettes: whether tubular, bell, bustle, or some modification of these.
Dark-light value arrangements: whether strong or moderate in contrast, dark or light in value.
Colors: whether warm or cool, bright or dull.
Texture: whether employed for reducing or extending effects.

The following optical illusions can be created when one has learned to manipulate line, space, and value for purposeful control.

Line movement (Figure 2) encourages the eye to travel vertically over the figure thus giving the impression of greater height. Note the suggestion produced by each of the forked ends *a* and *b*.

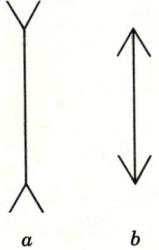

Figure 2. Vertical line movement.

224 *The Arts of Costume and Personal Appearance*

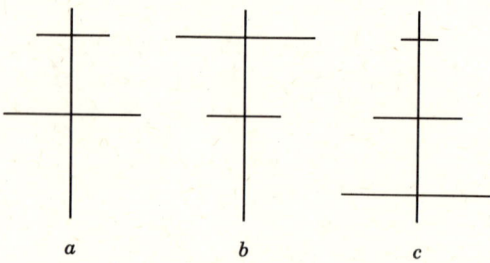

Figure 3. Dominance-subordination.

Emphasis draws attention to the most desirable point (Figure 3) by making it dominant and thus helps to control impression.

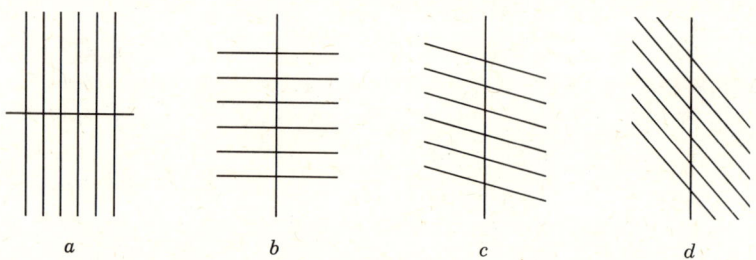

Figure 4. Emphasis through repetition of line direction.

Line direction given the most emphasis (Figure 4) controls eye movement. Note the stabilizing influence of the one line that holds all others together.

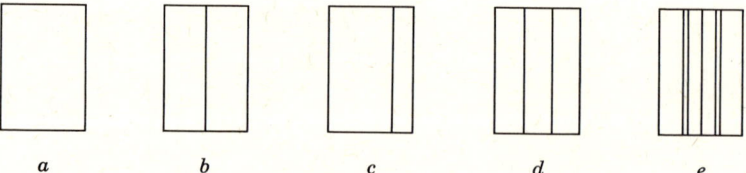

Figure 5. Space and control of center of interest.

A large, unbroken area (Figure 5) seems larger than one in which space is divided into smaller areas. The slenderizing effect of *b*, *c*, and *d* is less than that of *e*, which has small broken areas concentrated vertically in the center of the figure.

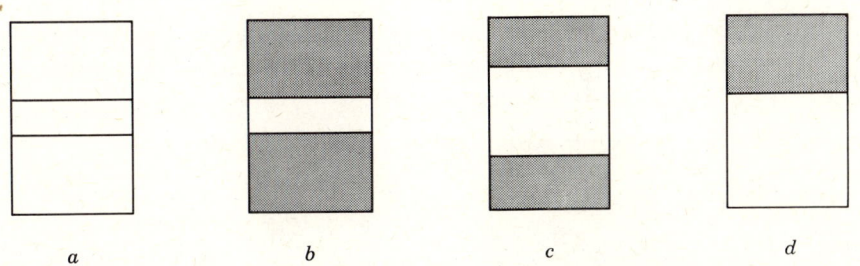

Figure 6. Contrast and horizontal line movement.

Contrast in value or color (Figure 6) focuses attention upon the area in which the change occurs. The value contrast in *b*, *c*, and *d* draws attention to the light section. The lack of contrast in *a* makes undesirable features less noticeable; but there is at the same time a horizontal movement.

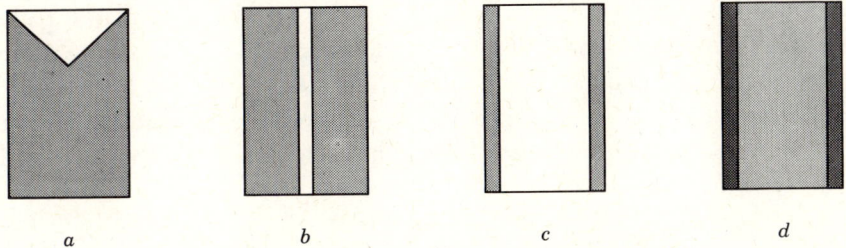

Figure 7. Contrast and center of interest.

Emphasis may be controlled by shape and contrast (Figure 7). Interest is centered at the top in *a*, and the lower part of the figure is made less conspicuous. In *b* attention is drawn to the center in narrow vertical spacing. A more narrow effect is given in *c* by tending to obliterate the sides. Successful illusions, as in *d*, depend on carefully chosen closer values.

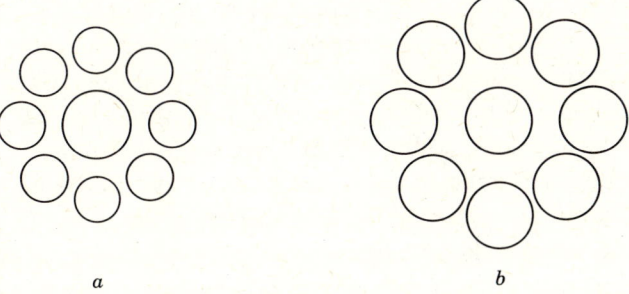

Figure 8. Proportion and scale.

226   *The Arts of Costume and Personal Appearance*

Scale and proportion may control apparent size (Figure 8). The central circle in *a* looks even larger in contrast to the small scale of the surrounding circles. In *b* the center is dwarfed because of the larger surrounding circles.

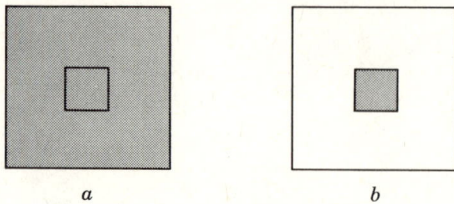

Figure 9. Contrast and apparent size.

Dominance-subordination is controlled through contrast (Figure 9). The power of attraction is greater in *b* because of stronger contrast.

These are the principles used to create the illusion of better proportioned bodies, and to assist those with figure irregularities. Fit does play a part in the artistry of illusion and cannot be underestimated. Tight-fitting clothes on the stout figure emphasize size; garments fitted too loosely accentuate the overly thin body. All other aspects of fit—waistline placement, hem length, armscye line, shoulder seams, and neckline—should be evaluated critically. Garments which appear to belong to the body are most graceful.

The Short, Stout Figure

The stout woman, with her heavy bosom and arms, her thick waist, and swelling curves, is the most difficult of all figures to costume beautifully. It is true that a "fat" woman can have a distinction all her own, provided she is meticulously groomed, suitably attired, and carries herself superbly. The charm of such a figure is often in a pretty neck or hands or perhaps trim ankles and feet. Every possible means should be used to emphasize any excellent features and to increase the impression of grace, dignity, and slenderness.

Lines in continuous, unbroken vertical movement or upward slanting diagonals give the illusion of greater height. Very restrained curves will give added grace, whereas severe, straight lines tend to emphasize rotundity by contrast. Seldom should rococo movement of any kind be used.

Silhouettes which are graceful and flowing, modified tubular versions, and those which give the impression of being draped on the figure are suitable. Easy, comfortable perfection of fit is imperative; any tight-fitting foundation or outer garment makes the figure appear larger. Emphasis should always be contained within the body silhouette, and should be placed near the center of the figure with the most dominant area near the face. Avoid all details of garments and accessories which dangle, float, or sway.

Sleeves cut on the bias will give a slimming effect when carefully but not too tightly fitted. The size of a large forearm may be camouflaged by use of a sleeve length which extends to or terminates several inches above the wrist. Wide, loose sleeves tend to make the figure appear wider by adding to horizontal line movement. Heavy upper arms should never be entirely exposed in evening dress but should be partially concealed by draped sleeves or a graceful stole.

Bodices should be designed with slightly draped fullness or ease but never be revealingly smooth and tight. Waists which are broken by vertical or diagonal movement are also slenderizing. A well-fitted brassière is most important, especially if the bust is low.

Waistlines, usually thick in this figure, are less conspicuous when undefined by a belt. Some irregularity of line which does not precisely define the waistline will minimize width. This may be accomplished by seams or panels which carry the eye upward and outward at the shoulder and inward as it approaches the waistline. Half belts or narrow, inconspicuous belts of self material may be used. Avoid wide belts and those of contrasting color, value, or texture.

Skirts should be simple, easy, and flowing in line, never tight and narrow. They should be worn long enough to break the effect of heavy calves. The sides should be nearly straight, a plumb line; when they are cut on straight grain, some fullness needs to be introduced near the bottom to give grace in walking and to balance the figure. This fullness may be introduced through pleats or low-placed gores in front and back. The princess line and the coat-style dress draw attention away from the broad outline of the silhouette and break up the width into vertical areas.

Coats may be full length, either straight or semifitted with easy, loose-fitting sleeves. Avoid double-breasted styles and coat lengths shorter than the skirts worn under them, because both designs produce horizontal movement.

Spacing should be broken by long narrow verticals and upward-slanting diagonals. Emphasis is always contained within the silhouette.

Necklines are cut close to the sides and back of the neck and have a strong vertical line movement. Draped necklines without bulk and properly designed dickey insets may be used.

Collars, if any, should be narrow and relatively flat and based on restrained curves rather than circles or sharp angles. The shawl collar is one of the most flattering.

Pocket-like details, if used, should be placed high above the bustline to create the illusion of greater length below.

The proportion of all individual parts of the costume must be in keeping with the size of the figure. Scale in accessories, as heavy jewelry and large flat bags, should be of sufficient size to appear to dwarf the figure. Shoes must be carefully selected. The spike heel and pointed toe make feet too slender to support the body, and the figure appears top-heavy.

Values which are medium to dark in tone help to reduce apparent size. Dull black has a slenderizing effect. Close values in fabric combinations or in prints camouflage and obliterate lines.

Colors which are dark in value and soft and grayed in tone are wise choices. Cool hues and those that are cool-warm give the illusion of smaller size. Color choice, however, will be dependent on personal coloring. Bright colors, warm or cool, create the illusion of greater size. Use of close value will produce a head-to-toe look for the stout figure. Hats, hosiery, and shoes of little contrast are in keeping; contrasting skirts and blouses should not be considered.

Texture is the one factor that is of prime importance in clothing the heavy person. Without the right texture, the illusory impression resulting from suitable design is destroyed. The right texture may sometimes make it possible to apply principles less rigidly. One important rule is to buy only materials with body, those which have a good fall, and those which will hang in fairly heavy, limp folds. Do not use fabrics which are flimsy, fluttery, bulky, wiry, hard, stiff, or shiny. Materials which have substantial draping qualities are seldom inexpensive, but in the end they are wise investments.

Shiny or stiff textures increase the apparent size of the wearer and accent the silhouette; dull-surfaced textures decrease the size of the wearer and conceal the silhouette.

Transparent fabrics are figure-revealing unless used in several thicknesses. Opaque sheers in neutral tones and darker values cause figures to recede.

Heavy, wiry, bulky or thick fabrics add to apparent size; light weight, smooth textures tend to reduce bulk.

Prints that direct the eye in an up-and-down movement, such as stripes or geometric designs, are slenderizing if their values are close and they are compactly spaced. Prints that lead the eye in a circular or swirling movement suggest obesity. Widely spaced prints and those of strong contrast attract attention to size.

Furs must be short-haired, such as broadtail, caracul, galyak, and mole. These are possible in full length coats if the person is not too heavy and if the garments are carefully designed. The use of fur in smaller amounts is often more judicious. Bushy, bulky, or long-haired furs must never be considered.

The Thin, Angular Figure

The physical opposite of the stout woman, the tall, thin, angular girl, has her problems also. This is not the tall, slender girl of ideal proportions. The angular person has no curves; she is flat front and back; she has prominent shoulder blades and a bony neck; her arms and legs are thin; and her posture is often poor. For this type, devices are needed to expand the figure and transform angular, sharp contours into a semblance of the graceful curves of our present ideal. In an age that insists on stark, streamlined simplicity, considerable shopping may be required to find appropriate garments.

Lines should direct the eye in a horizontal movement. Restrained curves soften angularity; large, full, round, buoyant curves cover or break up the thin figure. No garments based on straight, severe lines, such as mantailored clothes, should be worn. Princess lines add undesirable height and reduce apparent width.

Silhouettes which are adaptations of the bell or bustle give the effect of flowing grace. Tubular silhouettes softened with pleats, pockets, peplums, or tunics are possible, as these details add dimension. Bouffant effects are helpful when they are in agreement with the personality. Close-fitting, tubular garments are to be avoided.

Necklines which cover up are flattering (Figure 10). The cowl, scarves, soft bows, and rolled or flared collars with curved edges add width to thin necks. If filled in or masked with scarves or camouflaged with space-filling jewelry, the deep, round décolletage is possible. Dickeys and vests worn as underblouses and revealed at open necks are effective.

Bodices which are soft, full, and draped vertically or slightly on the diagonal add softness (Figure 6 Chapter Seven). Waists which are fitted loosely over the bust and more snugly through the midriff give the effect of a well-rounded bosom. A padded bra, combined with soft bodices, is helpful.

Figure-expanding sleeves such as the dolman, bell, or full bishop gathered into a band or deep cuff effectively cover and add width to long, thin arms. When in fashion, wide, full sleeves of chiffon, other sheer fabric, or embroidered organdy soften angular contours. Sleeveless garments are not flattering. Shoulders that are narrow, angular, or thin can be filled out and covered by the simple means of a well-shaped pad which conforms to the current shoulder silhouette.

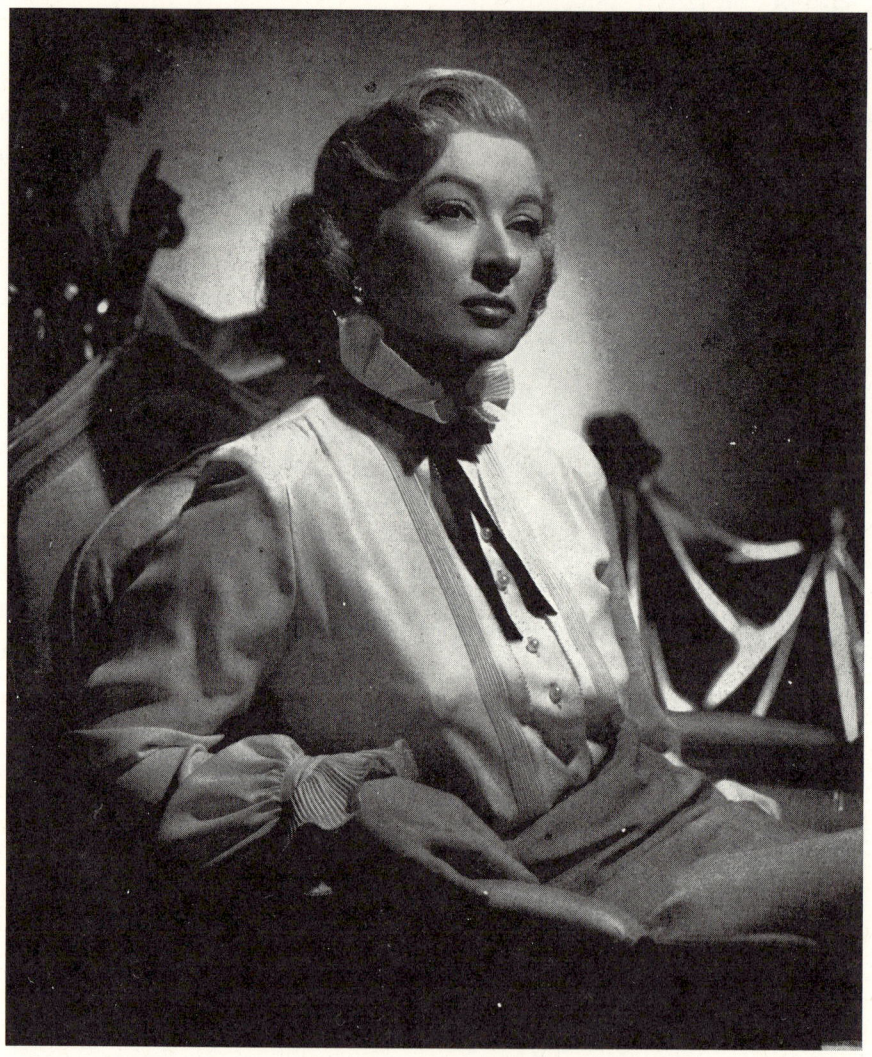

Figure 10. A charming suit blouse with exquisite detail. Courtesy of Greer Garson.

Waistlines which are casual, easy, or bloused are pleasing; wide belts are effective with skirts such as the dirndl. Contrast at the waistline, if not too strong, is good for this figure, as it draws attention to the area and thereby cuts the apparent height. Overblouses, peplums, and tunics, in lengths adjusted to figure proportions, introduce horizontal movement.

Jackets are best when full or boxy rather than figure revealing. The length, hip length or longer, must form a pleasing proportion to the total figure height. Rarely are the bolero or spencer good for this figure, as either makes the legs appear too long. Capes of all lengths tend to reduce height. Full coats may be worn by this type.

Space should be broken into dominantly horizontal areas with some minor vertical forms. Important emphasis may be at one side of the body or outside the silhouette rather than at the center of the body. Bulky pockets, thick buttons, and trimmings which stand out may be used to break space.

Scale should be related to the figure. Large handbags and chunky, colorful, costume jewelry are correct.

Values which are advancing add to size; consequently, light values are best. Close or moderate contrast will add interest and extension without being sharp and severe.

Colors which are warm and cool-warm, but of soft, grayed intensities, do most to increase apparent size. Color contrast is also effective. Strong intensities increase apparent size, but personal coloring and temperament must be considered.

Texture needs to fill out and flatter a thin figure. However, crisp or bulky textures are not the answer to the problem. The thin and angular person needs the flattering effect of soft, napped, or pile materials, rich trimmings, soft drapable fabrics in unpressed pleats, tucks, and other forms of flowing fullness. Avoid fabrics which are too stiff, severe, wiry, coarse, sharp, or lustrous.

Prints may be chosen to give life, color, and animation to the thin, angular body. Prints with smaller scale motifs may make the figure seem larger by contrast; but medium or large floral motifs, when not bold in contrast, are becoming. Widely spaced floral motifs will be flattering, but large-scale geometric patterns are too sharp in effect.

Furs which are long-haired, rich, and expensive are wise choices. Fox, lynx, marten, skunk, opossum, kolinsky, mink, raccoon, sable-dyed muskrat, persian lamb, and beaver may be used in capes, stoles, jackets, and coats and as trimming.

The Nordic Type

The tall, muscular, heavy-boned Nordic woman is another for whom the present fashions are not designed. Her problem is difficult in that she is too tall to resort to the vertical line direction best for the stout figure and too broad to emphasize horizontal movement, which reduces the height of the tall, thin, angular person. She must compromise with designs in which a balance of both horizontal and vertical line is employed, never one without the other. She must also break up the expansiveness of large surfaces into smaller areas.

Correct textures are her greatest aid in keeping down the impression of bulk and expansiveness. Shiny surfaces will catch the light and be reflected in rounded folds; dull, broken-surfaced fabrics such as heavy crepes will absorb the light and make shadows, which reduce apparent size. Bulky fabrics will make her appear massive; napped and pile fabrics add inches through their thickness and rounded folds. Clinging jerseys tend to be too figure revealing. In other words, this type of person needs lightweight tweeds and sheer woolens, pliable worsteds, heavy silk or wool crepes, semi-sheers, and prints in large vague designs. Like the stout person, she should wear nothing stiff, crisp, bulky, or clinging.

It is possible for this type to be most compelling, suggesting the splendid figures of Grecian and Roman matrons in their sweeping classic robes. At night the Nordic type can look superb in classic drapery that trails and accents the movements of a vigorous body. Colors must be subdued, with brighter hues reserved for accessories. She can be regal wearing large heavy jewelry with rich stones. On the street she should be inconspicuous and conservative, yet striking. This is accomplished through neutral tones, handsome fabric, and excellent cut and workmanship, rather than ornamentation.

There are many individual variations and combinations of physical characteristics. The three types most frequently encountered have been analyzed in detail. The devices suggested may be adapted to fit similar problems.

Individual Figure Faults

The previous discussion of the contemporary figure ideal pointed out that good proportion and correct posture are the major factors contributing to style and beauty. For those who possess certain deviations from this ideal, means of creating the illusion of more perfect proportions are given below.

Sloping shoulders may be built up with shoulder pads to conform to the prevailing fashion silhouette. A wide high lapel may be used to create the illusion of a straighter line.

Narrow shoulders may be extended by the use of shoulder pads. Garment lines which direct the eye outward toward the tip of the shoulder are effective, as is fullness in the sleeve cap when it is in fashion.

Rounded shoulders are a posture fault which may be corrected by improving body alignment. The defect may be minimized in dress by placing the shoulder seams slightly back of the normal position. A soft rolling collar also tends to straighten the upper curve of the shoulder; a bodice back which is bloused tends to fill in the curve below the shoulders and straighten the line (Figure 7 Chapter Six). A bolero, boxy jacket, or cape will accomplish the same effect. This figure fault is frequently accompanied by a hollow chest which needs filling out with soft details. Raglan sleeves accentuate round shoulders and a hollow chest.

Heavy hips which are large in comparison with other parts of the body may be minimized through the use of long vertical and diagonal lines. Several carefully spaced vertical lines are more effective than the single vertical. Emphasis should be placed high on the bodice of the garment to direct the eye away from the figure irregularity. The youthful person may cover heavy hips with a flared skirt (Figure 11 and Figure 7 Chapter Seven). If the torso is not too large, a semblance of balance may be achieved through soft fullness in the bodice. Conversely, the heavy bust needs to be balanced with a larger skirt area.

The prominent abdomen can be minimized by directing the eye to areas above and below the fault or away from the center front of the figure. This may be accomplished through easy fitting blouses and interesting necklines. A skirt with some fullness in the lower part will help to balance the irregularity. Slight fullness in the skirt at either side of the protrusion gives the appearance of a more normal contour. Hip length jackets should be avoided; longer ones cut on straight lines help to conceal.

Sway back results from poor posture and may be corrected, as can round shoulders. Dipping the waistline slightly in the back and filling in the hollow above with a bloused bodice is effective (Figure 7 Chapter Six). Peplums, bustle effects, and long jackets may also be employed to conceal this irregularity (Figure 1 Chapter Eleven). The sway back often is accompanied by a prominent posterior (Figure 13 Chapter Seven). Fullness at the back of the skirt, falling gracefully from hip to hemline, minimizes an excessively protruding derrière.

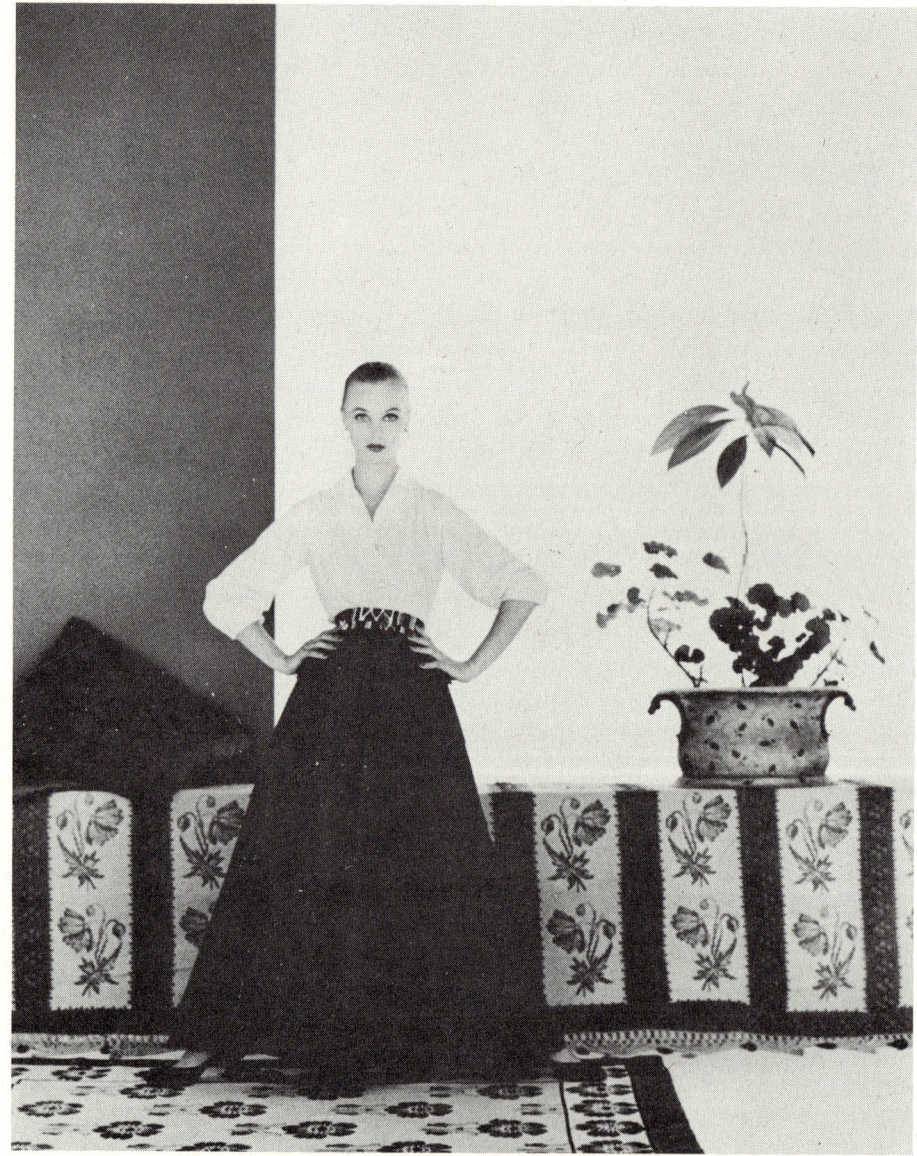

Figure 11. A red canvas skirt for evenings at home or at a college fireside, worn with a shirt of creamy wool jersey, studded with rhinestone buttons. By Toni Owen. Multi-colored belt from Pan American Shop. Photo by Scavullo. Courtesy of Harper's Bazaar.

Bowed legs frequently result from incorrect walking habits and can be improved through corrective exercises and learning to place the weight away from the outside of the feet in walking. The length of the skirt is important in minimizing this figure problem. Skirts should be kept inconspicuous, and all emphasis centered on the upper part of the body through making the bodice, head, or hat the center of interest.

A thick neck, heavy arms, full bust, or large waistline may be minimized by adapting the suggestions given in the section for stout figures. Other figure irregularities such as a thin neck, hollow chest, prominent clavicles, flat bust, or thin arms may be minimized through application of the devices for the thin person. Ungraceful hands should not have attention called to them through wearing elaborate rings and bracelets. Likewise, attention should be directed away from square, wide feet; shoes should be kept inconspicuous in color and most simple in line and free of decoration.

Becoming Necklines

The face is nearly always the center of interest in costume; detail is centered about the neckline to draw attention and to act as a transitional device to lead the eye to the face. In this function it is important that necklines and collars form an enhancing frame.

Necklines which are formed of hard, harsh lines tend to accentuate facial irregularities, and throw even the perfection of an oval face and the most regular features into sharp relief. Softened lines are much more flattering to most people, as they do not intensify irregularities. In evaluating neck details, remember that lines which repeat facial contours emphasize them through repetition; lines in opposition, through strong contrast. In nearly every instance the transitional line which bridges the gap between facial lines to be minimized and the desired line direction is effective.

The silhouettes of necklines and collars are composed of lines, and it is essential that the line direction of the forms and the shapes themselves be evaluated in relation to the face. Shapes which repeat and those which are too dissimilar give importance to facial contours. The overall silhouette and the details of the design such as the ends of collars must be taken into consideration. The square, circle, and triangle are not as interesting nor as flattering as shapes derived from an oval or alteration of stark, regular, geometric patterns. The interest of the neckline is attributable to the costume designer's creative ability in developing something above the ordinary. Necklines and collars need to be related to body contours, which are never harsh, straight lines or mechanical shapes. In this era of mass-produced clothing, aesthetic expression must be sought. All too frequently repeated are the round, close fitting jewel neckline, the regularity of Peter Pan collars, the straight rectangle of the convertible collar, or the deep, unadorned, sharp angle of necklines earmarked for the stout woman.

The apparent weight and the texture of fabrics are important in giving the correct effect and must relate to the texture of hair, skin, and eyes and to temperament. Harsh, lustrous, and stiff fabrics stress facial features; softer ones are flattering. The correct texture can reduce size or add softness to angles.

Scale and proportion of necklines and collars should be related to the face; when necessary, they should create a transition between it and the rest of the body.

Accessories such as the scarf, necklace, clip, and earrings may enhance or detract from the artistry of framing the face. The shape of perfectly round, large beads in a single strand may underline both the angularity or the roundness of faces. Graduated sizes are not quite as emphatic and produce a leading line. Reduction of the size of round beads and the combination of several strands into a rope produces a softer mass. Beads and other necklaces composed of more irregular, individual forms are flattering, as are earrings and pins in free forms generated by body contours. Scarves and necklaces worn close to the base of the neck shorten facial length and set up a horizontal line movement; accessories which are worn longer produce a transitional or vertical line, dependent upon their exact length. Button earrings and pins worn symmetrically placed on either side of the neck set up horizontal movement; long earrings foster vertical movement.

Covering the skin about the base of the neck will shorten lines (Figure 11); exposing it produces a longer line. A neckline with a dominant horizontal line encourages the eye to travel horizontally; a dominant vertical line in a neck opening adds length.

An appropriate hair style and skillful application of cosmetics, together with the correct neckline, can do much to create the illusion of a more ideal facial contour. In evaluating neckline details consider them in relation to neck, shoulder width, and total body impression (Figure 11 Chapter Three).

A small face combined with a small, dainty body is a matter of proportion; choose face-framing details in scale with both (Figure 12). When the face is small in relation to shoulder width and the rest of the body, it is necessary to create the illusion of a larger facial area. The line direction chosen

CREATING ILLUSIONS 237

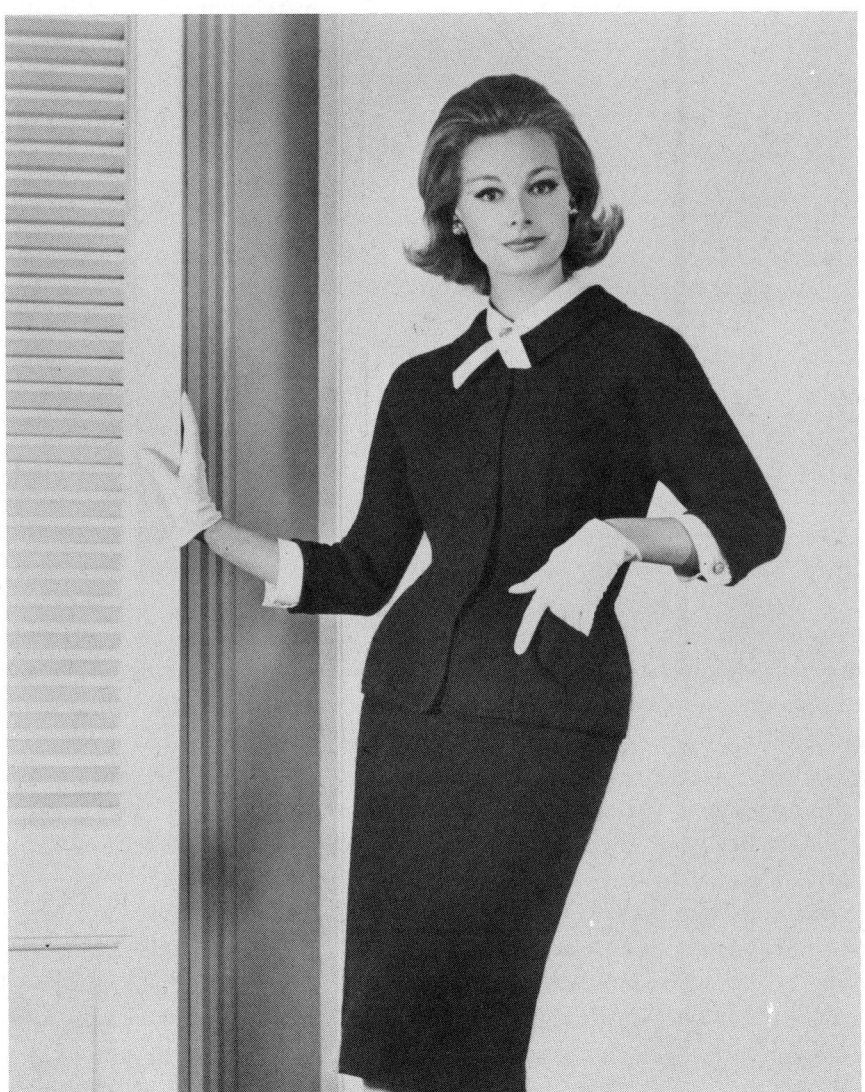

Figure 12. Hand-loomed navy wool suit by Ben Reig. Courtesy New York Couture Group, Inc. The scale of the neckline detail is suitable for a person with a small face.

will be dependent upon the facial outline of the individual, but lines should not accentuate the breadth of shoulders. The shapes chosen should be medium to medium small, but not small or large in relation to the individual. Necklines with some depth expose a larger area of skin, which increases apparent size; the plunging décolletage is a poor choice, because the contrast is excessive. The width of the neckline and the collar should be of medium scale. The texture and treatment of the neckline or collar and the accessories such as jewelry and scarves need to be transitional in character.

A large face combined with a large body also requires selecting neckline details of proper proportion (Figure 13). In creating the illusion of a harmonious relationship between a large face and a seemingly smaller body, shapes and spaces of moderately large scale give the required transitional size. The head needs to be kept in proportion to the shoulder width; do not overshorten the shoulder line. Fabrics should not seem to add thickness and bulk to the face, nor should they be so delicate as to be out of character. Necklines and accessories must not fit closely or seem tight; thus the jewel neckline and the choker necklace are eliminated. Details may be comparatively large and more dramatic; repetition of fine details such as multiple dainty pleats and pintucks accent largeness.

For the round face it is necessary to create the illusion of less width and greater length, and thus minimize its full circle contour. The dominant movement should be a transitional vertical, which is a line suggesting a restrained curve but directing the eye vertically. Necklines and collars fitting closely at the back and the sides of the neck are correct. Details lead the eye vertically, but the neckline does not terminate in nor the collar contain shapes based upon round, square, or acutely angular forms. When necklaces or scarves are worn, they should be fashioned about the neck to add some length. Bateau and jewel necklines as well as scarves knotted closely about the neck are unattractive. Choker length beads, especially of baroque shapes in a single strand, are incorrect, as are earrings and symmetrically placed pairs of pins. Instead study carefully the placement of a single clip in relation to the face and the neckline design. If the round face is accompanied by a large bust, necklaces should not terminate at the fullest part; nor should a clip be added to a deep neckline at this point. It is important that textures not intensify roundness, as would fluffy furs.

The square face, like the round, needs to be made longer and less wide. There is the additional problem of reducing the angularity in the square face. Essentially vertical line movement with a transitional element is needed. The

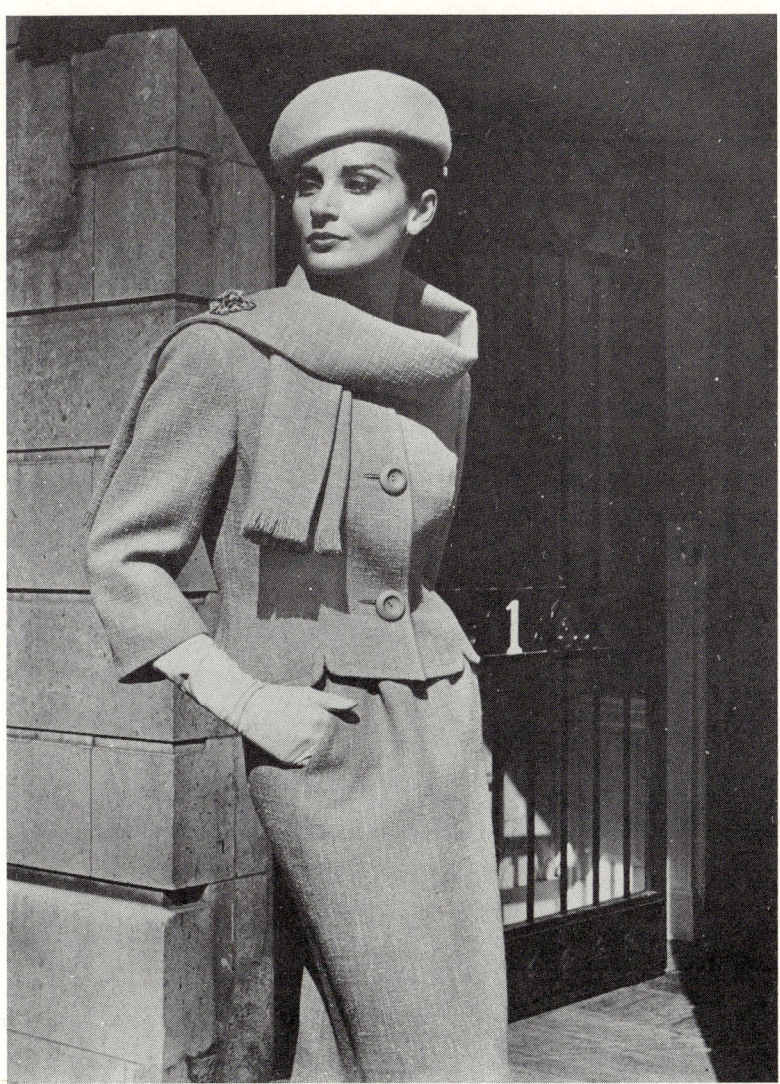

Figure 13. Flat-textured wool suit by George Carmel, hat by Lilly Dache. Courtesy New York Couture Group, Inc. The stole is in harmony with her facial features, body build, and personality.

shapes of details likewise should be transitional without sharp angles or full roundness. The jewel and bateau necklines, chokers, and earrings are to be avoided.

The triangular face requires that the illusion of less width in the lower part of the face and greater breadth of forehead be created. The angularity of the jaw line needs softening. Correctly applied cosmetics, a hair style that clears the forehead or covers it to give the impression of greater width, and hair brushed forward over the lower cheeks are effective when combined with the proper neckline details. Design lines that produce a vertical movement are the proper choice. Round or square shapes and very sharp angles, close fitting necklines and accessories, and earrings are to be avoided.

The oblong face tends to form a rectangular pattern and is usually comparatively thin and angular. Necklines that have a dominant horizontal movement, but never straight and harsh, should be selected. Shapes based on restrained curves rather than the circle or square are good. Collars and necklines should fit the base of the neck flatteringly, but should not be the shape of an unadorned circle or square. If the oblong face is accompanied by a long, thin neck (Figure 11), it may be desirable to cover part of the neck with a collar of high, soft roll, or the softness of a sheer scarf knotted at the base. Stiff fabrics may take on lines which are too harsh. Repetition of the basic length line of the face in long ropes of beads is unattractive; but the shorter lengths, including the choker, and earrings that do not dangle can create the illusion of a more oval face.

The inverted triangle or the heart-shaped face frequently has a sharp, thin chin and a broad forehead. The problem is that of making the chin appear wider and reducing the sharpness of the angle when it is present. Necklines and collars with horizontal line movement are complimentary, as are those based on short oval forms; deep plunging necklines terminating in a sharp angle or long oval are not. Necklaces of matinée length are attractive, as are earrings if the hair is brushed back from the lower part of the face. Restrained curves in the design of collars and necklines are becoming.

The diamond-shaped face is most challenging, as the width of the cheekbone area is excessive and the forehead and chin are both narrow. Much can be achieved through skillful use of make-up and the correct hair style to increase forehead and chin width, and to minimize the cheek area. Details for softening the angularity of jaws given in previous discussions may be used. Frequently this face is quite short and needs devices to create the illusion of greater length together with greater breadth in the forehead.

Creating Illusions with Cosmetics

Cosmetics correctly applied can create the illusion of more perfect facial contours. It is essential to study the shape of the face and the individual features before cosmetics can be applied effectively. This should be done in a good north light before a large mirror. The ideally shaped face is an ovoid (Figure 11 Chapter Three). To review, the face has four planes to be considered: the frontal plane, the forehead, and the two areas on either side of the face. The value and intensity of cosmetics is the determining factor in giving prominence to one plane over another. Dark values reduce apparent size by serving as a shadow; light values accentuate fullness, attract attention, or make highlights.

Cosmetics used to create illusion are chosen, as are all others, to enhance personal coloring. The contrasting value used to produce the semblance of change should be selected in the same color path as the basic make-up, but one or two tones darker. The areas to which they are applied, however, must never be defined by sharp lines indicating the termination of a color. Make-up from each area must be skillfully and gradually blended into the next without the slightest hint of a line of demarcation.

If the face is too wide, the centering of attention on the frontal plane will make the side planes less important; if the face is too narrow, the centering of attention out as far as possible on the side planes will create the illusion of greater width. Thus the face with a very broad forehead and narrow chin line, the inverted triangle, may have the wide forehead narrowed and the jaws made to seem wider by using foundation cream in the correct light tone for the skin on the lower part of the face and using a darker tone for the temple area of the forehead. For heavy jaws, as found in the round, square, or triangular face, use a light foundation on the frontal planes of the face and a darker value over the jaw line to make the heavy jaw recede and highlight the frontal planes. This principle can be used to camouflage a prominent forehead, receding chin, short or long neck, hollow cheeks, an oversized nose, or eyes too closely spaced. Another technique of illusion is that of using slightly more make-up on especially attractive features to call attention to them.

The use of dark and light rouges works similarly. A dark rouge on the cheek plane of a square or round face creates a shadow and causes width to be less prominent; conversely, a light or bright rouge magnifies the width. It must be remembered that light rouges belong to light, fair skins and hair, and dark shades to dark-toned complexions. A rouge too dark on a fair skin tends to stand out as a spot. Bright rouges belong to people of strong value contrast and more vivid personalities. Apply rouge so lightly that it is not obvious and blend the outer edges to nothing. Illusion may be created by the application of rouge:

> The oval face needs rouge applied in the center of the cheek and carried up to the temples in a circular, triangular area. The triangle is marked by a point in line with the center of the eye on the cheekbone, straight down to a point in line with the ear, and up to a point in line with the outer corner of the eye. Never apply rouge closer to the nose than the line indicated.
>
> The long, narrow face needs lighter rouge blended in a circular area in the center of the cheek and light foundation to highlight the entire face.
>
> The triangular face needs to have dark rouge applied on the outer half of the cheek and shaded up to the temple and down very faintly to the jaw line. A lighter foundation should be used on the forehead.
>
> The fullness of the square face accompanied by a straight hairline is broken up by applying darker rouge in a circle starting at the center of the eye and down over the jaw line.
>
> The round face should not have rouge applied in a circular area; dark rouge should be applied on the outer portion of the cheeks and carried up faintly to the temples.
>
> An inverted triangular face with a narrow jaw can be made to seem wider by light rouge applied at the highest point of the cheek.
>
> The diamond-shaped face should have light foundation on the lower part of the face and darker rouge in a circular area on the highest point of the broad cheek bones to create shadows. It should not be carried to the narrow temples or lower part of the cheeks.
>
> A full jaw will be apparently reduced when the mouth is made up to its fullest extremity of width.

Attempting to radically change the shape of the mouth through use of lipstick will be unsuccessful; observe its natural outline. Only slight and almost imperceptible alteration should be attempted, and then with utmost skill. If you lack the skill or get carried away, stop. For the mouth which is too short, extend the lipstick to the corners of the lips or ever so slightly beyond. For lips which are thin, color should be applied to the very limits of the lip line. To make lips appear less full, apply lipstick just inside the natural line, and perhaps extend it slightly at the corners to give the appearance of more ideal proportions. A long mouth may be shortened by not carrying lipstick to the extremities of the corners. If lipstick is extended beyond or applied just short of the lip line, be certain that your individual lip contour does not make it obvious.

Eyebrows likewise should not be altered appreciably in contour. They usually need to be plucked to give a neat line, and this must not be overlooked for a well-groomed appearance. Ideal brows begin in line with the inner corner of the eye. If the brows tend to grow across the bridge of the nose, remove them to the point of the ideal. Only straggling hairs should be removed from the top of the brow. Leave the width as it grows at the inner corner of the eye, and shape as necessary the outer two-thirds of the brow. Do not overthin the brows in this area; the width needs to relate to the width near the inner corner. Do not attempt to fashion a straight line or a decided arch. Brows which slant downward add age to a face. Brows, bone structure, and eye shape were well-planned by nature to be harmonious without undue intervention.

Choosing Cosmetics

Cosmetics today have come to be essential to young women. They help to point up the best we have, to create an idealized version of oneself, to put a little drama into life. A streak of bright lipstick or the faintest tinge of eye shadow may stiffen morale and often make the simplest white dress become something special. Some people who lack value contrast in brows and lashes are transformed with eyebrow make-up and mascara. Others need the glow that rouge can give the skin or eye shadow to accent fine eyes or put more color into dull-looking ones. From the professional standpoint, consider the hue, value, and intensity of rouges and lipstick, foundation and face powder, eye shadow and mascara. Every young woman probably does not need all these beauty aids every day, but everyone will use some of them at some time. Fashions change in the use of any one cosmetic, but good taste discourages the following of unnatural-appearing fads.

Make-up should always be used with the utmost discretion; it should never be obvious. The purpose of heightening illusion is defeated the moment the use of cosmetics becomes apparent. They should be applied with a light hand, except for lipstick, and utmost skill and perfection. It is better to err on the side of not using enough. There are those who believe that if make-up harmonizes with an otherwise unbecoming color, the color may be worn.

However, a basic principle is that cosmetics should harmonize with the natural coloring, and there are very narrow limits within which make-up color may stray from one's own. This also applies to changing hair coloring. Nature has given each a harmony of skin, eye, and hair coloring; when one part of it is changed appreciably, not merely enhanced, it becomes something unrelated to the natural unity.

The foundation or powder base may be considered to form the substructure for whatever make-up one needs to apply. Foundation may be colorless or tinted. The young may elect not to wear it, or probably will choose one that is colorless. The right foundation color can do almost miraculous things to the appearance of washed-out-looking skin, as well as to minor blemishes, lines, ill-proportioned features, and irregular contours. Apply foundation in a very light film and blend it into the hairline; carry it under the chin and down and back on the neck. It should be chosen to match the skin tones or in a shade darker and warmer; it may range from cream to rose, peach-bloom, terra cotta, or suntan, depending on one's skin coloring or the effect one wishes to achieve. A rosier tint may add a look of health to pale features; a darker, richer foundation may give a more subtle, vibrant glow of warmth. Some forms of foundation eliminate the need for face powder.

Lipstick and rouge should harmonize; and nail polish, if used, should be in the same color path. Rouges and lipsticks may be chosen from three different paths or color ranges.

> Those with an underlying blue cast, such as rose, orchid, and raspberry tones.
>
> Those with an underlying orange cast, such as peach, geranium, and poppy shades.
>
> Those of definite, clear red in lighter or darker tones.

It is obvious that rouges and lipsticks having a blue cast are best for those with blue and red-purple overtones. A slight shift of hue to the more definitely red or orange-red may add to the look of health and vitality which the red-violet rouges do not help to give. On the other hand, skin pigmentation which has yellow-orange or red-orange overtones needs the accent of the rouges of the red-orange or red range. The degree of vividness will depend on the brightness of the coloring. An ivory or olive skin usually does not require rouge on the cheeks but needs red-purple lipstick, sometimes in medium value, sometimes darker, depending on whether the general impression of the individual skin coloring is light or dark.

Rouge should be used with care; use only enough to seem natural. Too much or wrongly placed rouge may give a hard or old appearance. Lipstick is applied preferably with a brush. Carefully outline the natural contours of the lips and then fill in the rest of the area. Let it dry for a few minutes before blotting and it will stay in place longer. For a velvety appearance the lips may be powdered; for a gloss the lipstick is applied again very lightly.

Powder should be transparent, but mask the shine. Face powder of the same color and a little lighter value, never darker, than the powder foundation will usually give a more transparent effect to the skin. Press powder generously on the face with a clean cotton ball or pad, and cover the entire area to which foundation was applied. Permit it to remain for awhile, and then with a soft baby brush, remove the excess paying special attention to the hairline.

Eye shadow is optional and may be reserved for evening wear. It is used to deepen the eye socket, increase the size of the eyes, and emphasize the eye coloring. It should not be worn by those with deep-set eyes. Eye shadow must always be less intense than the eye coloring or it will defeat its purpose. One may want to repeat the color of the iris or complement it. Blue shadow is nice with blue eyes, and brown shadow with brown eyes helps to emphasize their color. But violet might be lovely with brown eyes, especially for a fair-skinned, light-haired brunette. A blue-violet shadow would do lovely things to blue-gray eyes. Green shadow will change hazel eyes to green; silvered blue for gray- or white-haired ladies will make them more beautiful. Apply eye shadow sparingly to the upper lid beginning close to the lashes. Blend it upward for about one-half the distance of the lid; do not carry it too close to the nose, as it will make the eyes appear closer together. Too prominent or puffy lids may be made to recede by the judicious use of eye shadow.

Mascara is required by those with little value contrast in their personal coloring. Those with very dark lashes and brows may not find it necessary for daytime or for evening. Mascara is used to accent lashes and brows, or eyebrow pencil may be used to define the clean line of eyebrows. Mascara may be black or brown to match the lashes and brows. It is applied from the lid to the tip of the lashes. Learn to use it so that each lash is separate. Using a small stiff brush after the application will separate lashes and give a more natural look.

Brush the eyebrows toward the nose to remove all powder, then smooth them outward and upward. They may be touched lightly with mascara or an eyebrow pencil. With a well-sharpened pencil build the eyebrows out with fine hairlike strokes. Never draw in a solid line. Brown is flattering to most people; a lighter brown may be better for very light coloring. Only those of very dark personal color wear black well. A person with black brows may touch them with the smallest amount of oil rather than color. Eye liner is in poor taste except for very special evening occasions.

All these factors enter into the selection of cosmetics. It is advisable to purchase cosmetics in shops where there are demonstrators to assist, and it is possible to try out different tones until the right one is found. Selecting by appearance only may be most disappointing and expensive.

One should test the effect of rouge, lipstick, and eye shadow through half-closed eyes to decide whether it blends or stands out sharply as a spot.

An attempt has been made in this chapter to reveal some of the devices for improving the face and figure through the technique of creating the illusion of beauty. Study carefully the appearance of garments and combinations of garments on each individual; line, space, and proportion and scale must be exactly right. Herein lies the artistry in being able to see and judge subtle differences which are so important in creating illusion.

You will enjoy reading these books to further assist you in the creation of the illusion of a more perfect figure and face.

Marion S. Hillhouse, *Dress Selection and Design,* The Macmillan Company, New York, 1963.

John Robert Powers, *How to Have Model Beauty, Poise and Personality,* Prentice-Hall, Inc., Englewood Cliffs, N. J., 1960.

Exercises

1. Sketch, trace, or clip interesting designs for the backs of dresses and suits to create illusions (a) of slenderness, (b) of added width.
2. Make a collection of sketches, tracings, or clippings to illustrate unusual necklines and collars which are right for the short, thick neck; the long, slender one.
3. Make a similar collection of sleeves for short, heavy arms; long, thin ones.
4. Select several suitable fabric combinations in the right values for reducing and expanding figures.

Thirteen

Hats and Hairdressing

A DISCUSSION of personal appearance would not be complete without a reference to hats and hairdressing. The face has been called the "reflection of the soul" and forms the center of interest of the personality. Most of us notice the face first when we meet someone for the first time; and in fact, it is discourteous to fasten the eyes on any part of the person other than the face. Hats and hairdress form a frame for the face; if hats are to be becoming and are to give the wearer style, the coiffures which accompany them must be right for the hats as well as becoming to the wearer.

Hats and hairdress probably reflect fashion changes more rapidly than do any other parts of the costume, as can be seen in looking over old fashion magazines or photograph albums. Women sometimes make the mistake of clinging to the hairdress which they used at a period of their girlhood when they were the most beautiful. In the eyes of the younger generation this habit serves to "date" the person rather than to preserve her youth. Current fashions in hats and hairdressing are too fleeting to be treated in detail in this book, but certain principles may serve as a helpful guide.

THE COIFFURE

In any age, a perfect oval face with regular features is the ideal of feminine beauty; but this does not mean that faces that do not conform to this mold may not be both beautiful and interesting. It does mean, however, that any great deviation from the oval shape, such as a very square jaw, should be camouflaged if a woman is made to look her most attractive. The ideal silhouette of the head, including the coiffure, is also an oval shape; and whenever the hairstyle becomes exaggerated and ceases to follow these natural lines, it becomes a passing fad which looks odd as soon as it is out of fashion.

In striving for the illusion of a perfectly proportioned ovoid head, there are certain principles that apply. By arranging the hair with fullness where needed, by bringing it over parts of the face to camouflage a too full line, or by brushing it away from the face to highlight certain features, we can often create a very pleasing effect. The kind of balance that is right, no matter what the changes in fashion prove to be, can be attained by following certain guides.

> The distance from forehead to nape should approximate the distance from chin to crown. If one distance is noticeably shorter than the other, there is a lack of balance and consequently an unpleasing contour. Thus the person with a heavy jaw or a prominent chin will never wear a style that is entirely flat at the nape of the neck, such as a mannish cut or a part down the center back with the hair drawn tightly away from the part. She will bring the hair low on the neck and forward toward the jaw line for balance.
>
> The distance from ear to chin and from ear to nape should also balance. The girl with a small, receding chin will avoid a full, long hair style brought forward over her cheeks at the jaw line. A prominent nose may be made less conspicuous when the hair has soft fullness over the forehead rather than being drawn severely back.
>
> If the neck is short and plump and the head round, the hairline should be tapered to a point at the neckline to make the neck seem longer; the hair may be parted on the side and arranged diagonally. A center part or any circular movement should be avoided.
>
> If the head is flat at the crown, this area needs to be covered or filled out with a coiffure so designed as to build out the flat part with fullness and to dress the hair at the forehead and nape rather close to the head.
>
> If the head bulges at the crown, the hair should be dressed flat over the crown and built out wider and higher below and above the bulge. If the head is narrow and the neck long and thin, the hair should be brought away from the temples and cheeks to highlight the face as much as pos-

sible and dressed with a large, soft wave movement partially covering the ears and the back of the neck. Earrings of a soft luster may help to add width to the face.

For the person having a thick, muscular neck and broad, athletic shoulders, the square line in back needs to be broken by the use of a soft curved or diagonal line. A mannish clip exaggerates the squareness of the shoulders.

The shape of the face itself can often be made to seem in more perfect proportion by the way the hair is dressed (Figure 11 Chapter Three). If one is fortunate enough to have an oval face with a normal hairline, she may use simple, classic arrangements (Figures 1, 12, and 13); or she may have the pleasure of experimenting with rather exotic styles. In any case, each girl should learn the lines which are most becoming, in order to have some originality in dressing her own hair or to be able to tell a hairdresser how to achieve the effect she wants. Some suggestions for hair styles for different facial shapes follow.

> A face with rather heavy, large features should have the hair dressed loosely with swirling waved lines, not small, tight curls.
> A round face may be helped by having the hair conceal part of the hairline at the forehead, temples, and ears. Building some height on top is often becoming.
> A square face needs hair dressed softly near the jaw line to minimize the angle of the jaw with some fullness and softness at the forehead and temples to balance the wide jaw.
> A long, narrow face can be foreshortened by wearing the hair flat on top and drawn back from the temples and ears to provide a highlight at the temple line, and with some fullness and softness at the sides.
> The triangular face with a narrow forehead needs to have the upper part of the face highlighted by bringing the hair back from the temples, thus giving more width at that area. To narrow the line at this point the hair should be dressed softly at the jaw line but not fluffed.
> With the diamond shaped face, the hair should be dressed forward at the cheekbones and brushed back above and below the ears.

Many other devices for creating illusions of perfect contour can be worked out by one who has grasped the principle of smart and becoming hairdress. The photographs on the following pages (Figures 1 to 13) will illustrate

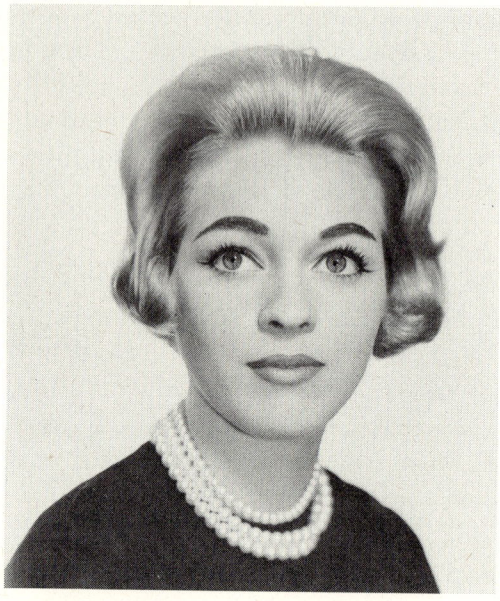

Figure 1. A woman with an oval face and regular features may use a simple coiffure which is entirely bisymmetrical, or she may experiment with more exotic styles. She will do well to keep a natural look, avoiding tight curls or a fussy effect.

Figures 1–11 courtesy of Mr. Ben Myers, Lincoln, Nebraska.

some of the points mentioned. Since the faces are those of models, they may not show decided defects in proportion; but the hair style will be suitable for a person of the facial type for which it was suggested.

THE HAT—COMPLEMENT TO THE COSTUME

The hat is more than a protection. It is a frame for the face, a trim for the dress, the single most important accessory to a smart appearance, the culminating note by which drama is given to the *tout ensemble*. A hat may need to be gay and a bit frivolous, young and casual, or dignified and sophisticated.

A hat should be an adornment. It should give its wearer a lift. Unless it actually does something for her appearance, it should not be purchased. It should be chosen with the same care used in selecting a dress; and perhaps with more care, as a hat is often worn with several different costumes.

HATS AND HAIRDRESSING

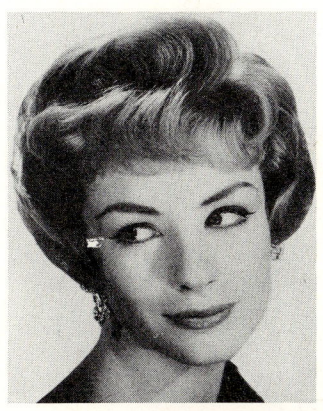 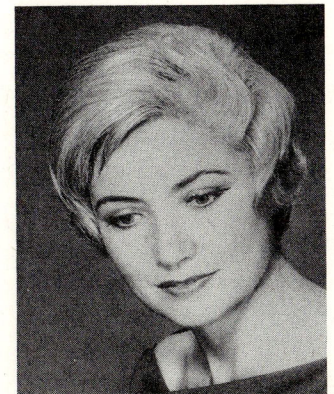

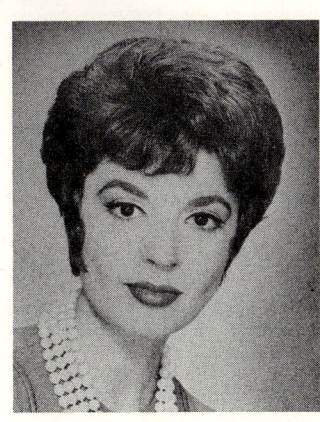 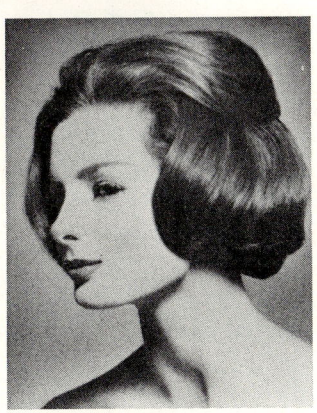

Figure 2 (upper left). An oblong face may be made to seem more nearly oval by dressing the hair so that it is fairly flat on top, but waved softly at the sides to increase the general effect of width. The forehead is partially concealed, and the side part and asymmetric shape soften the facial contours.

Figure 3 (upper right). A round face is made to appear less broad by using a short side part and partially covering the temples and cheeks.

Figure 4 (lower left). A hairdress for a square face. Waves are brought forward onto the cheeks, partially concealing the highlight of the jawline. The hair is dressed rather full to increase the impression of width at the top.

Figure 5 (lower right). Another suggestion for a square face. In this case the face is rather short in proportion to its width. The forehead is highlighted at one side by brushing the hair away from it, thus lengthening the line from chin to forehead. The hair is swirled softly over the cheeks, narrowing the face by covering the highlight of the jaw.

252   *The Arts of Costume and Personal Appearance*

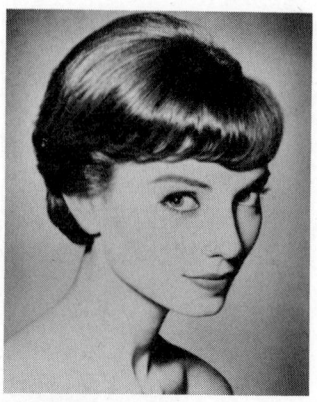 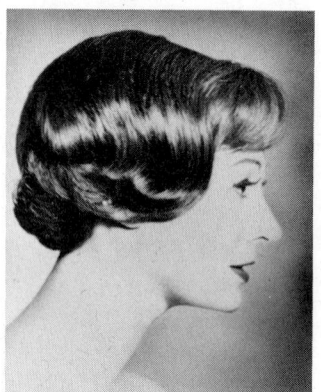

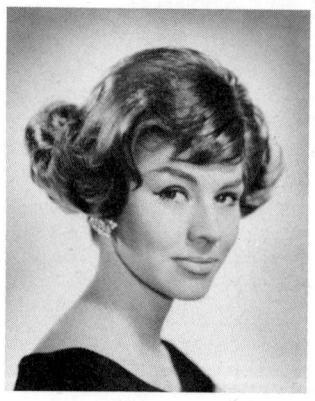 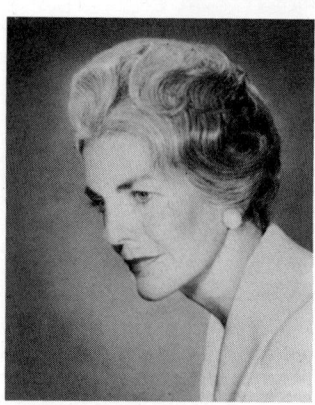

Figure 6 (upper left). An inverted triangle (wide forehead and narrow chin). The forehead is concealed by bangs, while the lower part of the face may be broadened by brushing the hair back to reveal the ears and highlight the lower part of the face.

Figure 7 (upper right). For a receding chin and forehead, the hairdress is kept fairly close to the head, in order not to overbalance the small chin. The forehead is partially concealed with bangs, and the line from chin to ear is made to seem longer by a proportionately shorter line from the nose to the hairline.

Figure 8 (lower left). When the hair grows too low on the forehead, it may be brushed across in a half bang so that one is not conscious of the actual position of the hairline.

Figure 9 (lower right). A prominent chin and long jawline are softened by dressing the hair so that it is full in the back and has height on top to give a more perfect balance.

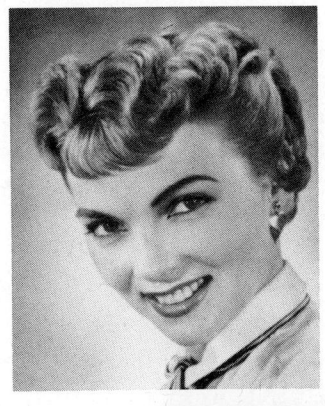
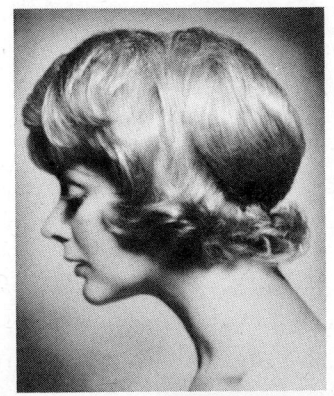
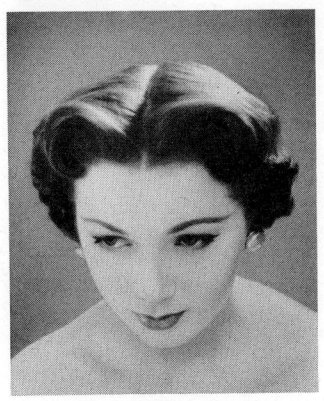
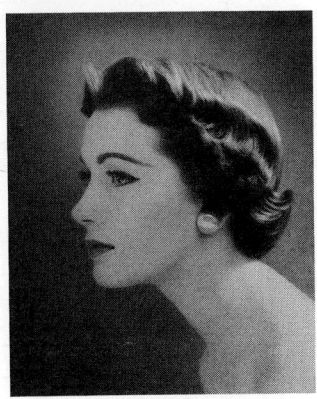

Figure 10 (upper left). A forehead narrow in proportion to the lower part of the face may be broadened by the use of bangs parallel to the brows, but brushed away to highlight the sides of the forehead.

Figure 11 (upper right). A rather full hairdress will help to conceal a high forehead and long neck, and will help to balance a prominent nose and chin. If too full or bouffant, however, it will be out of proportion for a face with small, delicate features.

Figures 12 and 13 (lower row). Two views of a hair style from Elizabeth Arden's studios, about 1953. Beauty of line outlasts many minor changes of fashion.

Christian Dior said, "Hats, especially on a dull winter day, make for gaiety. The color of a hat must harmonize with the rest of your clothes but not necessarily match. In fact, it's better if it doesn't match. But accessories like a scarf or gloves must go with the hat to 'team' it with the rest of your appearance. . . . Hats must look smart or be entirely inconspicuous. The woman who knows she is not pretty loses badly by wearing 'pretty' hats at indecisive angles. They must be sharply straight or at an acute angle. You don't want a very dull frame for your picture!" [1]

Many young women, and older ones too, do not know the types of hats that are becoming to them or right for their needs. They do not know their own shortcomings with respect to facial irregularities; or if they do, they are bewildered in attempting to find the right hat to overcome these defects. The situation is not improved by many millinery saleswomen who know the fashions but have little more knowledge than the customer as to the right lines to enhance features.

As women so often lack essential knowledge about the lines that are right for facial contours and for occasions, their headgear too often is a reflection of their state of mind at the time of purchase. They buy on impulse, or because of some happy association, or because they desire to be chic at all costs, and sometimes because they are carried away by a ravishing color or an adorable shape.

On the other hand there are those who have very definite notions of what they can wear and are not willing to adjust their pet ideas to the changing fashions. Consequently they cannot find in the shops what they think is right for them. Furthermore, many are unwilling to pay the price for a good hat. They may go hatless on many occasions, or perhaps they dress their hair so elaborately that a hat may not be worn. Thus they think of a hat as an expensive accessory, and do not realize the artistry that can be shown in a really well-designed hat.

Hats Reflect the Times

The inspiration for some of the newest of our hats is borrowed from costume museums. Lilly Daché, Sally Victor, Mr. John and other milliners are constantly scouring the art galleries of our great cities for ideas to adapt to the tempo of today's clothes. It may be the *biretta* of a young noble lady of the Renaissance (Figure 14), or the double-brimmed flat *hatte* of an

---

[1] Christian Dior, "What Fashion Tells You," *Woman's Home Companion,* January 1953, pp. 17, 18. (Copyright by George Newnes, Ltd.)

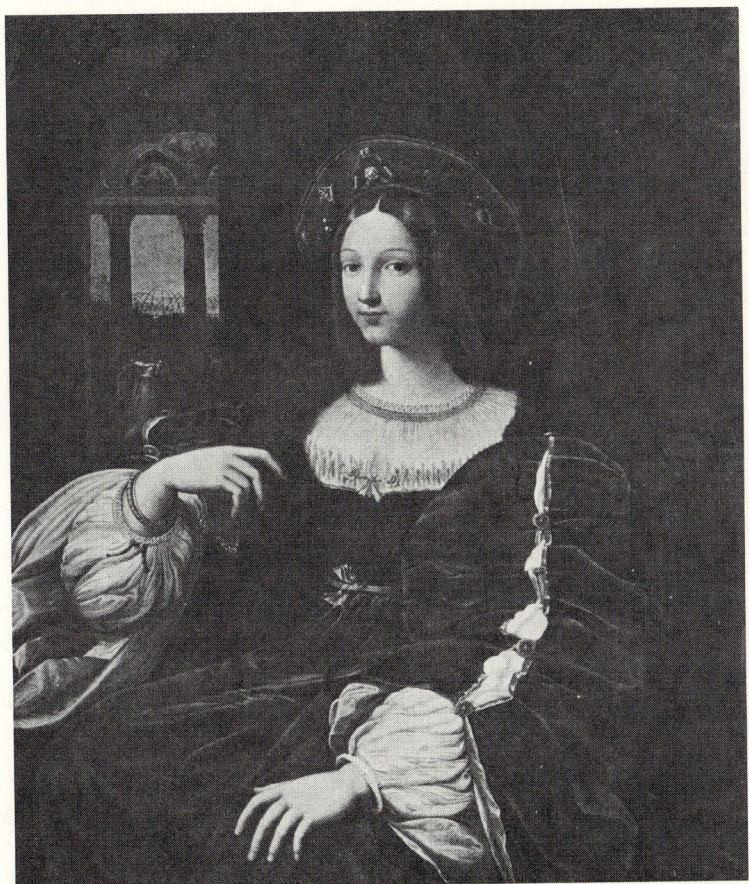

Figure 14. Johanna of Aragon (*sixteenth century*). By Raphael. *Italian Renaissance costume of rust-red velvet with gold satin facings and white gauze sleeves and yoke delicately embroidered. The hat is a wide biretta of velvet with jeweled ornaments, worn far back on the head.*

aristocratic Dutch lady (Figure 15). Or it may be the dashing brim of a cavalier, as in Frans Hals' *Portrait of a Young Man*, which suggested to Florence Reichman her large brown beret (Figure 16), or an adaptation of the snood and wimple of the Middle Ages (Figure 17).

Millinery in recent years has taken two divergent paths—the one to high-fashion hats, usually chosen to complement styles of a given season, or even to be worn with a particular costume; the other to all sorts of head coverings

256 *The Arts of Costume and Personal Appearance*

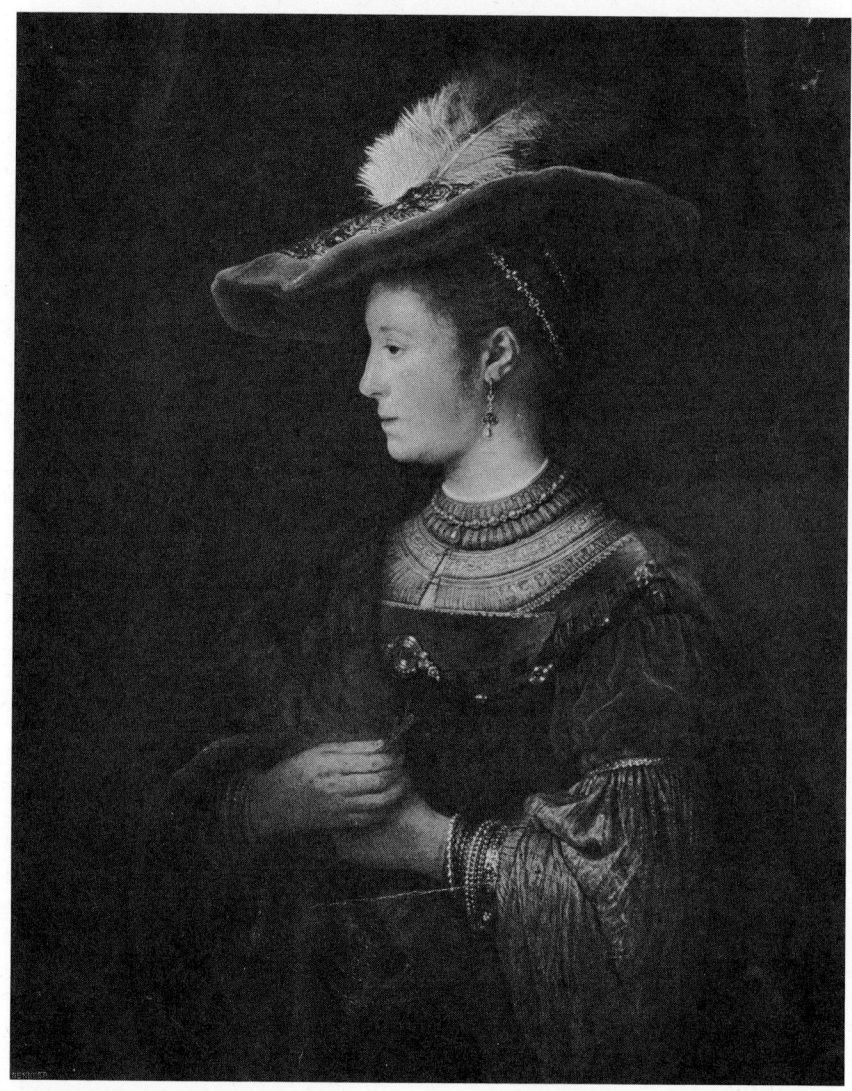

Figure 15. Rembrandt's *famous portrait of Saskia, seventeenth century Flanders. A wide, flat beret-like hat worn straight on the head, secured by two jeweled bandeaux.*

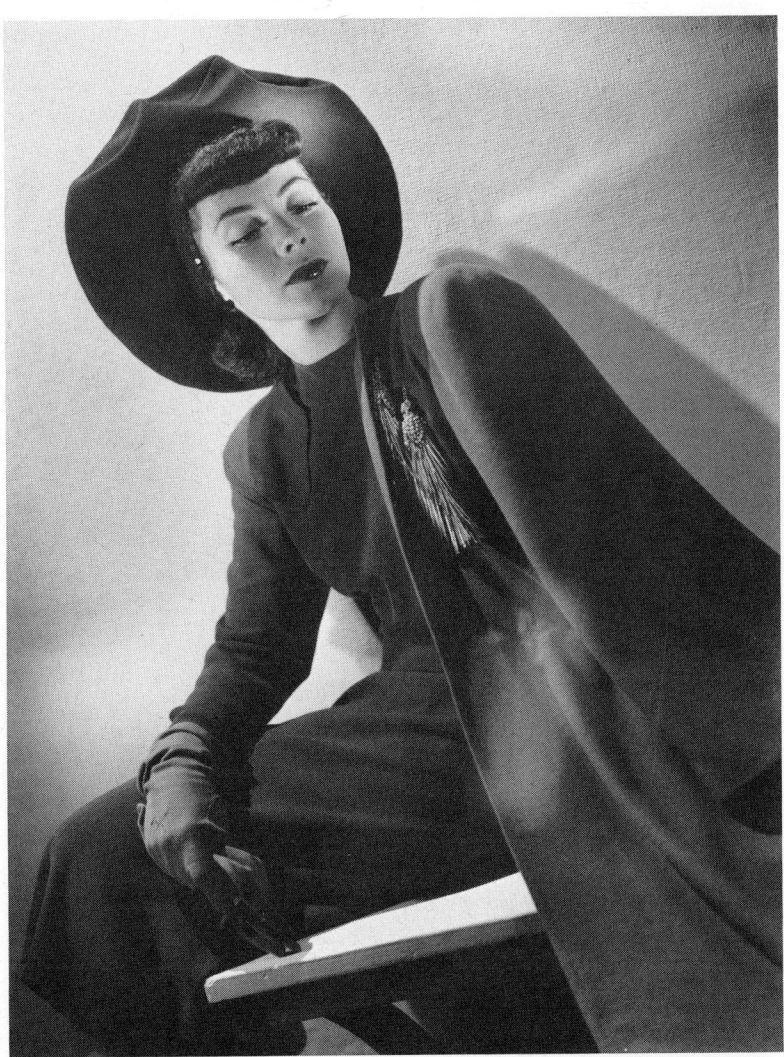

Figure 16. Beret designed by Florence Reichman for the Metropolitan Museum's Renaissance in Fashion, 1942. Based on Frans Hals' Portrait of a Young Man. Courtesy of Miss Reichman.

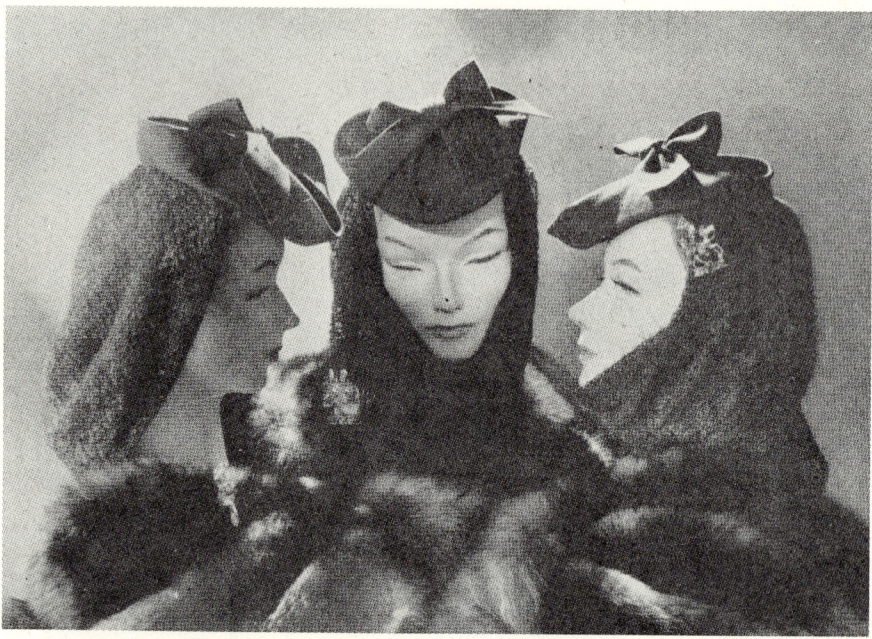

Figure 17. Tricorne with snood or wimple. A version of a fashion of the Middle Ages, adapted about 1943. Courtesy of Harper's Bazaar.

which we may not have thought of classifying as hats at all. They are the items, however, that have kept production in the millinery industry up to its customary level, in spite of the fact that women are seen hatless on occasions which in the past would have demanded a hat.

Women who know how to select becoming hats usually enjoy wearing them. They know how to put them on, and they get a thrill from wearing a hat that gives them a changed personality. They appreciate that the actual materials are not all that one pays for in a good hat; rather, it is the creative expression of some milliner that distinguishes a superb one from just another hat. The problem of finding a becoming hat requires both time and discrimination.

Women who know good hats are keen observers of millinery; they use fashion magazines and the shops to keep themselves informed. They know that there are few things that can be more ephemeral and transitory than a hat fashion. But they know, too, that millinery is the vanguard of our fashions and that millinery designers have a primary influence on silhouette. Hats are a kind of closeup reflection of the mood of the times. This fact is often very difficult to recognize, because we are too near to our own times to see them in perspective. Anatole France once said that if he were allowed to choose one book out of all those published a hundred years after his death, he would choose a woman's fashion magazine to tell how women were dressing; and that these fripperies would reveal more than all the philosophers, novelists, and preachers of the times.[2] Out of our contemporary "millinery madness," as out of the experiments of modern painters, may emerge a style which will be the typical expression of our age!

The woman, then, who wishes to keep herself in tune with the times will be open-minded toward new concepts, wise enough to compromise with preconceived ideas, and quick to see the hat which is not a passing fad but will stand her in good stead longer than one season.

When the mood of today's hats seems frivolous, it may be a kind of singing in the dark, the expression of an effort to put a bit of gaiety into a world burdened with problems.

[2] John Carl Flügel, "Psychology of Clothes," *Golden Book,* December 1931, p. 435.

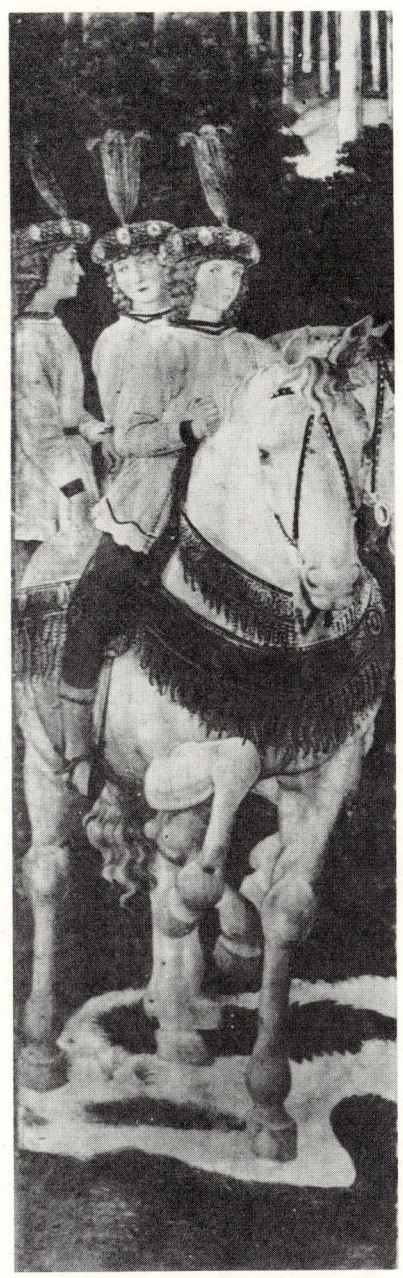

Figure 18. Detail from Journey of the Magi, *painted in 1459 by Benozzo Gozzoli. Ricardi Palace, Florence. Three young girls of the Medici family wearing the popular birettas of the time—with tall, exotic plumes.*

Hats to Convey Personal Expression

With hats, more than with any other kind of apparel, one has the opportunity to give expression to temperament. Good hats may be found to express the dramatic, the striking, and the sophisticated, or to embody daintiness, delicacy, and the elements of femininity. Extreme silhouettes, severely tailored textures that are heavy, stiff, or shiny, colors that are vivid or strongly contrasting are carried with assurance by the forceful or dramatic woman. By contrast, hats with dainty decorative detail, delicate colors, and fragile or soft textures are at once associated with the small, demure woman.

There is a manner of wearing hats which can impart style to the wearer or leave her spiritless. We remember the young aristocrats in fifteenth century portraits because of the way they wore their French *bonets* and *birettas* (Figure 18). Likewise, we remember the tilt of the wide brim which gave dash to Van Dyke's and Frans Hals' cavaliers and swashbucklers. The very feminine hat such as the one worn by Romney's *Mrs. Davenport* (Figure 19) suggests a summer afternoon at an English country house in the eighteenth century.

Good Design Important in Hats

All the principles of design are embodied in a good hat; we should judge it as a design as well as for its possible becomingness to certain facial contours, individual scale, and temperament. The silhouette of a hat should be clear cut and definite, with a certain significance which etches it on the memory. The fact that people tend to remember outlines of hats may explain why changes of fashion in hats are more rapid than in dresses. A good hat should have a relationship to the shape of the face and head based on the principle of variety with unity.

By the very nature of their essential function and structure hats are made up of curved lines and shapes. But some hats have a severity due to starkness of line, stiffness of texture, the severe mode of ornamentation, or the absence of trimming. Other hats are given the effect of softness and grace by a more undulating quality of line, flattering textures, or the daintiness of their trimming. Stiff-tailored cartwheels and sailors belong to forceful individuals, to young faces, or to those so blessed with natural beauty that the hat becomes a foil for their features. These same types of hats are becoming to more faces when softened with trimmings that relieve their severity, and particularly when they are worn tilted at exactly the right angle to conform, somewhat, to facial contours.

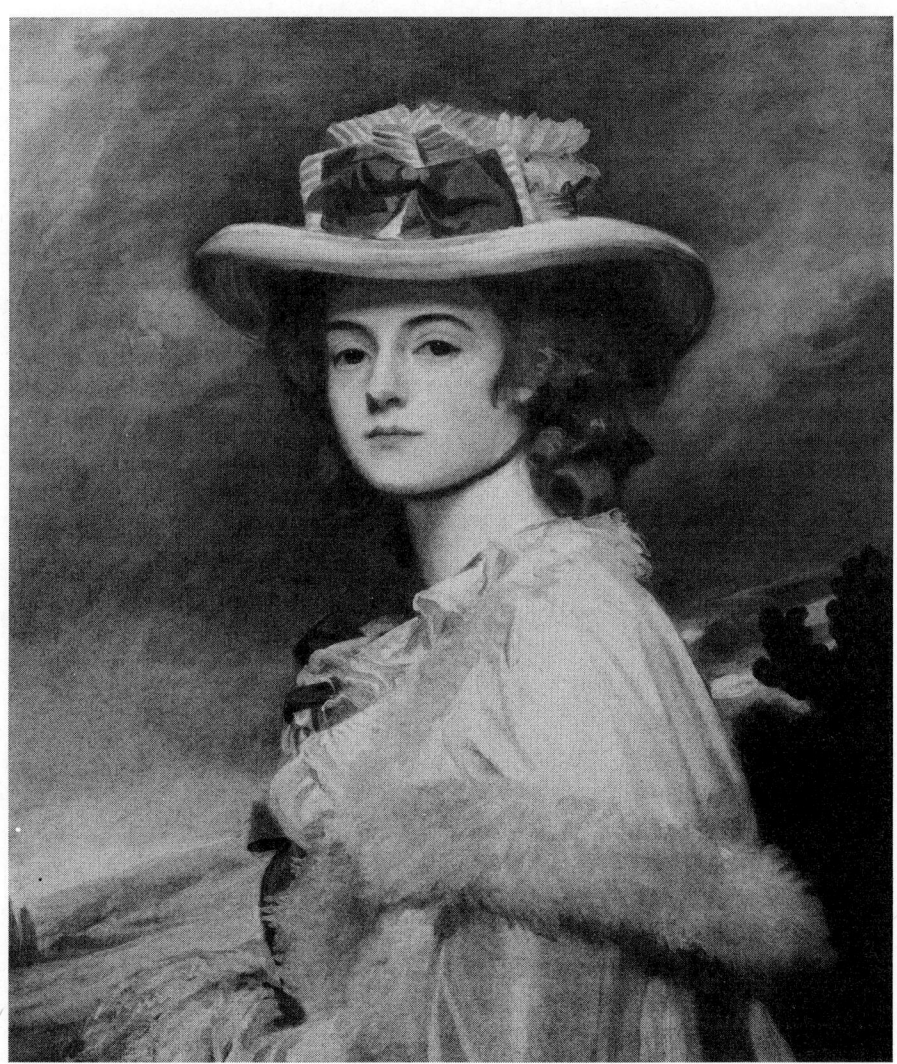

Figure 19. Mrs. Davenport *by* George Romney *(1734–1802)*. *Courtesy of* National Gallery of Art, *Washington, D. C. Mellon Collection.*

A severe hat (Figure 28) demands beautifully coiffed hair, perfection in make-up, perhaps earrings for softening, and an excellent carriage of the head and body. It is not a pretty hat but is the embodiment of style when worn with sleek street suits by smart, sophisticated women. We appreciate such hats also because they illustrate the elimination of all nonessentials. This same sophisticated quality is also expressed in a wide beret (Figure 16) which frames the face.

Another essential of good hats, as of costume, is that they embody but one idea in their structure and decoration; their trimming should be an integral part of the structure and enhance it.

The rhythm in good hats is fascinating to observe; it is seen in the dip of a brim, in the manner a scarf is draped, or the way the trimming repeats a line of the silhouette. Sometimes the movement is in wide, forceful curves (Figure 41); or it may be a circular movement, as when a curved feather swirls about and rises from a round crown, or the staccato movement produced by certain angles. Regularity of feature is usually necessary for a rather severe hat worn straight on the head (Figures 16, 30, and 36). An asymmetrical shape (Figures 20, 38, and 39) is usually more flattering. Fashion, also, dictates whether hats are to be worn straight, slightly tipped, or decidedly to one side; whether they are worn off the face or forward; and whether they cover the hair or perch on top of a coiffure.

Hats Are Suited to Occasions

Many women find it difficult to distinguish between hats that are right for sports and street and those intended for more formal wear. It is all a matter of the fitness of things, of holding to the laws of unity, not permitting oneself two ideas out of harmony. There are hats which by the nature of their texture or line or color belong to afternoon or evening; others seem versatile enough to be right for a variety of occasions, provided that the costume is not definitely of one type. For example, the beret (Figure 21) and the casual hat (Figure 29) suggest a youthful wearer and an informal occasion such as spectator sports or street. Another beret (Figure 20) could be of velvet and suitable for wear to luncheons or teas.

The bonnet (Figure 31) and the breton (Figure 25) suggest the ingénue and are flattering types for a youthful face, whereas the cloche (Figure 40) in several tones of satin suggests maturity, sophistication, and occasions such as luncheons or matinées in the city.

The derby (Figure 28), with its severe lines made more feminine by the use of a perky veil, can be very smart on a youthful looking woman of fine features who likes a clean-cut look in her tailored street and travel ensemble. It is not for the woman whose features are mannish or severe or for the one who depends on one street hat for all occasions.

Hatlets, bandeaus, and decors (Figures 32, 33, and 34) can be flattering and feminine, and have the added advantage of keeping the coiffure under control for late-day occasions.

The picture hat (Figure 41) can be one of the most flattering and feminine of modes; it may appear in straws, felts, velvets, stiffened nets, and laces. It suggests such glamorous summer occasions as afternoon weddings, garden parties, and formal teas. This hat is best worn by a woman who is at least average in height. In informal straw versions it may be a beach or gardening hat.

Types of Hats

Even though we think of hat fashions as the most evanescent of the styles in a clothing wardrobe, there are certain shapes which can be identified and named, whether they appear in portraits of a past day or, with subtle changes, in the current mode. Not all of these types will appear in any one season, but variations of certain styles can be recognized in current modes.

BERET. A round shape developed in infinite variations, ranging from a little flat circle covering the top of the head and perhaps pulled down slightly over the hair, to an enormous mushroom of felt or velvet or fur which shadows the face (Figures 20 and 21). Originated in the Basque province of southern France.

BICORNE. A hat with brim caught up on its two opposite sides; derived from Napoleon's great bicorne of hatter's plush.

BONNET. A scooped brim of straw or fabric encircling the face and attached to a form of hood or cap (Figure 6 Chapter Five); often enriched with flowers, ribbons, or feathers. They were the principal type of head covering worn in the first fifty years of the nineteenth century.

BRETON. Hat with a brim which rolls up all around; inspired by the hats of Breton sailors (Figures 24 and 25).

BUMPER. A small hat with a round brim which is rolled up and inward so that the edge of the brim is concealed (Figure 27).

CALOT. A tiny skull cap seamed or molded to the shape of the head; the Juliet cap is an example (Figure 26).

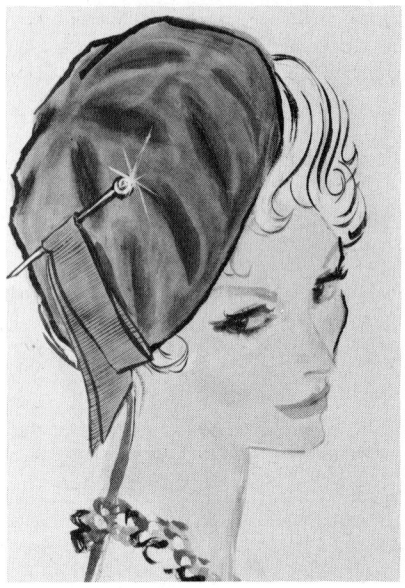

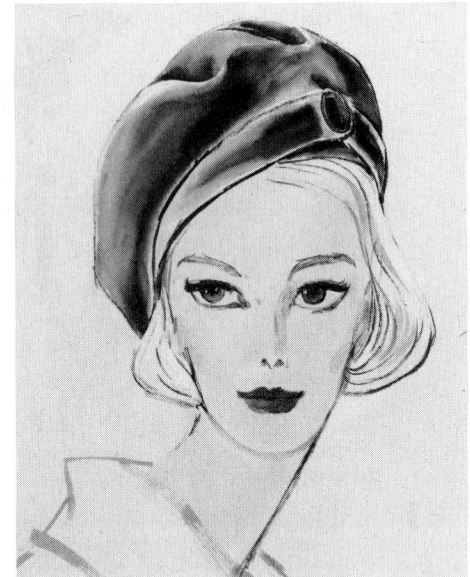

Figure 20. Soft beret of felt or fabric, capable of manipulation.

Figure 21. Beret of felt, velvet, or other fabric, with bandeau.

Figures 20–41 courtesy of Mr. James S. Heffley, Gold & Co., Lincoln, Nebraska.

CANOTIER. A narrow, straight-brimmed hat with low crown, resembling the sailor.

CARTWHEEL. A wide, flat, usually stiff-brimmed, low-crowned hat of straw or fabric.

CASUAL. An informal hat with soft brim and crown, suitable for sports wear or practical for travel (Figure 29).

COIF. A small, close-fitting cap; often combined with a veil or sheer draped fabric.

COOLIE. A hat sloping downward in an unbroken line from a peak at the crown, like a Chinese coolie's hat.

CLOCHE. A straw, felt, or fabric hat of deep crown and narrow mushroom brim, usually turned down, covering most of the hair (Figures 30 and 40).

DERBY. A very stiff felt hat with round crown and narrow, curved brim (Figure 28); worn by women with formal hunting costume; or occasionally appearing in current fashion in fabric hats.

HATS AND HAIRDRESSING 265

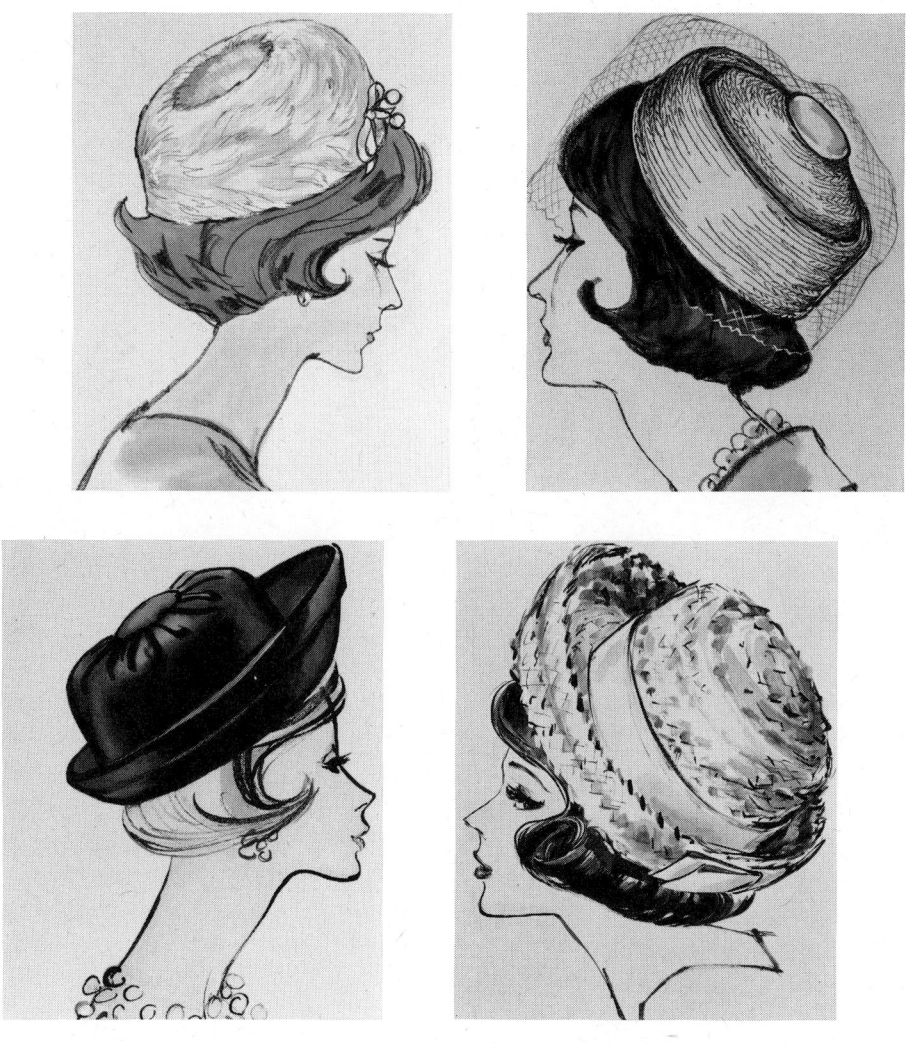

Figure 22 (upper left). Feather-trimmed pillbox, suited to dressy occasions.

Figure 23 (upper right). Low-walled pillbox of straw with stiffened veil.

Figure 24 (lower left). Breton covered with a fabric such as a matte satin.

Figure 25 (lower right). Breton of rough paillasson straw.

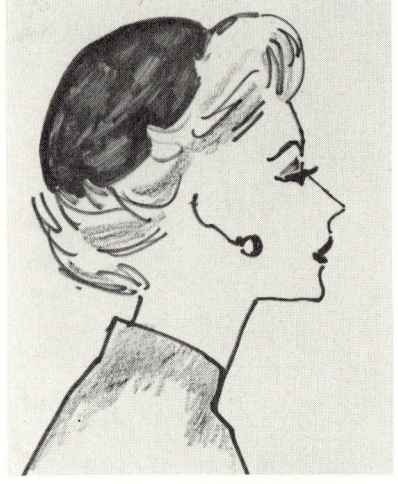
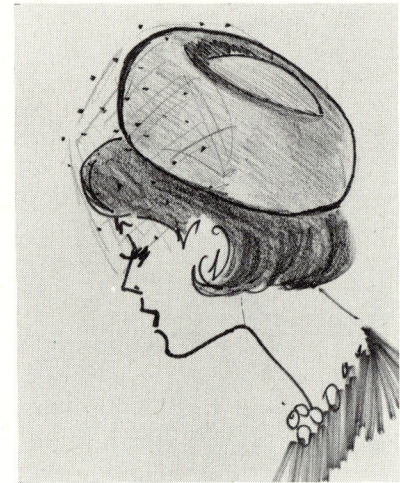
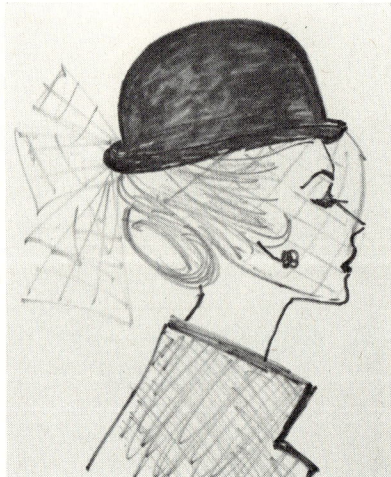

Figure 26 (upper left). Calot of feathers or fabric; sometimes called the Juliet cap.

Figure 27 (upper right). Bumper; a very round hat with rolled brim, usually of felt.

Figure 28 (lower). Derby; a very stiff and tailored hat, usually of felt, or fabric-covered.

HATS AND HAIRDRESSING 267

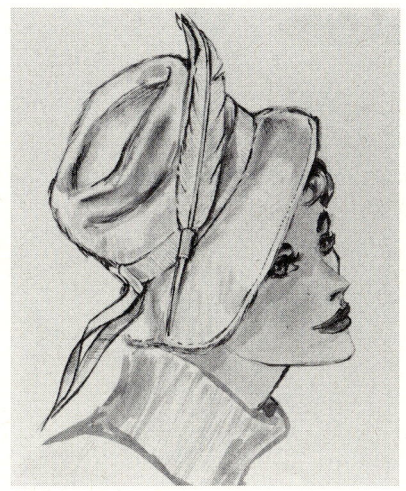
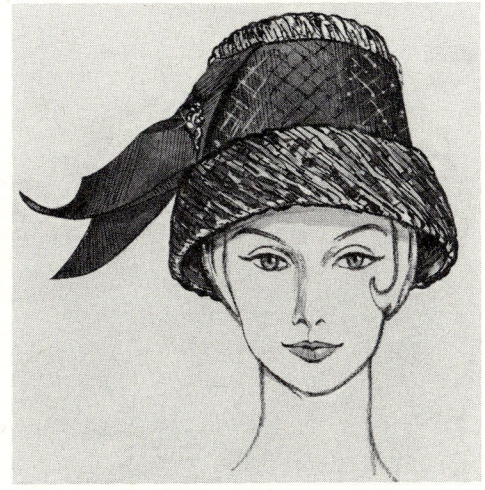
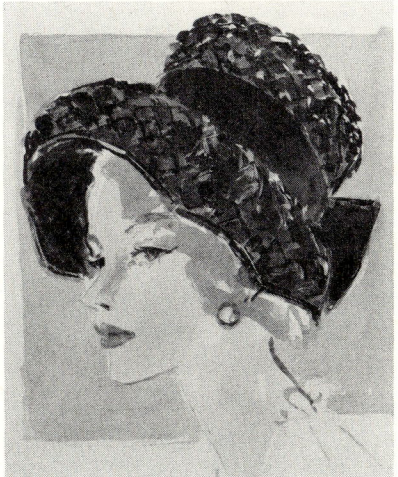

Figure 29 (upper left). Brimmed casual hat, allowing some manipulation of crown and brim, and worn at various angles.

Figure 30 (upper right). One form of cloche, in straw with wide grosgrain ribbon trim.

Figure 31 (lower). A flattering bonnet of rough straw. A bonnet, with a more flaring brim, reveals more of the face and hair of the wearer than does the cloche.

268 *The Arts of Costume and Personal Appearance*

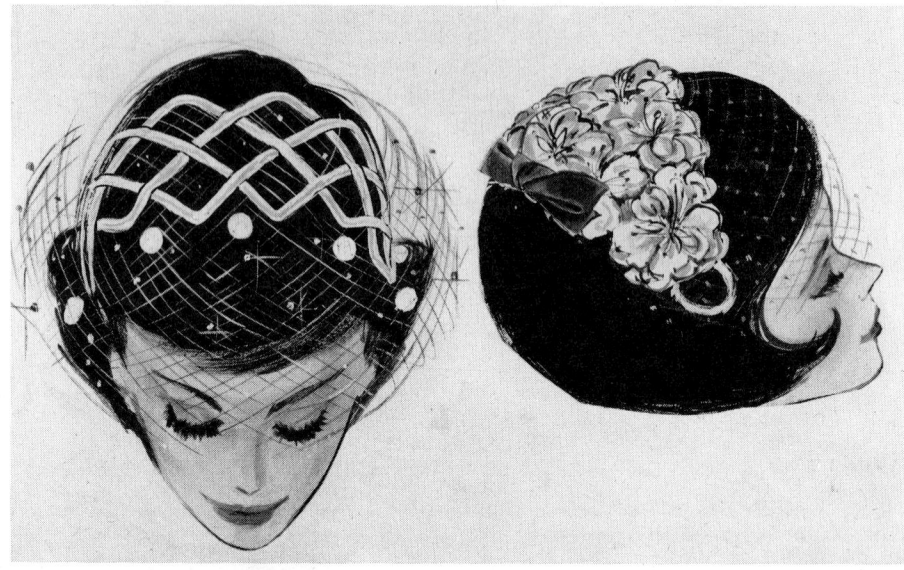

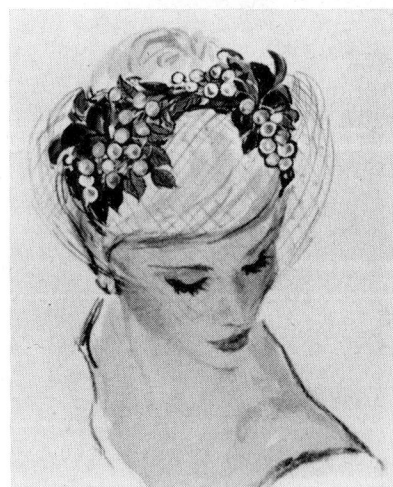

Figures 32, 33, and 34. Various forms of dainty and dressy little hatlets or decors. Wired forms with velvet, flower, or fruit trim, and usually with a stiffened veil.

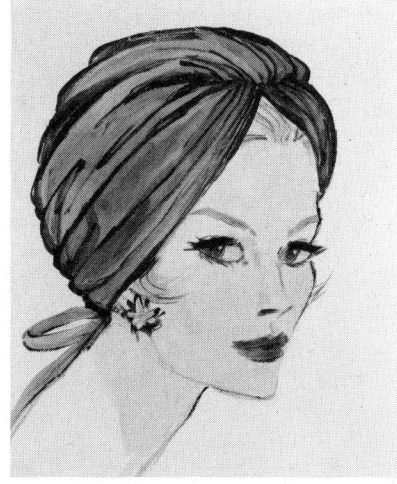
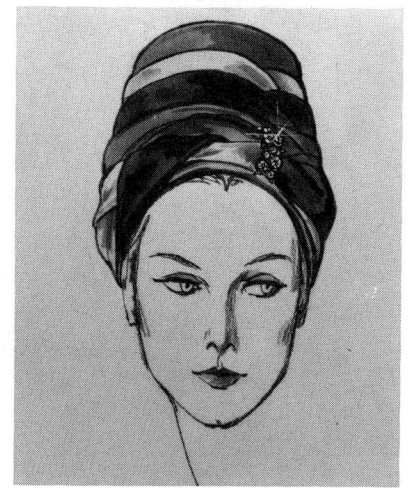
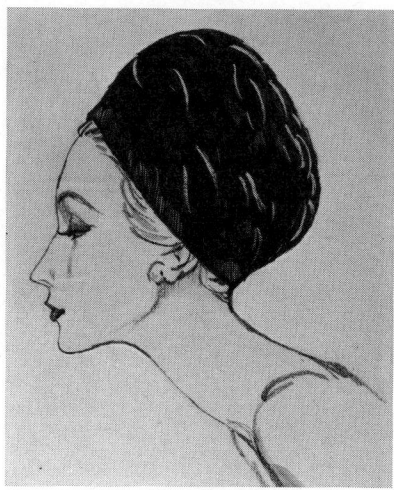

Figure 35 (upper left). Softly draped turban of silk crepe or chiffon.

Figure 36 (upper right). Turban in various shades of satin. More formal draping on a shaped crown.

Figure 37 (below). A feather toque. Toques include many types of small hats, usually of fabric, which fit down more firmly on the head than a pillbox. In softer types, flattering to older women.

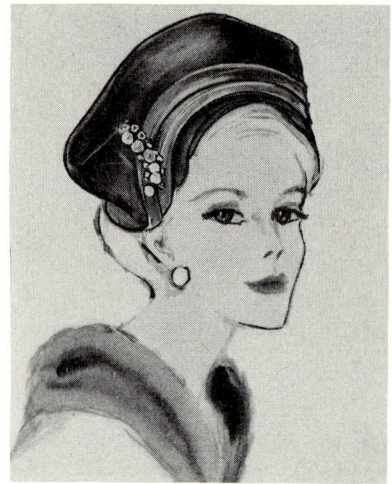
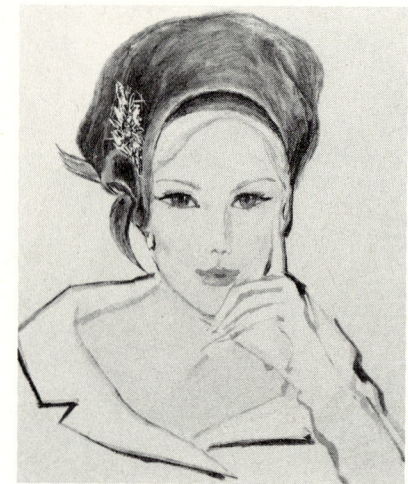

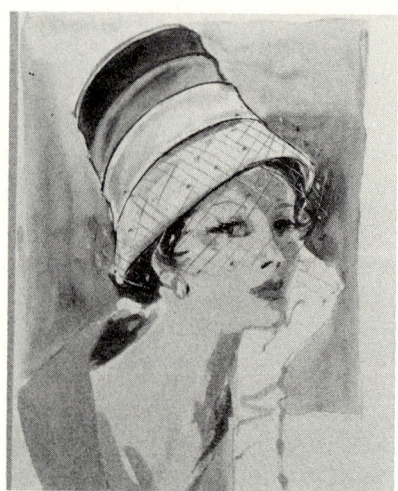

Figure 38 (upper left). Profile hat of manipulated felt with satin trim.

Figures 39 (upper right). Another version of the profile hat in beaver or soleil felt. The asymmetric shape of the profile hat is becoming to many wearers. Avoid the extreme type that entirely conceals the face and hair on one side.

Figure 40 (below). A cloche in a sophisticated version, in varying shades of satin.

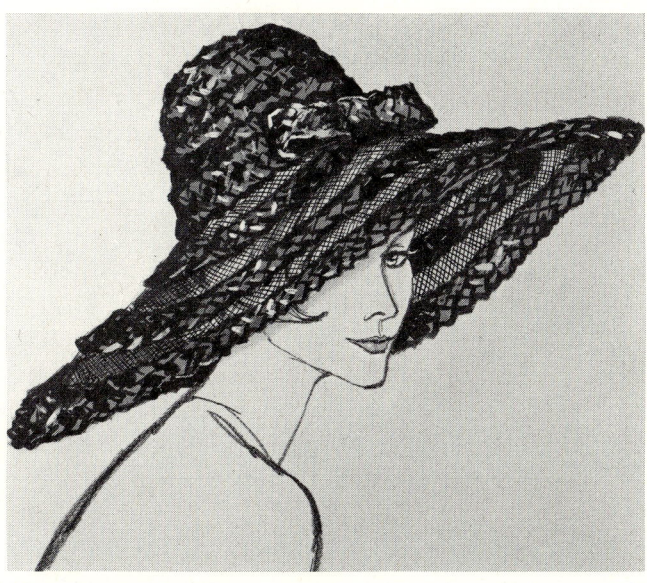

Figure 41. A picture hat in stiffened net and straw braid. The brim of a picture hat has a graceful undulating line, in contrast to the stiff-brimmed sailor. A flattering and romantic style, which drifts in and out of current fashion in many versions of felt, straw, and the filmiest of fabrics.

FEDORA. A soft felt or straw casual with lengthwise crease in the crown and a side roll to the brim.

HALO. A round, flat hat similar to a stiffened beret, attached to a fitted bandeau and worn somewhat back on the head.

HATLETS. Various confections in tiny hats, including circlets, decors, headbands, flower or feather whimsies, stiffened veils (or cages), and small coifs.

LEGHORN. A hat of fine straw braid, usually with a small crown and flexible wide brim (Figure 5 Chapter Five).

MUSHROOM. A small, round crown, with a brim which turns down all around.

PICTURE HAT. A general term to describe a graceful hat with a broad brim which forms a flattering frame for the face (Figure 41).

PILL BOX. A small, round, straight-sided, brimless hat; shallow or high wall (Figures 22 and 23).

PROFILE. A hat, usually with a narrow or medium brim, shaped to conceal one side of the face and form a frame for the other side (Figures 38 and 39).

ROCKER. A small hat curving up at both front and back, suggesting the shape of a chair rocker.

SAILOR. A straight-brimmed, shallow-crowned hat with varying widths of brim; associated with hats of the Gibson Girl era, having its origin in the hat traditional in the British navy. A *padre* sailor has the sides of the brim turned up like the headgear of certain churchmen.

SNOOD. A cap or fillet of open-meshed material used to confine the hair in the back; one of the lovely feminine fashions of the early Renaissance, seen in modern guise in daytime and evening versions (Figure 17).

SOMBRERO. A tall-crowned, wide-brimmed felt hat which can be manipulated in all manner of dashing ways. Casuals in many forms are based on the sombrero. Of Spanish origin, seventeenth century, and seen today in Mexico.

TOQUE. A small, round hat, brimless or with upturned brim; the term covers a variety of small hats with interesting fashion features or unusual cuts (Figure 37).

TRICORNE. A hat with low, flat crown and a brim which is caught up in three places to form a triangle with a point in front; originally a masculine fashion of the eighteenth century.

TURBAN. Of Oriental derivation; a close-fitting headgear made by skillful draping of yards of soft material about the head or by simulating the effect of draping (Figures 35 and 36).

VISOR or CHUKKER. A cap with an eye-shading brim in front, or front and back.

WATTEAU. A small, flat, crownless plaque set far forward over the face with the high back filled in with flowers and feathers; worn by Watteau's ladies in his paintings of eighteenth century France.

WIMPLE. A scarf worn to cover the head, with ends draped about the shoulders; originating in medieval times.

The basic materials for hat bodies are generally felts or straw braids, though many hats are made of fabrics such as velvet, tweed, satin, velour, crepe, or such novelties as wool yarn or wool braid. In some seasons, fashion decrees fur hats, which may be of short-haired furs like mink, seal, or leopard, or long-haired furs like squirrel or opossum. Furry effects are given by hats of maribou or ostrich feathers or by fur-fabrics with soft pile of man-made fibers like the coating materials.

Felt bodies may be made of rabbit fur or wool noils. Bodies of rabbit fur are often imported from Europe, or they may be made in the United States from imported fur fiber. Hat bodies from wool noils are made in the United States, although the noils are sometimes imported from Australia, New Zealand, or Argentina. Felts may have a soft, polished finish, a lustrous, hairy nap (as in soleil felt), a soft velour finish, or a long furry nap, as in the hats called beavers.

Straw hats may be imported as straw bodies or made in this country of imported or domestic straw braids. Traditionally, we have imported straws of the milan type and fancy straw braids from Switzerland, leghorns and raffia braids from Italy, balibuntals from the Philippines, panamas from Ecuador, and bakus and toyos from China. Now, however, the majority of our "straw" hats are made from man-made fibers, stiff and tough and lustrous. The American Viscose Company makes a strawlike fiber called "Visca," and many synthetic straws are imported from Switzerland, Italy, Formosa, and Japan. These often imitate the textures of the traditional straws but may also introduce many novelty effects. They may be made in chalk-white or in bright colors, in bright or dull luster. Purses and shoes are made from the same straw braids.

One essential step in the manufacture of the hats for a new season is that of making the wood blocks on which the hats are shaped. Every variation in crown or brim in any but a soft hat must have its own block; and these must also be made in different head sizes. A solid block of wood is carved to correspond to the season's hat shapes and a plaster model made from it. Then aluminum blocking dies are cast, and the damp hat bodies molded over them. So important is the role of the blockmaker that it is often his firm that sends representatives to Paris to bring back models which will become the patterns for the blocks for the coming season. The little "hatlets," of course, do not require this kind of foundation; but because they do require handwork, we are finding many of them on the milliners' shelves labelled "made in Japan."

Hats to Camouflage Shortcomings

The purchase of a hat should be made thoughtfully and not in five minutes as some women proudly boast of doing. One should stand before a full-length mirror and study the effect of profile and back. This enables a person to see that the hat goes with height, length of torso, and width of shoulders and hips, as well as to make sure that its angle and the position of its trimming are right.

Many women's hat problems are due to oversized heads; however, this difficulty actually may be caused by too much hair—long hair, thick hair which should be thinned, or a very bouffant coiffure. The crown in these instances is of particular importance; if it is not right, no brim or trimming can correct it. Hats that are not intended to fit down over the crown, if not too diminutive, or hats of adjustable head size may be a solution, as they cut down size by illusion.

It is essential to have a clear concept of the ideal figure and of the classically oval face and head when selecting a hat. Listed below are some rather common problems. General suggestions have been made in each case for creating the illusion of perfect contours.

- Repetition of irregular facial contours in hats serves to emphasize them; a Roman nose under a mushroom brim will become more prominent. One solution is to counterbalance the prominent nose with an irregular brim or soft trimming slightly out over the forehead.
- A round face is made to seem more so when its lines are repeated in round hats; severe, straight brims and stiff, off-the-face toques emphasize it too, by creating a sharp oppositional effect.
- A long, thin face is accentuated by stiff shapes (Figure 30) by tall-crowned, narrow-brimmed hats, or by close-fitting turbans (Figure 36). The remedy is to use hats with irregular lines and softened edges (Figures 15 and 41).
- Angles of a square face are emphasized by angles in shape and trimming. Soft, full hairdressing about the jaws, undulating lines in brim, and fullness in hats help, by contrast, to make full jaws seem narrower.
- Heavy chins are reduced by highlighting the forehead with heavier effects in turbans, and with berets or sailors worn with some degree of tilt.
- Oval faces can wear hats straight on the head (Figures 30 and 36); nearly all other faces need the softening effect of undulating dips and tilts to camouflage shortcomings.

Proportion and scale in hats is of extreme importance; there is need for a sense of weight for the heavy person and a sense of lightness for the small, slight, feminine person. Generally speaking, large people need larger hats, if not in brim then in crown or trimming (Figures 29, 31, and 39); conversely, women of small scale need small hats (Figures 20, 22, and 26). And the dramatic beret (Figure 16) demands a slender face and smooth brow, sufficient height to carry its wide brim and close-fitting headband, and a flair for wearing hats smartly.

Heavy bodies and heavy faces need thickness such as cushion-edged brims or heavy trimming close about the crown. The wide, low-crowned cartwheel or sailor with its horizontal movement is not for those who need a hat with bulk and upward movement.

Delicate features and slender bodies are overpowered by hats with too much brim, crown, or trimming. A fairly wide brim is possible if the crown is small and the material and trimming delicate or seemingly light weight.

Hard lines in features and planes of faces need softening with flattering textures and graceful lines.

A round face and pug nose are given piquant, interesting angles when the brim is tilted.

Weak chins are made less so by letting the forehead show and wearing dashing, lively hats with upturned brims.

Wide, drooping-brimmed swaggers cast flattering shadows over long necks and slender faces when the hair is worn loose and full around the neck.

The roughness of paillasson straw smooths out complexions and makes their texture seem fine.

The heart-shaped dip in the brim of a wide leghorn is often becoming to a girl with a short and broad face, because it produces an effect similar to the widow's peak so much admired.

Feather and flower toques do very flattering things to white- or gray-haired women for afternoon, and are good even on large women when the hair is full at the sides and the toque is worn slightly tilted.

The older woman usually looks better in hats with some brim, or with irregular undulating lines, or with a soft trimming such as folds of chiffon. She should usually avoid large, drooping brims which repeat the downward lines of wrinkles.

Large full turbans of heavier materials worn forward on the head make features seem smaller.

Halo hats are best worn by a person with an oval or heart-shaped face. They accent a high, smooth, unwrinkled brow.

Tiny sailors or *canotiers* with shallow crowns and narrow brims, unless they are heavily trimmed or have heavy edges, are for small faces.

Skull caps and calots are for young faces and placid brows and are usually more becoming when there is a softening effect of hair about the face and back of the head.

Colors which one cannot wear in dresses can often be worn in hats because of the transition made by the intervening hair. Red worn above the face often gives a flattering glow.

The rapid changes of fashion in both hats and hairdress probably account for the dearth of writing about them. A study of hats of the past several centuries can be amusing and enlightening, for we see reflections of old styles in hats of today. The following references give illustrations which will help us in recognizing basic types of hats.

Mary Brooks Picken, *The Fashion Dictionary,* Funk and Wagnalls, New York, 1957.

R. Turner Wilcox, *The Mode in Hats and Hairdress,* Charles Scribner's Sons, New York, 1945.

Fourteen

The Wardrobe

Making a careful plan for a season's wardrobe and carrying it through as a part of a longer-range plan for seasons to come is a test of skill, knowledge, and sagacity in practical affairs. It is not only proof of our understanding of design, color, and texture, but it also tests our character in regard to discernment, organization, and the self-discipline required to hold unswervingly to principle and purpose. You may look like a million on more taste than money.

The culminating skill in the art of wardrobe building is complete integration. It is important to correlate all items in one ensemble, and to be certain that these items are in harmony with the entire wardrobe plan. A completely coordinated wardrobe should be the aim of every modern woman, especially those who want to hold to a high standard in appearance on a limited allowance.

After carefully assembling a basic wardrobe, one may then be entitled to a color splurge if one wishes and if one's budget will permit. This variety may be introduced in the choice of accessories and apparel for more specific occasions, such as jackets, sport dresses, and separates. Such accents of color or contrast in an ensemble often serve as a bit of spice in a tasty morsel.

PROCEDURE FOR PLANNING WARDROBES

You are an artist! Whether or not you will be remembered as an outstanding artist depends on how skillful you are in presenting yourself to those with whom you come in contact. The fundamentals are acquirable. This entire volume has been devoted to the elaboration of every facet of costume and appearance in order to help you develop your sense of what is becoming as well as how and when to wear it.

Analyze Yourself

It is hoped that at this point you have made a thorough analysis of yourself—your physical features, your intellect, your emotions, and your spiritual nature. It is essential that you be true to yourself and that you discover who and what you *are,* not what you would *like* to be. Do you know who you are? Do you know what you really look like? What kinds of things do you enjoy? Where do you go? What activities claim your attention? How are you different from others? Where do you live? These things you must know, and you must let them be your guide in planning your wardrobe.

Perhaps a final question or two will help to determine whether you have discovered yourself and whether you understand the place of clothes and appearance in the scheme of things. Do your clothes claim too much attention? The looks you get may imply contempt rather than admiration. The clothing you wear and how you wear it make the first impression on people with whom you come in contact. Your manners and speech are noted next, and last of all, your character. Does your wardrobe express the real person within? If you discover that the real person within has not cultivated qualities such as kindness, courtesy, a certain humility, and a sense of your own intrinsic worth, now is the time to begin anew. If you have a deep and abiding love for all mankind, then you will want the first impression and the lasting impression to be the real you and one to be admired.

Analyze Your Wardrobe

Regardless of how little or how much one may have to spend for clothes, the smart, intelligent, alert young woman will take stock of what is on hand at the beginning of each season. It is important to consider each item carefully. Note which items are wearable as they are, which ones need to be cleaned or altered, and which ones are of no further use to you. Make an individual clothing inventory comparable to that in Table 1. This will help you recognize your wardrobe assets and liabilities. You may be surprised at the quantity of items you find in certain categories and the dearth of articles in others. This may be explained by the fact that your particular activities do not require certain types of apparel, or it may indicate that you have made too many unplanned or careless purchases. After completing your inventory summary ask yourself the following questions:

> Do you consider your annual clothing expenditure high, medium, or low?
> Do you have certain basic costumes over which your coat is not suitable because of a pronounced discord of style, color, or trimming?
> Do you have suitable accessories for each costume or wardrobe area?
> Are your separates of such a type that they may be mixed harmoniously and worn for many occasions?
> Do you have certain costumes in which you never have a good time? If so, why?
> Do you have certain ensembles which you have worn for several seasons and each time you wear them you receive compliments? If so, why?
> Do you have certain needs which your present wardrobe does not supply?
> Do you have garments which require so much care that you hesitate to wear them?

Honest, straightforward answers to questions such as these in relation to your inventory of clothing will determine how skillful you really are in the selection, planning, and financing of your wardrobe.

Plan Your Expenditures

Observation and investigation indicate that there is little or no relation between being well-dressed and the amount of money spent on apparel. Studies show that some people get along on very little, while others put small fortunes into their clothing. Remember, it isn't the amount that is spent on clothing that reveals taste, but how much thought, skill, and artistry is demonstrated in the use of the clothing dollar.

There is no fixed standard concerning the amount of money one may legitimately spend on clothing. Costume expense is flexible; the amount you spend is determined by your income, your fair share of the family clothing dollar, individual or family interests, and standard of living. People who live richly and who have broad interests and activities, plan their expenditures so

TABLE 1 INDIVIDUAL CLOTHING INVENTORY

DESCRIPTION OF ARTICLE	NUMBER	COLOR	FABRIC	DATE PURCHASED	ORIGINAL COST	SERVICE EXPECTANCY IN YEARS	ANNUAL COST	RATING *

I. Coats and wraps
  Winter
    Tailored
    Dress
  Summer
    Tailored
    Dress								

II. Suits
  Winter
    Tailored
    Dress
  Summer
    Tailored
    Dress								

III. Separates
  Jackets
  Skirts
  Sweaters
  Blouses
  Others								

IV. Dresses
  Street, office, or school
  Afternoon or date
  Dinner
  Formal								

V. Sportswear
  Spectator
  Active								

VI. Lingerie
  Slips
  Bras
  Girdles
  Briefs
  Sleepwear
  Robes								

VII. At home wear
  Hostess gowns
  Pants and tops								

VIII. Accessories
  Footwear
    Shoes
    Hosiery
  Hats
  Gloves
  Handbags
  Others								

IX. Miscellaneous								

* Rate items in relation to use, serviceability, and becomingness from highest (1) to lowest (3).

that they may have more for education, books, travel, leisure, hobbies, home improvements, entertaining, and giving. With increasing claims on our financial resources, planning becomes a necessity if we hope to maintain an adequate and interesting wardrobe.

The wardrobe that demonstrates taste on a limited amount of money will have every article appropriate and functional, bearing the stamp of the wearer's individuality. The young woman with good clothes sense will not let herself be carried away by anything which can be worn only on a particular occasion or to satisfy a certain rare mood. She will keep herself up-to-date by taking time to study the best fashion magazines, by consulting the best authorities, and by analyzing the displays in good shops. She will not be the "first by whom the new is tried," but she will be quick to see the possible changes that can be given to face and figure by the ingenious adaptation of current fashions. She will buy clothes of excellent quality that may be worn many places through different seasons rather than the kind intended for one specific purpose and one particular season.

Study your clothing inventory to determine your most urgent needs, plan purchases that will correlate with existing wardrobe items, and shop until you find the right items for your wardrobe. In using the term right we are referring to the application of all principles of costume selection. This process takes judicious thought and evaluation and is not a result of impulse or whim of the moment. Decide sanely, not permitting any deviation as to wardrobe needs and what can be spent for them. Clothes should be chosen for the places you go, the things you do all day, and the people you are with, not for the places you would like to go.

Garments such as coats, suits, and basic dresses which are worn longest and are most expensive should be purchased first and used as a core around which other wardrobe needs are harmonized. It is important to keep to one basic color path or one dominant hue for practical, daytime clothes. This color should be dark, practical, but becoming, such as black, navy (dark violet-blue), midnight (dark greenish-blue), brown, gray, or tan. This of course does not mean adherence to one hue, but a harmony of tones developed around one dominant color path. Wardrobe items such as expensive hats, shoes, and handbags usually should be the same in color as the basic garments. Variety in color can be introduced in smaller, less expensive accessories. Good leather bags, gloves, and shoes are marks of a well-dressed person and should be considered as investments that not only outlast several cheaper ones but also look well while they are lasting. The importance of choosing accessories with emphasis on good structure, with decoration of a very restrained character, and with functional design well suited to the individual and the occasion cannot be overstressed. Foundation garments and costume slips in tailored finish and substantial, durable materials and workmanship, without lace or frills, are the best types for very limited budgets. Since city clothes differ decidedly from country clothes or clothes right for small towns, locality becomes a factor in wardrobe building.

Consider the care each purchase will require; whether it is a wise choice for you is determined by the time and money you have or are willing to spend on its care. The wise use of your clothing dollar includes shopping for certain items when prices are most reasonable. This does not mean that one buys an article because it is on sale, but it does mean that one makes a planned purchase when that item is less expensive. Be very determined to be a wise shopper.

"I haven't a thing to wear!" This statement need not be yours if you adhere to what you know of yourself and carefully plan your clothing expenditures accordingly.

SOCIAL CONVENTION

Will it be appropriate? This is the most important question to ask yourself when buying clothes and accessories and of no less importance when deciding what to wear on each occasion. Whether or not it is right is determined by the climate, the area in which you live, the kind of life you lead within as well as without your home, and current fashion. The design, color, and texture of your wardrobe must express you, but social convention establishes the suitability of the elements of costume which are correct for a particular time. Your taste reflects you; if it is bad, it simply shows a lack of respect for yourself and is insulting to those around you.

This portion of the book will be devoted to proper attire for various occasions, and perhaps it will help you to sense the fitness of things.

For Street and Traveling Attire

Clothes for business, shopping, professional wear, or travel should be comfortable but with an expression of the reserve one feels among strangers. Details in violation of good taste are the too sheer blouse, décolleté neckline, and the too "fussy" costume. They should be practical, conservative, impersonal, yet distinctive. Clothing which resists soil and retains its original appearance saves time for the busy woman and assists her in maintaining a well-groomed appearance. Accessories should be in harmony with clothing worn for these occasions, simple yet distinctive. Gloves and hosiery should harmonize with the ensemble and not produce a striking contrast, as white gloves and too light hose often do. The street suit, if carefully selected with more than one purpose in mind and if properly accessorized, may serve more formal daytime occasions such as church, luncheons, and social affairs.

The coat is tailored and made of fabrics such as the heavier twills, fleeces, and tweeds; it may be fur-trimmed or worn with bright scarves. Fur coats of mink, muskrat, leopard, sheared beaver, or sheared raccoon are suitable. For spring wear one might select faille, ottoman, or hopsacking in redingote or straight, unfitted styles.

The suit is also tailored. It should be cut on classic lines; if it is conservative in color, line, and fabric, it can be worn for many seasons with only minor changes. The fabric may be selected from worsted, wool flannel, tweed, or firm double-knit jersey. Warm-weather suits may be made from linens, silks, cotton tweeds, or blends of these with man-made fibers.

The dress is tailored; if it is conservative in line and color, it lends itself to easy change with accessories. Jacket dresses are particularly suitable and may be made of lightweight wools, crepes, or shantungs. Warm-weather dresses are designed in cottons, linens, silks, and man-made fibers. Firm knitted fabrics and small textured weaves are particularly appropriate.

The hat must be in keeping with the tailored lines of the entire costume and selected according to the requirements of your facial shape and body build. Your choice may be a breton, a toque, a sailor, or a coolie hat. Your hat may be of felt, velour, fur, or of fabric matching the costume. Spring and summer hats may be made from straw or straw-like braid, or of starched linen or piqué.

The shoe must be very plain and uncluttered. The walking pump of calf, alligator, patent or suède is a good selection.

The glove may be made from cape, washable doeskin, suède, cotton, or nylon. The fabric, whatever it is, must be a firm weave and not the see-through variety. The glove is made in a simple, conservative style; the length will be determined by the length of sleeve.

The handbag may be relatively large but in proportion to the person carrying it. The plain, conservative bag that can be hung over the arm is practical for street or travel. Lizard, calf, or suède are used for winter wear; early spring calls for patent, and later on bags of straw, leather in lighter tones, or fabric.

Jewelry must be worn in moderation. Matching sets of bracelet, earrings, pin, and necklace are very boring; the imaginative use of harmonizing pieces will express your individuality. Interesting shapes and colors in metal, ceramic, or wood are good choices.

For Spectator Sports and Campus Wear

Good taste for campus or any spectator sport calls for clothes which are casual and nonchalant. Textures should be sturdy and practical, without glint or sheen. The girl on a limited budget will choose coats and suits which can do double duty as street clothes by change of accessories.

The coat may be a boy-coat, an all-season coat with water-repellent finish and zip-in lining, a bulky knit coat of fingertip or shorter length, or a fur-lined cloth coat. It may be fashioned from tweed, cheviot, camel hair, bouclé, fleece, suède, or leather; plaids, stripes, and plain colors are used. Warm weather calls for short coats or jackets made of wool or heavy textured cottons.

The suit that is tailored of sturdy tweed or a similar fabric is an excellent choice. Warm-weather suits made of hopsacking, seersucker, Tarpoon, cotton tweed, or cotton cord are appropriate.

The dress suitable for spectator sports and campus wear may be one from wool jersey, washable flannel, cotton jersey, or corduroy. Separate skirts of denim, seersucker, hopsacking, cotton tweed, cotton cord, and linen suiting are correct when worn with matching or contrasting shirts and blouses. Often material to match the skirt is used for an overblouse or waistcoat.

The hat in keeping with this casual wear will be a fabric or felt cap, beret, cloche, or any narrow-brimmed hat. Gay wool or silk is used in scarves or hoods. Your creativity will be expressed in the manner in which you wear your scarf; find an interesting way to wear it.

The shoe is generally flat. One may choose saddle shoes, brogues, moccasins, oxfords, or ghillies; they may be made of calf, pigskin, or buckskin. Pumps with low or medium heels and made of leather, straw, or linen are also proper choices.

The glove worn for spectator sports or campus wear will be of capeskin, pigskin, or cotton suède. String gloves, gloves with leather palms, or gay woolen or angora mittens are other possibilities.

The handbag that is carried may have shoulder straps; the clutch or wallet may be more desirable at times. Calf, novelty fabric, or saddle leather are often thought of in relation to this type of costume. Bags of reed, straw-like braids, or washable fabric are appropriate in warm weather.

Jewelry must be very restrained in design. Metal, wood, or leather will express a harmonious relationship to the attire for these occasions.

For Afternoon Occasions

Clothes that are worn to luncheons, matinées, daytime receptions, formal teas, and bridge parties, and which the college girl calls "date" dresses, are street length. They are less décolleté than dinner and evening dresses and usually have some sleeve. These costumes are designed with an air of sophistication, and the textures are softer and more elegant than those used in street dresses.

The coat will be of wool velour, duvetyn, or fine broadcloth; often it will have a fur trim manipulated to bring out unusual lines. Straight coats of silk or linen are appropriate, as are fur coats, jackets, capes, or stoles in marten, mole, mink, or squirrel.

The suit or jacket dress will be cut on softer lines and will have beautiful workmanship. Appropriate fabrics might be matelassé, damask and brocade in monotone effects, wool with satin or velvet, taffeta, faille, bengaline, ottoman, moiré, and velveteen.

The dress will be cut on softer lines too and may be of black silk crepe or sheer jersey, soft wool, or fabrics mentioned for the jacket dress.

The hat of velvet, fur, antelope, or soleil felt in a small toque, turban, or pill-box shape will be entirely proper. Wide-brimmed picture hats or small flower-trimmed straws are worn during warm weather.

The shoe selected will be the pump of patent, kid, or suède; for warm weather, linen or lighter-colored leather.

The glove will be an eight-button length or longer when sleeves are not wrist length. They may be white, bone, or black in doeskin or fine kid. Cotton gloves in white or colors are also used. A woman need not remove her gloves when shaking hands but must do so when accepting food.

The handbag may be a small clutch in black suède, kid, broadcloth, faille, or other fabric.

The jewelry may be a little more ornate in design to be in harmony with the richer textures.

For Informal Evening and Dinner Attire

Clothes for company dinners at a home or in a restaurant express sophistication, elegance, richness, and individuality, but demand a certain amount of reserve. The activity which follows—cards, the theater, dancing—will modify or determine the apparel worn. The length of the dress is dependent on the formality of the occasion, and only rarely is it designed without sleeves. In a large city a more formal type of clothing is demanded, whereas in many smaller communities leeway is permitted. We sometimes forget that family dinners, too, are more enjoyable occasions when all members appear at the table suitably dressed.

The coat, cape, or stole of a more elegant fabric or fur may be worn. Generally it is designed with softer lines.

The dress will have either short cap or long sleeves; rarely are the arms and shoulders completely bare. It will be cut on body lines; and although not necessarily evening length, it is often longer than daytime wear. The crepes, moirés, satins, velvets, and lamés will be used in neutral colors such as beige, taupe, moleskin, amethyst, and blue. This dress is not worn before six.

The dinner suit is entirely proper any time after four-thirty in the afternoon.

The hat may or may not be worn. It would be a small toque, turban, or bandeau.

The shoes, cut on pump or sandal lines, will be fashioned of satin, crepe, faille, or kid. They are often dyed to match the gown.

Gloves of white glazed kid or black suède in longer lengths are proper.

The jewelry will be handsome and decorative. Pearls, rhinestones, gold, semiprecious jewels, or real jewels, if one is fortunate enough to own them, are in good taste.

For informal, at-home gowns that express friendliness and originality one might choose vivid color contrasts, exotic prints, or rich textures. The fashion silhouette may include long and flowing or fitted trousers with matching or contrasting tops; or at other times, gowns with simple draped effects.

For Formal Evening Attire

Gala occasions such as formal balls and the opera afford the greatest opportunity for women to dress up, to express through their clothes gaiety and romance, luxury and sophistication. Besides glittering jewels, magnificent furs, sophisticated color, and the loveliest of fabrics, it is the place to wear the *robe de style* as the best expression of the *grande toilette;* or the gown may be more closely molded to the silhouette, depending on the dictates of fashion.

The coat or cape for this occasion may be a rich napped woolen in a beautiful pastel or white. An evening wrap of a fur such as chinchilla, ermine,

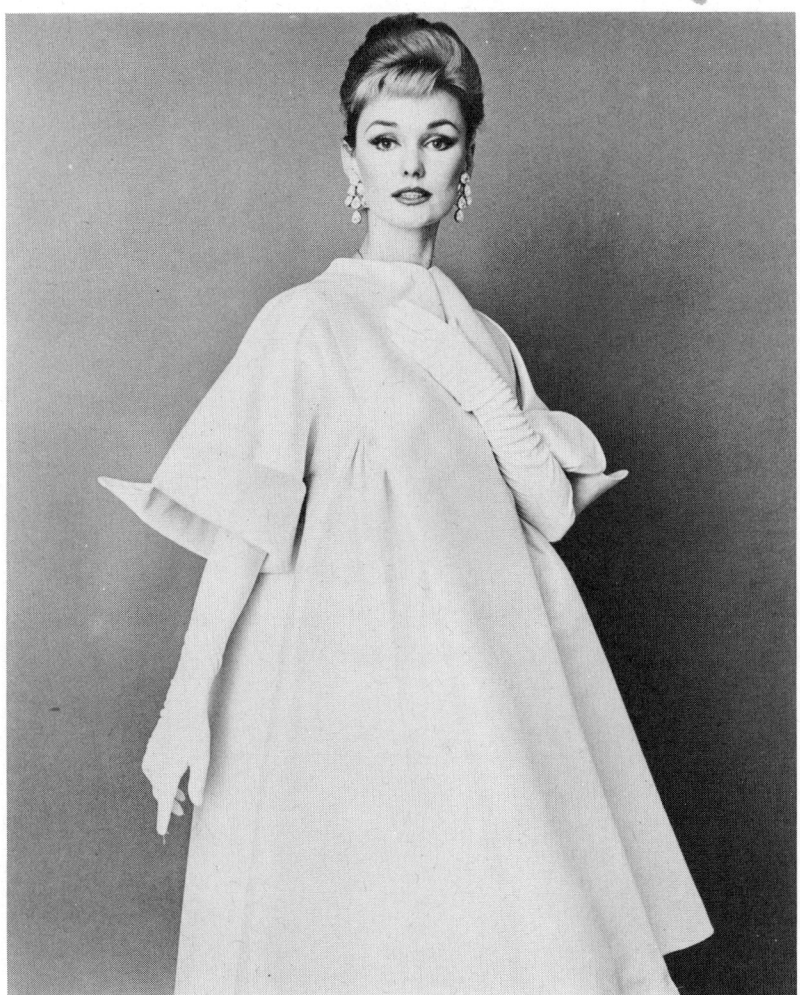

Figure 1. Evening wrap by Pauline Trigere. Courtesy of Lord & Taylor. Harmony of design and texture for formal wear.

or mink is the ultimate in elegance; but others of formal fabric might be even more distinctive (Figure 1).

The dress is sleeveless, floor length, and often décolleté. Bouffant dresses are lovely in slipper satin, *peau de soie,* taffeta, Lyons velvet, brocade, sequin-embroidered tulle, or organza with Chantilly lace (Figure 2). For dresses of

288 The Arts of Costume and Personal Appearance

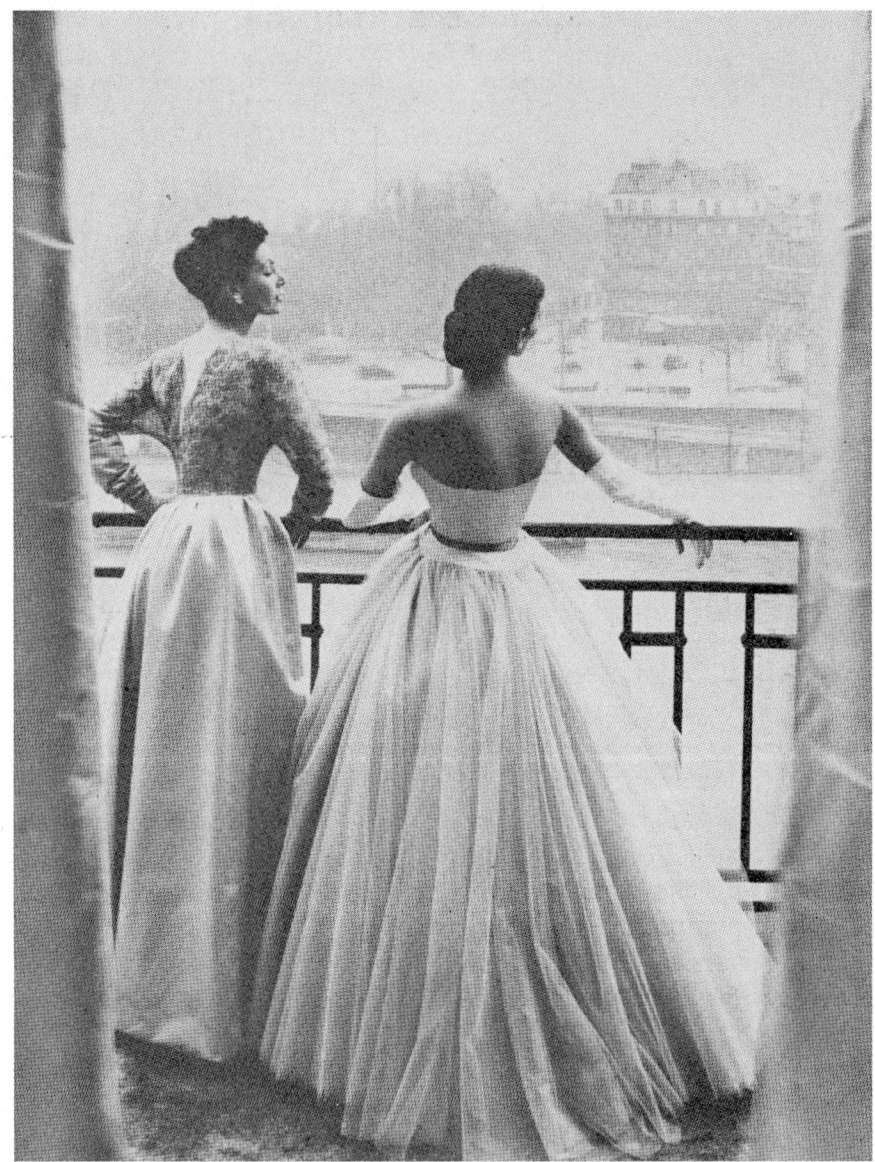

Figure 2. Right: Pink satin bound close and dropped below waist level to join swirling layers of tulle in many pinks. *Left:* An ice-blue lace melting into a stiff satin skirt. Designed by Balenciaga. Photo by Derujinsky. Courtesy of Harper's Bazaar.

more subtle design, fabrics such as chiffon, georgette, lamé, or silk jersey are demanded.

The shoe will be gold or silver kid, satin, or faille to match the gown. Pumps or sandals will adorn the foot.

The glove will be elbow-length or longer in doeskin, glacé kid, or fabric in colors to match the gown. These gloves are a part of the costume and are not removed during the evening except when one accepts food. The gloves are removed entirely at the dinner table.

The handbag carried is always small and of brocade, gold or silver kid, velvet, satin, or a beaded fabric.

The jewelry is more elaborate than for daytime wear. Rhinestones, pearls, crystal, diamonds, rubies, emeralds, and other precious stones may complement the costume, but exercise discretion in their use.

For Leisure, Relaxation, and Active Sportswear

The freedom, comfort, sturdiness, weather resistance, and adaptability of well-designed wear for sports such as tennis, golf, and swimming appeal to the modern young woman. She has carried over many of these costumes, such as shorts, slacks, pedal-pushers, Bermudas, tapered pants, and play suits, into her daily life and made these items acceptable for at-home wear. They are entirely improper for street wear.

For tennis the correct attire is a dress with a round or *V* neckline, short or no sleeves, and a knee-length or shorter pleated skirt. Sometimes shorts are preferred. The garment will be of cotton piqué, broadcloth, linen, or sharkskin. Generally the costume is white rather than colored, to keep from distracting other players on adjoining courts. White canvas shoes and white anklets are suitable footwear; and a tennis cap, a visor, or a simple ribbon will keep the hair in place or shade the eyes.

For golf the classic shirtwaist dress with action-pleats is functional. Most often it is made of flannel, gabardine, or linen in white, pastel, or neutral shades. Traditionally the golf shoe with rubber soles or cleats is worn; however, a rubber-soled oxford or any sturdy brown leather walking shoe and either anklets or service-weight hose may be selected. The hands will be more comfortable if the golfer dons brown leather gloves, fabric gloves with leather palms, or doeskin golf gloves.

For riding one will wear cream or woodsy brown breeches or jodhpurs in whipcord, cavalry twill, or gabardine. The shirt will be tailored in white cotton, linen, or lightweight wool. A turtleneck sweater in neutral colors is acceptable, and it is worn without the coat. The riding jacket is single breasted, cut on man-tailored lines; tweed is the best choice. Brown leather, chamois, or heavy string gloves are a necessity. Ankle-high jodhpur boots or flat-heeled riding boots which hug the calf and come just below the knee will be worn. And finally, a felt hat, a derby, or fabric cap will hold the hair in place. Riding for special occasions such as the hunt or for horse shows may require other habits.

For swimming the one-piece bathing suit is superior to any other for someone with a less than perfect figure. A very heavy person appears to better advantage wearing a dressmaker draped suit in a fabric with body. For others, stretch fabrics are possible. Rubber caps, thong sandals, beach coats, shifts, bulky sweaters, hats, and dark glasses are sometimes needed at the beach or pool. Bathing suits should not take the place of play clothes; they belong only at the beach or swimimng pool.

For skiing the trousers are a most important item. They are cut to fit the ankle snugly, have elastic under the foot, and permit complete freedom of movement. The water- and wind-resistant fabrics and stretch fabrics are popular. Bright colors in sweaters and shirts, wool and suède jackets, ski caps with ear tabs, warm gauntleted mittens or gloves, leather ski boots, and wool socks are needed. Two pairs of wool socks are used, the outside one worn over the trouser leg and turned down over the top of the shoe.

For skating the person with a young and shapely figure might choose the ballerina-type costume; others should choose wool skirts or slacks or ski pants. Gay turtleneck sweaters, colorful scarves, wool stockings, and warm caps complete the costume.

The Arts of Costume and Personal Appearance has presented the basic principles for aesthetic individual expression. The tempo of the times changes, and each individual matures and fills different roles in life, but the fundamentals still serve as guideposts. Being an attractive person is a matter of never-ending attention to detail, objective evaluation, and continuing study and development of aesthetic discrimination.

The following books will help you in your study of wardrobe building and social convention.

Helen G. Chambers and Verna Moulton, *Clothing Selection,* J. B. Lippincott Company, New York, 1961.
Anne Fogarty, *Wife Dressing,* Julian Messner, Inc., New York, 1959.
Edith Head, *The Dress Doctor,* Little, Brown and Company, Boston, 1959.

Household Finance Corporation, *Money Management—Your Clothing Dollar,* Chicago, 1959.

Dora S. Lewis, Mabel Goode Bowers, and Marietta Kettunen, *Clothing Construction and Wardrobe Planning,* The Macmillan Company, New York, 1960.

Claire McCardell, *What Shall I Wear?,* Simon and Schuster, New York, 1956.

Harriet T. McJimsey, *Art in Clothing Selection,* Harper & Row, New York and Evanston, 1963.

Emily (Price) Post, *Etiquette,* Tenth Edition, Funk & Wagnalls Company, New York, 1960.

Amy Vanderbilt, *Complete Book of Etiquette,* Doubleday & Company, 1963.

Exercises

Select wardrobe problems from the following list. Consider in each case the design, color, and texture which will be appropriate to physical irregularities, temperament, coloring, and social and practical needs.

Campus wardrobe for college girl of forceful, businesslike traits, small stature, and light coloring
Date ensemble for self with possibilities of changing its aspect
Limited wardrobe for a winter vacation in Florida
Wardrobe to wear and take with you to New York City in one suitcase and a dressing case
A spring trousseau for a bride, consisting of three blouses and three skirts which could be teamed in such a way as to make nine outfits

Appendix A

Color Terminology

ACID COLORS. Colors with the sharpness of chemical solutions: carmine, magenta, violet, ultramarine, cyan- or green-blue, blue-green.

ANALOGOUS COLORS. Neighboring colors, those which have adjoining positions on the color circle, as Y, YG, G.

CHROMA. The degree of intensity, saturation, or purity of a color; brightness or dullness.

CLOSE VALUES. Small interval, subdued or weak contrast between values in a composition, such as between values three steps apart or less on the value scale.

COLOR PATH. A series of colors exhibiting a gradation in one or more dimensions, such as a gradation of hue with constant value and intensity or a gradation of value with constant hue and intensity.

COMPLEMENTARY COLORS. The strongest possible contrasts to each other, having nothing in common; opposites on the color wheel; when mixed in proper proportions they produce a neutral gray.

EARTHY COLORS. Colors suggesting earth tones and consequently partly neutral: umbers, siennas, terra cottas, ochers, mustards, olive greens, and other colors originally made from vegetable dyes.

HIGH COLORS. In commercial usage, bright colors.

HIGH KEY. A composition in which the prevailing tone or dominant value is approximately 7, 8, 9 of the value scale, light.

HUE. A color name.

INTENSITY. The brightness or dullness of a color.

JUXTAPOSITION. Placing colors near together or side by side.

LOW KEY. A composition in which the dominant tone or value is approximately 1, 2, or 3 of the value scale, dark.

LUMINOSITY. That quality which gives the impression of lightness with brightness.

LUMINOUS HUES. Range from yellow-green through yellow to red, red-purple, and magenta, and give the impression that they are light and bright as distinguished from grayed or earthy colors.

MODERATE CONTRAST. Extremes of value no more than 4 or 5 value steps apart.

MONOCHROMATIC COLORS. The colors of the spectrum, which in their pure state are composed of but one wave length. This distinguishes them from colors of nature, which are impure and composed of different wave lengths.

NEUTRALS. Strictly speaking, black, white, and the complete range of grays between black and white are the only true neutrals, but browns and beiges are extremely neutralized hues frequently used as neutrals.

PASTEL. Hue of low intensity raised to high value.

PRIMARY COLORS. The basic colors appearing in the spectrum, which cannot be produced by mixture, but from which all others are derived. Primary colors mixed in proper proportion produce white light.

SATURATION. Complete impregnation with one hue only.

SHADES. Dark values of any hue.

SOFT COLORS. In commercial usage, grayed colors.

SOMBER COLORS. Blues, violets, and purple in darker values and low chroma.

SPECTRUM. Color spectrum, the band of successive colors which appears when a ray of sunlight is passed through a prism or crystal, breaking up the light into a sequence of strong colors.

STRONG CONTRAST. A large interval between values in a composition, such as 6, 7, or 8 steps.

TINTS. Light values of any hue.

TONE. The prevailing effect of a color brought about by blending or veiling.

VALUE. The degree of light strength in a color, also called luminosity.

VALUE KEY. The relationship of values in a composition, specified according to its dominant value as affecting its darkest and lightest values.

Appendix B

Popular Color Names

APRICOT. A tint of orange like the flesh of the fruit.
BEIGE. The natural color of unfinished cloth, in the gray before dyeing or finishing.
BONE IVORY. A neutral that is deeper and richer than bone.
BRONZE. A dark brown with a greenish cast.
BROWN. A dark neutral made with varying amounts of red, orange, and yellow reduced to value approaching black.
CARMINE. Red with a bluish cast of pure intensity and medium value.
CERISE. Vivid purple-red of above middle value.
CHARTREUSE. Yellow-green or green-yellow of high value and strong intensity.
CHERRY RED. A chalky red, blended with magenta-cobalt.
CINNAMON. Color of the spice of that name.
CORAL. Red-orange of natural coral, light, medium bright.
CORNFLOWER. Purplish blue of the flower, in medium value and intensity.
CREAM. The pale yellow-orange of rich cream.
CRÈME DE MENTHE. A cool green warmed with a touch of yellow ocher.
CRIMSON. Bright red with bluish cast in medium value.
EGGSHELL. Similar to cream.
EMERALD. Bright green of medium value, the color of the stone.
FLESH. A tint of red-orange.

GOLDEN ASH. The clear, deep gold of oakwood and autumn leaves.
IVORY. White with a yellow-orange cast.
LEMON ICE. A cool and frosty yellow.
LODEN GREEN. A dark, very neutralized yellow-green.
MAGENTA. Vivid red-purple above medium value.
MANGO PINK. Pink with overtones of apricot.
MAPLE GOLD. Coppery in tone; think of sunlight on the maple leaves in autumn.
MARINE BLUE. Dark, warm, uniform blue.
MAUVE. A pale red-purple.
MIDNIGHT BLUE. Dark, grayed green-blue.
MUSTARD. A green-yellow with an earthy tone like prepared mustard.
NAVY BLUE. A dark purple-blue of grayed intensity.
OCHER. A yellow of medium value and intensity found in clay and ranging from pale yellow to brown.
OLIVE. The dark grayed green of the olive.
OYSTER. A light, grayish white with a blue cast.
PEACH. A bright tint of red-orange.
PEACOCK. The bright, dark blue-green or green-blue, like the feathers of the peacock.
PERIWINKLE. A light blue-purple, as of delphiniums.
PINK. A tint of red with a bluish cast or with an orange cast.
PLUM. A soft, dark blue-purple, like the fruit.
RED CEDAR. Red with a rich, strong, luminous tone.
SAPPHIRE. The color of the stone, medium light and bright.
SCARLET. Intense orange-red of medium value.
SHELL PINK. Pink with an orange-red cast.
SHRIMP. The bright red-orange of the fish.
SIENNA. A clay color used "raw" as a yellow-brown pigment, "burnt" as a reddish brown pigment.
SILVER BIRCH. A silvery gray.
SPRUCE BLUE. A deep, powder blue.
STONE GRAY. A neutral warmed with purple.
TANGERINE. Yellow-red hue, high saturation and medium brilliance.
TAUPE. A very dark, warm gray.
TERRA COTTA. One of the clay colors of medium-value red-orange.
TURQUOISE. The light value blue-green or green-blue of the jewel.

ULTRAMARINE. An intense dark blue with a purple cast, which, according to the Munsell System, makes it the complement of yellow, not orange. Lapis lazuli is ultramarine in tone.

UMBER. A brown pigment, after heating becomes "burnt" umber, a reddish brown pigment.

VERMILION. An intense red at middle value or above.

WALNUT. A deep, rich brown.

WEDGWOOD. The dark-valued purple-blue of Wedgwood pottery.

Appendix C

Glossary of Costume Textures

The glossary on the following pages is for the convenience of the reader who may not be familiar with a wide variety of fabrics, furs, and leathers. The reader should become familiar with the labelling rules which are in effect in the United States, and should learn to watch for these labels in purchasing fabrics or garments.[1]

Over the centuries, spinners and weavers have developed variations in texture and pattern in using the natural fibers—cotton, wool, silk, and linen. As the man-made fibers have been introduced, they have made available a wider variety of fabrics than were ever dreamed of in previous centuries. Research by the large textile firms has developed more and more new fibers; and textile manufacturers have had to learn new techniques in using them. It has frequently been found that blends or mixtures of fibers widen the scope of fabric properties. Fibers and fabrics can be "engineered" for certain specific uses, and new finishes have enhanced many fabric properties. For example, some of the advantages of these new developments may be seen in improved crease resistance and dimensional stability, wash-and-wear properties, and variations in texture.

As purchasers of textile materials we should become familiar with names

---

[1] Federal Trade Commission, *Rules and Regulations Under the Textile Fiber Products Identification Act,* 1960, *Rules and Regulations Under the Fur Products Labelling Act,* 1952, *Rules and Regulations Under the Wool Products Labelling Act,* 1939, Government Printing Office, Washington 25, D. C.

of man-made fibers, such as acrylics, nylon, modacrylics, polyesters, olefins, and others as they appear. But in the final analysis, we want to know how to use these various textures. The producing of beautiful fabrics and the creation of pleasing costumes from them are still arts which give satisfaction to both the creator and the consumer.

In grouping the fabrics in this glossary, we have used the names *cotton, wool, silk,* and *linen* as categories representative of the type of texture associated with these fibers. The actual label on the fabric might read:

Batiste: 65% polyester fiber, 35% cotton.
Flannel: 50% acrylic fiber, 50% wool.

Since man-made fibers may be as smooth and lustrous as silk, as dull and strong as linen, or as soft and bulky as wool, we will group the fabrics irrespective of fiber content under the heading which most nearly describes the material as traditionally constructed. The headings should really read: "Cotton and similar textures"; "Wool and wool-like textures."

New developments are making possible all sorts of fabric variations never thought of before; and each year will no doubt add to these developments. For example, *stretch fabrics* have made possible a closer fit and greater comfort, especially in clothing for sportswear. The property of elasticity (ability to stretch and to return quickly to the original size) may be given to fabrics in many ways. Probably the oldest of these methods was *knitting,* which produced a fabric far more stretchable than woven fabric. The use of natural or synthetic rubbers forming the core of a yarn and covered with cotton, rayon, silk, or other fibers made possible fitted bathing suits and girdles of figure-controlling strength. Special rubberlike synthetics called *spandex* have introduced much finer yarns which may or may not be covered and which have excellent elastic and holding properties.

Stretch yarns, developed first in the 1940's in Switzerland, may revolutionize garment fitting. Using no rubber but only various methods of treating yarns by twisting, heat-setting, and chemicals, a stretch yarn may be developed for use in either knitted or woven fabrics; the stretch may be developed lengthwise or crosswise or in both directions; and the stretch can be regulated from a slight elongation to a very great extension as needed. Some of the woven fabrics being made with stretch yarns are denim, terry cloth, corduroy, bedford cords, and tweeds. It is said that the introduction of trim-looking, flattering ski pants gave a great boost to women's interest in skiing.

Other new developments include: *pile fabrics,* resembling furs and sometimes called fake furs, made of acrylic and modacrylic fibers, and used as coats, coat linings, jackets, robes, and trimmings; *foam laminates,* giving warmth without weight and greater stability to fabrics for coats and jackets; *metallic threads* with plastic coatings, washable and nontarnishable, adding glitter to fabrics for evening wear; *double and triple knits* in wools, cottons, and other fibers, which are firm and stable enough to be tailored like woven fabrics.

THE FAMILY OF COTTONS

BATISTE. A very lightweight, soft, semisheer cotton of plain weave made from very fine cotton yarns, with a luster due to mercerization. Adaptable to gathering, shirring, and draping where straight, limp folds are desired. Plain colors or prints.

BROADCLOTH. A fine, firm, closely woven cotton, highly mercerized, resembling fine poplin. Plain or striped. For shirts, tailored blouses, and summer skirts. Crease resistant finishes have enhanced the advantages of this material.

CHAMBRAY. A smooth cotton of plain weave and fine yarns with warp threads of one color and filling of another color or white, producing iridescent effects. Chambrays are adaptable to soft-tailored summer suits and dresses and to soft dirndl styles.

CHINO. A firmly woven cotton fabric with a very fine, steep twill weave. Used for cotton suits and jackets and for sports clothes.

CHINTZ. A drapery, slipcover, and upholstery cotton with a permanently crisp, glazed finish, which produces a stiff but pliable hand and a lustrous, polished surface. Printed or plain colors. In lighter weights and suitable patterns, it is adaptable to summer sleeveless dresses with little jackets and to play clothes cut full and gathered or circular. Sometimes quilted.

CORDUROY. A pile fabric with rounded ridges or cords of pile in narrow or wide wales. Adaptable to tailored suits, coats, and negligees.

CORDS. Heavy yarns spaced at intervals in warp or filling give body and texture interest. Used primarily for summer suits and sports clothes.

DAMASK. Fine, highly mercerized cottons in the types of Jacquard patterns formerly reserved for silks. May be used for cocktail and evening gowns for spring and summer.

DENIM. A heavy, twilled cotton familiar in white filling and navy blue warp for slacks and jeans, but high style for sportswear in multicolored effects, stripes, plaids, and iridescent colors.

DIMITY. A crisp, plain, semisheer dress cotton with small cords running in bars or stripes. Suited to frilly blouses, gathered skirts, and little girls' dresses.

GABARDINE. A fabric of mercerized yarns in a weave of raised diagonal cord-like twill. A very compact weave, firm, and suited to severely tailored suits and sportswear.

GINGHAM. A dress material of medium-weight cotton in plain colors or in checks, plaids, or stripes. Best grades are fine, soft, dull-surfaced, closely woven in beautiful colors. Adaptable to soft-tailored dresses and suits or to soft silhouettes of the dirndl style.

HONAN. A fine cotton in soft colors and prints with slub yarns, imitating an ancient silk weave.

HOPSACKING. A rather coarse cotton in plain weave, dyed or printed, popular for sports clothing.

JERSEY. Knitted cotton for sportswear, summer suits, and tailored dresses. Double knit constructions and shrink-resistant finishes help to insure permanent shape and good tailoring qualities.

LAWN. Fine mercerized cotton with a crisp but not stiff hand. Lends itself to many different finishes; often printed or embroidered.

MADRAS. Indian madras, a rather coarse yarn-dyed cotton in plain weave, usually in bright plaids, stripes, or checks. Used for sportswear for men and women.

ORGANDY. Fine, transparent, dull-surfaced crisp cotton in plain weave. Suited to crisp lingerie trimming and details and to formal afternoon and evening dresses. Quality depends on fineness of yarns, clearness of weave, and permanence of finish. Swiss organdy often has small printed figures, giving a shadow effect, or dainty embroidered figures.

OTTOMAN. A fabric with very heavy crosswise ribs. Originally a silk fabric but recently a popular fashion in cotton for spring and summer suits and coats.

PIMA COTTON. Long-fibered cotton used in the finest of mercerized materials.

PIQUÉ. Cotton fabric in white and colors, plain, striped, or printed. Narrow or wide wales running warpwise, or novelty piqués such as cloque and birdseye. Suited to flat tailoring, to crisp lingerie details on tailored garments, and to summer formals for younger girls.

POINT D'ESPRIT. A fine, dull-surfaced, somewhat crisp cotton net with design in dots of snowflake effect. White and pastel colors. Suitable for bouffant evening frocks and bridal gowns.

SEERSUCKER. A dull-surfaced medium-weight cotton with crinkly stripes alternating with plain surface. Seersucker gingham has yarn-dyed checks or plaids. Suitable for tailored dresses and suits and sport skirts. Interesting rough textures, particularly becoming to coarse skins.

SUITINGS. Firm cottons with the look of heavy linen, serge, or tweed; usually yarn dyed and with a crush-resistant finish, and often styled with the importance of fine worsteds.

SUÈDE OR DOESKIN. Firmly woven cotton with a fine napped surface that conceals the weave; often treated for water repellency. For sportswear.

SWISS. Transparent, crisp, plain woven cotton, frequently made with dots or small embroidered figures. Coarser than organdy and suited to summer frocks for afternoon and evening, cut on straight, gathered, or circular lines.

TERRY CLOTH. Soft fabric with uncut loops on one or both sides of the cloth, in gay colors, prints, or yarn-dyed stripes. Absorbent, warm, and bulky. It is popular for shorts, shirts, beach coats, and sport jackets.

TICKING STRIPES. Firm twill weave, used for summer suits, sportswear, and travel.

VELVETEEN. Cotton with a dull surface and short, dense pile. Suitable for suits and dresses made in a softly tailored style for street, afternoon, and evening.

VOILE. Plain open weave with fine, tightly twisted yarns. Quality is dependent on fineness of yarns, and a clear surface is made by singeing away fuzzy ends. Cotton voile has a hard feel and finish, and is at its best when draped by gathering in straight, limp folds.

THE WOOLEN AND WORSTED FAMILY

BOUCLÉ. Wool fabric of a novelty yarn, often with such tightly curled loops that it looks like needlepoint. Used in knitted or woven coatings or suitings.

BROADCLOTH. A soft, lustrous, medium-heavy woolen, with a nap which has been sheared, then pressed flat and polished to a beautiful luster and smoothness. Firm but pliable; adaptable to softly tailored, dressy suits and coats for women. Unfinished broadcloth has a soft nap which has not been pressed down and polished, so that it is duller and less elegant than the finished broadcloth.

CAMEL'S HAIR COATING. Natural-colored hair from the camel made into a thick, fleecy, napped fabric. Best grades are very soft, springy, and light in weight, with great warmth for their weight. Other specialty fibers which are used alone or with wool in coatings and suitings include rabbit's hair, cashmere, vicuna, llama, angora, alpaca, and mohair. Many of these fibers are used in their natural colors, from creamy white to gold to dark brown. Most of them are more expensive than wool, and are used for their softness, warmth, texture, or color to enhance the qualities of the wool material.

CHALLIS. A lightweight wool in plain weave and small printed design. Soft, smooth, too light for tailoring, but adaptable to soft, straight folds in dirndl styles and evening gowns.

CHEVIOT. A heavyweight monotone twilled woolen or worsted with wide wale; coarse and wiry. Rough, heavy-surfaced, hairy, unsinged. Suited to tailored sport coats and suits.

CREPE. Wool crepe made of woolen or worsted yarns comes in different weights and degrees of sheerness; it is dull and pebbly, with a slightly harsh, dry feel. In fine grades it drapes beautifully in straight folds. Suitable for softly tailored dresses and suits.

DUVETYN. Very softly napped, elegant wool fabric, for dressy coats, jackets, and suits.

FLANNEL. A soft, somewhat fulled woolen of medium weight with slightly singed surface, pressed down; comes in plain and twilled weave. Suited to tailored dresses and suits.

FLEECE. Bulky woolens for casual coatings. A fairly long, soft nap conceals the basic weave. Fleece coats are usually cut straight or flared, with little seaming. Extra long nap is sometimes referred to as brushed woolen.

FUR FIBER BLENDS. Seal, raccoon, mink, muskrat, rabbit, and similar fibers are sometimes blended with wool for novelty effects. Usually the fur fibers are on the surface or in the nap of the material, giving a soft hand or luster and a furry feel.

GABARDINE. Worsted with a twilled construction and dry feel; dull, firm, resilient, enduring. Excellent tailoring qualities for men's and women's suits, coats, uniforms, and riding habits.

HOMESPUN. Plain or twilled woolens, hand loomed, or resembling hand-woven materials. Many tweeds are called homespuns.

KNITTED WOOLENS. All wool or blends of wool with other fibers; available in a variety of stitches, from plain jerseys to ribs, lacy effects, Argyles, and fancy Jacquard patterns. *Double knits* are made with two sets of needles, creating a fabric of double thickness. They are stable, snag proof, and adaptable to a more strictly tailored treatment than most knitted fabrics.

MELTON. A smooth, firm wool with a low nap and excellent tailoring qualities, for tailored coats in straight lines or semifitted.

NOVELTY WOOLENS. A broad term used in reference to all sorts of unusual fabrics, often of too short fashion duration to be given a recognizable generic name.

SCOTTISH PLAIDS AND CHECKS. Woolen or worsted fabrics with the traditional Scotch plaid designs or District Checks, or modifications of these. *Glenurquhart, Gun Club, Hound's Tooth,* and *Tattersall* are terms describing certain definite patterns. For coats, dresses, and suits in plaids or in plain and plaid combinations.

STRETCH WOOLENS. Textured yarns of all wool, or stretch yarns of other fibers used with wool in woven or knitted fabrics, give comfort and shape-retaining qualities, allowing a better fit.

TROPICAL WORSTED. Fine, firmly woven, lightweight cloth of tightly twisted yarns and dry hand. Long wearing, crush resistant, and suited to fine tailoring; for spring or summer suits and coats such as redingotes or straight coats to be worn over silk or silklike dresses.

TWEED. Firm, rough-surfaced, and nubby, with a homespun effect. Monotones or varied colors, usually dyed in the fiber before spinning the yarn. In weights from coarse homespuns for suits and coats to softer, lighter weights for dresses or evening coats.

VELOUR or VELOURS DE LAINE. High grade woolen with a soft nap and a warm feel. Some are very thick and fulled, suited to dressy afternoon and evening coats and wraps. Others in a lighter construction, closely sheared and drapable, may be used for afternoon suits and dresses.

WHIPCORD. A worsted similar to gabardine but with a steep and pronounced twill; compact, strong, and springy. Suited to riding habits and sharply tailored coats.

ZIBELINE. A coating with a long, rather wiry nap of straight fibers, laid over in one direction. Often of llama or camel hair. Less bulky looking than the raised fleeces.

FABRICS IN THE LINEN GROUP

BUTCHER LINEN. A plain weave in a rather heavy fabric of coarse yarns; suited to sportswear and summer coatings.

CREPE LINEN. Semisheer linen with creped yarns and cool, harsh feel; resistant to crushing. Suited to both flat and soft tailoring and to small tucks and pleats.

HANDKERCHIEF LINEN. Lightweight, thin, smooth fabric with the natural surface irregularities of linen fiber. Plain colors and prints. Suited to dresses draped on soft but straight vertical lines and to tailored blouses.

HOPSACKING. A plain weave, more open than suiting or butcher linen, of coarse or textured yarns. Suited to sportswear and summer coatings.

SUITING. Heavy, lustrous yarns in plain and various twill and herringbone weaves, and in plaid and striped mixtures. Best grades resist crushing. For tailored street wear and sportswear.

TWEED. Linen suiting woven of stock-dyed yarns with colored slubs, similar to wool tweed. For summer dresses, suits, and coats.

SILKEN FABRICS

BENGALINE. Heavy, fillingwise ribbed fabric, often with cotton or wool filling yarns entirely covered by fine silk or rayon warp. Ribs are round and raised. Suited to dressy suits and afternoon wraps.

BROCADE. A rich, heavy fabric with an elaborate raised pattern in gold and silver thread or a pattern woven in relief against a foundation of another weave such as a satin, twill, or plain weave. Some varieties are rather stiff, best treated in silhouettes with crisp effects; others are very pliable and drapable when used on diagonal grain of material.

CHIFFON. Fine, thin, gauzelike fabric in plain colors or prints, with a soft, bodiless finish. It gives beautiful texture interest when shirred, corded, ruffled, pleated, or draped. Often printed in lovely designs, the color softened and made more subtle because of its sheerness when worn over slips of black, white, or color. Used in double thickness, it can be made into semitailored dresses with wide tucks or pleats.

CREPE. Interesting textures obtained by the use of tightly twisted yarns in warp or filling or in both directions. The size of the yarns and degree of twist produce many variations. Fashion dictates the type of crepe suited to current lines in a given season.

Canton crepe. Filling crepe with a fairly heavy fall and pebbly surface.

Crepe de Chine. A semisheer crepe, plain or printed, suited for lingerie, blouses, and dresses. Soft, drapable; enough body for straight vertical fullness but not for diagonal grain.

Flat crepe. A crepe with slightly twisted filling yarns. Fine, close weave; smooth, lustrous surface; drapable on straight lines or folds. Unbecoming to coarse skins.

Georgette crepe. A sheer, semitransparent fabric of considerable body with a dull surface due to high twist in both warp and filling yarns.

Satin crepe. A rich, lustrous, adaptable, satin-faced fabric with a creped back, the untwisted warps appearing as floats on the face and the tightly twisted fillings appearing on the back, producing the crepe. Some grades have a definitely pebbly satin face; others are smooth. The combination of shiny and dull surfaces has many uses in dressmaking. Good quality satin crepe has much body and pliability, and is capable of draping on either the straight or diagonal grain of the material. May be used on crepe or satin side.

DAMASK. Jacquard woven fabrics, usually with a satin design on a crepe or corded background. Elegant fabrics for cocktail or evening gowns. Often used as the lining in fine fur coats.

FAILLE. A flat, firm, filling-ribbed fabric which has staged a revival from the old days of elegant rich silks which had a crisp stand-alone quality. Some qualities have stiff finish; many are soft and drapable. Suited to handsomely tailored afternoon suits and coats for mature women.

FOULARD. A soft, twilled silk usually printed in small figures. Good for tailored blouses and soft suits. Similar to tie silk, surah, or cravat silk.

LAMÉ. A fabric shot with metal threads or woven with a brocaded pattern in gold and silver. Very rich and luxurious. Some versions are stiff or crisp, adaptable to circular cutting or crisp silhouettes; others are pliable, with sufficient body for draping on the diagonal grain of the fabric.

MATELASSÉ. Jacquard woven fabric with a padded or cushioned effect, obtained by double-cloth weaving. When in fashion, used in cocktail or evening gowns by mature women.

MOIRÉ. A watered effect produced by a special engraving process on silks and acetates which have a corded or poplin weave. Has body and firmness, and a suggestion of dignity and maturity. Suited to afternoon suits and evening dresses and wraps.

ORGANDY, ORGANZA, MOUSSELINE DE SOIE. Very sheer, slightly crisp fabrics similar to cotton organdy but more fragile and of gossamer thinness. Suited to evening gowns in which effects are achieved with much fullness, through flounces, tiers, or full gathers, or for dainty trimmings. Available in plain colors, prints, or yarn-dyed fabrics with beautiful iridescent effects.

OTTOMAN. A crosswise ribbed fabric on the order of faille or bengaline, but with much heavier ribs, often spaced with finer ribs between. For dressy suits and for coats, either in duster style or with full skirts, fitted or belted at the waist.

PEAU DE SOIE. Firm and rather heavy dress silk, softer in finish than taffeta, and with a fine ribbed or grainy appearance. For cocktail and evening gowns, and for the *robe de style*.

SATIN. A smooth, highly lustrous fabric produced by long warp floats. Manufactured in light, medium, and heavy weights. Medium and light weights have good pliability and body suited to soft, clinging, and diagonally draped silhouettes. Slipper satin is a heavy, very lustrous satin, usually made of acetate, suited to flat surfaces in circular cuts for evening gowns and wraps.

SHARKSKIN. A medium-to-heavy, sleek, smooth, slightly lustrous suiting with firm, severe, unyielding surface. For sharply tailored suits, slacks and sports apparel. Usually found in man-made fibers rather than in silk.

SPUN SILKS. Rough textured silks, made from wild and waste silk fiber, with irregular yarns in a plain weave, producing a rough, harsh feel. They vary in weight from light to quite heavy, and from a flat to a very rough-textured surface. Similar textures appear in man-made fibers, and in various blends of these with silk.

SURAH. Twill or serge in plain colors, plaids, or prints, suited to soft-tailored dresses, blouses, and suits. May be of silk or of rayon, acetate, nylon, or other man-made fibers; coarser than foulard.

TAFFETA. A closely woven, smooth fabric of plain weave with crisp finish. In plain colors, prints, stripes, or plaids, or shot with metallic threads. Warp printed taffeta has a pattern printed on the warp threads before weaving, producing a blurred effect. Taffetas are suited to crisp afternoon and evening silhouettes and trimmings.

TULLE. A delicate and cobwebby net with a slightly crisp finish, suited to bouffant ball gowns and diaphanous effects such as evening stoles and bridal veils. Usually of silk or nylon.

TWEED. Characterized by coarse yarns of spun silk with noils of fiber in contrasting color. For spring and summer suits and dresses.

VELVET. An inclusive term for pile fabrics with plain or twill back, in which warp yarns form the pile. They may be of all silk, rayon, nylon, or cotton, or may have the pile of one fiber and the ground fabric of a different fiber; for example, a silk pile on a cotton back, or a rayon pile on a nylon or silk back. Many velvets are now treated with a crush-resistant finish, making them more serviceable.

Chiffon velvet. A very light silk velvet, lustrous, with an erect pile and elegant draping qualities.

Lyons velvet. A velvet with an erect, thick pile and a stiff back, suited to circular-cut silhouettes and millinery uses.

Panne velvet. A pile which has been pressed or steamed flat in one direction, giving a lustrous, satiny surface. It is used in diagonally draped or circular cut silhouettes.

FURS

BEAVER. A dense, silky fur in rich shades of brown; one of the warmest and most durable of furs. Long guard hairs plucked to reveal the velvety underfur. Practically all beaver is now sheared, as it makes the fur more pliable, keeps it from kinking, and brings out interesting shadings. Beaver is sometimes bleached and dyed in light gray, beige, and pastel shades. Suitable for slim or average figures, for dressy, general, or sportswear, or for trimmings.

CHINCHILLA. A precious, fragile, soft, silky, short-haired fur of gray-blue color. For evening wraps and trimmings.

ERMINE. A species of weasel from Russia and Canada, having a dense, delicate, creamy-white fur with tails tipped with black. One of the most aristocratic and expensive of furs, it has long been associated with royalty and court costumes. "Summer ermine" is used in its natural golden brown hue. White ermine is suited to formal evening wear, in capes, jackets, and trimmings.

FISHER. A species of American marten, scarce and expensive. Rich dark brown underfur with long black overhairs. Beautiful and durable. Suited to hats, scarves, and stoles for slender and average figures.

FOX. Long-haired, thick-furred pelts, soft and silky in better grades, coarse hair in lower grades. Natural colors include silver, white, blue, and red. Mutations, produced by careful cross-breeding, develop lovely shades of beiges, grays, and browns. Pelts also dyed in a variety of colors, including black. Used as scarves, coat collars, or for short or long jackets. The latter are dressy, but because of their bulk are suited only to tall, slender figures.

GUANAQUITO. (Pronounced wa-na-ki-to.) A medium to long-haired fur with straight, bushy hair; a young guanaco, related to the South American llama. Of a tawny camel-beige tone with white belly. Makes up best in bulky jackets for dressy afternoons, and becoming only to the tall slim or average figure.

KOLINSKY. A species of weasel from Siberia and China, closely resembling mink. Straight-haired, silky fur of medium length, often dyed in shades of brown to simulate sable. For trimmings for cloth and fur coats, or for dressy capes and jackets.

LAMB.

Persian lamb. A lustrous, tightly curled pelt from the skin of the young Karakul sheep. Pliable and versatile; used for all sorts of coats and trimmings for almost any type of wearer. Naturally a mottled gray and black; usually dyed black or dark brown. "Persian" in this case does not designate the country of origin, but the type of pelt.

Broadtail lamb. The skin of a prematurely born or very young Karakul lamb. The fur, usually black, has not yet begun to kink, and the lustrous, short hairs produce a characteristic moiré pattern. Thinness and pliability of the pelt allow it to be manipulated like cloth. Smart, sleek fur for town and dressy wear.

Broadtail-processed lamb. From the skin of young wool sheep (not of the Karakul family). Pelt is sheared, pressed, producing a moiré pattern. Naturally white, or dyed gray, brown, or black.

Mouton-processed lamb or mouton lamb. The skin of a lamb which has been sheared, the hair straightened, chemically treated, and thermally set to produce a moisture-repellent finish. Short, dense fur resembling sheared beaver, sturdy and inexpensive; suited to school or sportswear for young girls. Slightly bulky, so best for an average or slim figure.

LEOPARD. A short, flat, silky hair in pale fawn or light orange background, having spots with tan centers surrounded by dark brown to black rosettes or rings. Suited to sport and street wear for sophisticates; for coats and trimmings on large flat surfaces.

LYNX. The longest-haired fur of the furred world, except the monkey. Fine, silky texture. In its natural color, gray to orange-red and slightly mottled; used for trimmings for sport and street coats. When dyed black, resembles fox and becomes a dressy fur suitable for jackets, long stoles, and trimmings. For slim, young figures.

MARTEN. A weasel with beautiful soft fur of medium weight and medium length.

>Baum marten. Resembles Russian sable; yellow-brown in color, varying widely in shades, but distinguished by its yellow throat. Suitable for dressy capes and jackets, scarves, and trimmings for average or slim figures.

>Stone marten. Gray-white underfur with lustrous, coarse, dark brown guard hairs. Used in natural state or dyed to imitate sable. Uses, same as baum marten.

MINK. A very durable fur of the weasel family. Short, dense underfur with long, lustrous guard hairs; soft, silky, lightweight, in a rich brown color with darker center streak. Used for dressy coats, wraps, trimmings, and formal evening wear; it has become almost a symbol of luxury and fashion.

>Mutation mink. Developed by careful breeding; has introduced a lovely range of natural colors, from bluish gray and beige to white, in soft silky pelts.

>Japanese mink. Shorter guard hairs and a soft texture; usually dyed to imitate American mink, and less expensive.

>Pieced mink. Consists of gills, paws, and sides of mink pieced together for less expensive coats and linings.

MUSKRAT. A short, straight fur that is soft and silky. Used in its natural colors, silvertone to brown, or dyed to resemble sealskin, mink, or sable. An attractive and practical fur for coats and trimmings for dressy or general wear. For slim and average figures.

NUTRIA. A South American peltry resembling beaver, but with hairs about one-half as long. Dark brown, with coarse, long guard hairs usually plucked. Sport coats and linings.

OCELOT. A spotted animal from the Americas. Background of the pelt is bluish-tan, with black spots that are elongated. Suited to trimmings and sportswear.

OPOSSUM. A long-haired, bushy fur with grayish hairs and gray-white underfur. Adaptable to youthful jackets and coats of a sport type.

RABBIT. A very soft, tender, light fur, formerly called lapin or coney. Not durable, but inexpensive and extremely versatile. Can be sheared, processed, and dyed to resemble almost any other short-haired fur from beaver to ermine. For trimmings, stoles, evening jackets, or general wear.

RACCOON. A bulky fur with dense, light grayish brown underfur and long, stiff, coarse, upright silver guard hairs tipped with black. Makes bulky sport coats, collars, and stoles. A youthful fur for the tall, slender figure. Sheared raccoon is less bulky, and can be dyed and finished to resemble other short-haired furs, such as beaver.

SABLE. One of the most aristocratic and valuable of furs. Best skins are very deep, soft pile in medium brown with blue cast. Silky guard hairs sometimes with white tips. Of medium length and medium weight. Used for sumptuous wraps and trimmings.

SEAL.
Fur seal. A soft, dense, fine, even fur, very warm, rich, and beautiful. Mouse-colored, it is customarily dyed black or a golden or very dark brown. A supple fur, adaptable to coats and trimmings, and capable of considerable manipulation. The conservation of the Alaska seal, considered the best type, is under the control of the United States Government.

Hair seal. A short-haired fur with no underfur. Flat, sleek, silky fur in champagne, black, or brown. For trimming, and for short coats and jackets for sport or street wear. Slenderizing.

SKUNK. A very durable, bulky, long-haired, coarse, dark brown peltry with two white stripes which are often dyed black or cut away in the making. The quality of skunk is judged by the thickness of the underfur, which holds the lustrous guard hairs erect, and by a fresh, lively appearance. Makes smart bulky jackets and capes for casual wear. For slim or average figures.

SQUIRREL. A soft, dense, light fur, rather bulky and only semidurable. For dressy coats and jackets and trimmings. Gray squirrel, considered the choicest, is usually used in its natural color. Others are usually dyed brown.

LEATHERS

ANTELOPE. A fine, soft leather made from antelope skin, velvety in texture owing to suèding, and of a rich sheen. Extremely rare. "Antelope finish," a suèded finish, is applied to lamb, goat, or calfskin.

BUCKSKIN. A fine, close-napped surface. Porous, loose, and stretchy. Its napped surface is not produced by suèding, but is found underneath the top grain of the deer skin and removed by soaking in lime solution. Usually tanned to a creamy white, used for women's summer sport shoes.

CALFSKIN. Made from skins of young cattle. Characterized by hair cells so minute as to be hardly distinguishable with the naked eye. Strong, rigid, tight, even grained, supple. Suited to men's and women's tailored gloves and in heavier grades for shoes and handbags.

Smooth calf. Has a somewhat glazed surface like glazed kid. For general wear.

Suède calf. A shoe leather of uniform velvety nap in many colors and in black and white. Suited for general or afternoon wear.

CAPESKIN. A tight, close-grained, durable glove leather, coming from the skin of the South African haired sheep. Suited to tailored gloves.

CHAMOIS. A suède-finished undersplit of lamb or sheep skins in natural yellow color; a result of the fish oil process. A very porous, supple leather entirely washable and suitable for tailored gloves for town and country wear.

DOESKIN. A suède-finished leather developed from sheep- and lambskins. For tailored gloves in white or light colors.

EMBOSSED LEATHERS. Designs stamped or pressed on hides by plates or rollers. Usually done on calfskin, the designs often imitate the natural markings of other leathers, such as alligator, lizard, or pigskin, or employ other conventionalized motifs.

KID. Thin, fine, soft, smooth, flexible grain with glazed or matte finish. Made from very young milk-fed animals tenderly reared for fine glove leather. Suited to dressy evening gloves because of its tight, close grain and attractive finish.

Glazed kid. A finish made by polishing kid skins with a frosted glass cylinder which burnishes it to a desired luster and brilliance. Suited for dress wear only.

Gold and silver kid. Gilded or silvered; thin, pliable, metallic; sometimes embossed and dyed in many colors. For belts, shoes, and trimmings.

Matte kid. Fine kid leather finished with a smooth, dull surface of great beauty. Suited to general or afternoon shoes.

Patent kid. Kidskin finished with transparent lacquer or varnish. Smooth, shiny, pliable. Now available in many colors besides black and white. Suitable for afternoon wear.

Suède kid. A deep, velvety texture made by napping kidskin on the flesh side. Used for afternoon and evening gloves.

MOCHA. Sheepskin suède, finished on both sides of the leather. Soft, supple, velvety in feel. Suited to street and semiformal wear.

PATENT LEATHER. Any leather with a varnished finish, usually made from cattle hides, although horse, colt, and kidskins are also used. Now largely replaced for shoes, belts, and handbags by vinyl and other plastic materials. These may be called "patent" but not "patent leather."

PIGSKIN. A tough, durable leather with a very coarse, furrowed grain made from skins of wild hogs, obtained in Mexico and South America. It is marked with growth of bristle pricks by which it can be identified. Suited to sport and motoring gloves or heavier grades of sport handbags.

PIN SEAL. A fine-grained, semiglazed leather used for handbags. When the grain is imitated in sheepskin, calfskin, or goatskin, should be described as "pin-grain."

REPTILE. Alligator, snake, and lizard skins, with their original markings. Often imitated by embossing calf or other skins, in which case they should be called "alligator grained."

Index

Accessories, afternoon, 285
   campus, 284–285
   dinner and informal evening, 286
   formal evening, 289
   leisure and sportswear, 289–290
   selection, 281–282
   street and travel, 283
Acid colors, 200–201
Albers, Anni, on texture and weaving, 121
Analogous colors, 191, 195
Anderson, Donald, on texture, 123
Art terminology, 67–68
Ashton, Dudley, on physical fitness, 24
Auburn coloring, 214–216

Balance, formal, 68, 94–96
   informal or asymmetric, 97
   perpendicular, 97
   radial, 99
Baldinger, Wallace S., on space, 81, 86
Beauty, cultivating, 44
   standards of, 1–3, 19, 31–33
Bouffant silhouette, 132

Care of person, 20–21
Carpenter, J. Barrett, on dissonance, 188–189
Chandler, Albert R., on proportion, 82–83
Chroma or intensity, a dimension of color, 190
Cleanliness, first requisite of beauty, 20
Clothing and social values, 3–4
   evidenced in the past, 1–2
   psychological implications, 4–5, 7–8
   subjective aspects, 6–8

Clothing plan and inventory, 278–282
Coiffure, in relation to facial shapes, 247–250
Color, acid hues, 200–201
   associations or mood, 176–177, 202–203
   chroma or intensity, 190, 201
   circle or color wheel, 184–186
   custom in usage, 176
   design element, 68, 201–202
   dimensions, 184–191
   dissonance, 188–189, 198–200
   earthy hues, 200–201
   light, a modifier of, 177–181
   physical aspects, 178–180
   physiological aspects, 181–182
   primaries, 182–183
   psychological aspects, 175–177
   secondaries, 183–188
   spectrum, 179
   systems described, 182–189
   terminology, 293–297
   value, 187–188
   warmth or coolness, 176–177
   wave lengths, 178–179
Color combinations, analogous, 191, 195–196
   complementary, 191, 196–198
   dissonance, 188–189, 198–200
   harmonies, 194–198, 201–202
   monochromatic, 191, 195
   relationships, of hue, 200–201
     of intensity, 201
     of value, 201
   simultaneous contrast, 191

316 Index

Color in costume, analysis of personal coloring, 205–211
   auburn-haired, 214–216
   blondes, 212–214
   brunettes, 216–218
   choosing becoming colors, 209–220
   composite types, 217, 219–220
   gray and white-haired types, 219–220
   Irish blonde, 219
Color science, afterimage, 181–182
   chemistry of pigments and dyes, 180
   physicist's contribution, 177–181
   physiologist's contribution, 181–182
   psychologist's contribution, 175–177
Color systems, 182–189
   Carpenter's theory of discords, 189
   Ives' instrument for measurement, 183
   Maxwell's analysis of light, 182–183
   Munsell, 184–187
   Ostwald, 183
   Prang and Brewster, 182, 185
   Rood's table of values and laws of contrast, 188
   Young-Helmholtz, 182–183
Color terminology, 293–297
Complementary colors, 191, 196–198
Composition, principles of, 68
   balance, 94–99
   emphasis, or dominance-subordination, 111–113
   proportion and scale, 99–102
   rhythm, 102–107
   unity or harmony, 113–114
Cosmetics, choosing and using, 243–246
   creating illusions, 241–246
Cox, George, on line, 67–68

Dark-light (*see also* Value), 145–150
   in contemporary costume, 152–160
   in Japanese prints, 150
   in printed fabrics, 161–171
   in value schemes, 155–161
   meaning of, 145–148
   patterns of, 149–150
Dearborn, George, on clothing and social values, 4
   on subjective influence of clothes, 6
Design, achieving distinguished, 84–92
Design, elements, 67–68, 78–83
   principles, 68
   relationship of form and function, 92
   silhouettes, 84–86, 91–92
Dewey, John, on space, 83
Dior, Christian, on grain of materials, 127
   on hats, 254
Dissonance, in color, 188–189, 198–200
Dominance-subordination, meaning of, 111–113
Duer, Caroline, on wrinkles, 22
Durant, Will, on Cretan costume, 2

Earthy colors, 200–201
Economic society, changes in, 3, 10
Elements of design, 67–68
Emphasis, or dominance-subordination, 68, 111–113
Ensembles, suited to occasion, 282–290

Fabrics, glossary of costume, 298–308
Facial shapes or contours, analysis of, 42–43
   illusions created, by cosmetics, 241–246
   by coiffures, 247–253
   by hats, 273–276
   by necklines, 235–240
Fashion, compared with style, 12–13
   defended by Lawrence Langner, 13
   fads in, 12
   industry, size and scope, 10
Federal Trade Commission, 298
Femininity, *see* Yang-Yin
Fibers in textile fabrics, 298–300
Figure irregularities, analyzed, 40–41
   creating optical illusion, 221–226
   individual problems, 232–234
   Nordic type, 232
   short, stout figure, 226–229
   thin, angular figure, 229–232
Figure proportions, contemporary ideals, 31, 36–40
   height-weight tables, 38–39
   model measurement chart, 40
Fogarty, Anne, on good taste and money, 11
Form and shape, elements of design, 68, 78, 81
   in costume, 85–86
Foundation garments, 221–222
Furs, glossary, 308–312

INDEX

Glossaries, of color terminology, 293–297
    of costume textures, 298–308
    of furs, 308–312
    of hats, 263–272
    of leathers, 312–313
Graves, Maitland, on dark-light, 148
    on plans for value contrast, 160–161
    on texture, 121–122
Greenbie, Marjorie Barstow, on personal appearance, 6
Grooming, perfection in, 20–21
Guilford, Richard C., on personal appearance and self respect, 7–8

Hairdress, becoming lines in, 247–253
Harmony, the goal in costume design, 68, 113–114
Hats, to camouflage shortcomings, 273–276
    to complement the costume, 250, 254
    to convey personal expression, 260
    good design in, 260–262
    materials used in, 272–273
    reflection of the times, 254–260
    suited to occasion, 262
    types described, 263–273
Health, diet for, 23–24
    exercise for, 24
    relation to beauty, 23
    sound, healthy body, 23
Hoffman, Betty Hannah, on femininity, 55, 58
Hue or color, 184–185

Illusions, optical (*see also* Figure irregularities), 221–226
    becoming necklines, 235–240
    disguising figure irregularities, 226–235
    techniques of creating, 223–226
Intensity, *see* Chroma

Jakway, Bernard, on texture, 118
Jewelry, becoming, 235–240
    good design in, 236

Langner, Lawrence, on fashion, 13
    on role of clothing, 3–4
Leathers used in costume, 312–313
Lemmon, Robert S. and Sherman, Charles, on personality in flowers, 50–51

Leverton, Ruth M., on nutrition and weight, 37
Line, a design element, 67–69
    direction or movement, 78
    distinguished line, 86, 89
    nature of, 68–78
Lynes, Russell, on clothes and mores, 4

Make-up, choosing, 243–246
    creating illusions with, 241–243
Marcus, Stanley, on fashion, 13
    on modern trends in dress, 17
Masculinity, *see* Yang-Yin
Meiklejohn, Helen, on clothes and personality, 8
Millinery, *see* Hats
Monochromatic colors, 191, 195
Morgan, Clifford T., on personality, 46
Munsell, color circle, 184–186
    color sphere, 184
    color system explained, 184–187
Murphy, Gardner, on clothing and roles, 4

Necklines for different facial types, 235–240
Neutral value scale, 159
Nordic type, 232

Opdyke, George H., on line, 89
    on proportion, 100
Ostwald color system, 183

Personal appearance, affecting inner feelings, 6–8
    related to behavior, 4–5
    social aspects, 3–4
Personality, and personal expression, 46–47
    expressed through costume, 47
Personal traits, affecting costume selection, 47, 63
    characteristics, 48–49
    costume features of Yang-Yin, 65
    expressed as Yang-Yin, 49–51
    noted among contemporary women, 52–55
    physical aspects, 63
    recognized in history and art, 48–50
    temperamental aspects, 63
Physicist's contribution to science of color, 177–181

318 Index

Physiologist's contribution to science of color, 181–182
Poise, aided by grooming, posture, 44
Posture and health, 25–26
   correct sitting, 29–30
   correct standing, 26–27
   correct walking, 27–29
Powers, John Robert, "golden rules of glamour," 19
   model measurement chart, 40
   model weight chart, 38
   personal appearance and mental health, 6–7
   personal appearance and social behavior, 7
Prang color system, 182, 185
Prints and patterned fabrics, characteristics, 167
   criteria for judging, 165–167
   dark-light patterns in, 161–164
   influenced by texture, 167
Proportion, Greek, 82–83, 99–101
   law of relationships, 68, 99–102
   scale in dress, 101–102
   scale in hairdress, 248–249
   scale in hats, 273–275
Psychologist's contribution to science of color, 175–177

Rhythm, a design element, 68
   forms of, 102–107
Ries, Dorothy W., on Yang-Yin balance, 51
Rood, Ogden, on value level of hues, 188
Roosevelt, Eleanor, on attitudes, 55
Roosevelt, James, on Eleanor Roosevelt, 55

Sabin, Robert, on Martha Graham, 50
Self-made beauty, facial expression, 21
   grooming, 20–21
   ideal proportions, 31–40
   posture and carriage, 25–30
   sound, healthy body, 23–24
   voice quality, 22–23
Shape or form, element of design, 68, 78–81, 85–86
Silhouette, as shapes in costume, 84–86
   bouffant, 132
   bustle, 136
   circular, flared, 132
   crisp, 132
   draped, 129–132

Silhouette, dressmaker-tailored, 128
   judging a good, 91–92
   tailored, 128
   textures affecting, 127–136
   types of, 127
Silverman, Milton and Margaret, beauty treatment for the mentally ill, 7
Social convention and wardrobe planning, 282–290
Space, element of design, 68, 81–83, 85–86
Style, and individuality, 13, 16–17
   and quality, 15–16
   and sense of values, 13–14
   and social convention, 14–15
   attainment of, 10–11
   compared with fashion, 12–13
   definition, 11
   in past periods, 12
Subordination, *see* Dominance-subordination

Taste, and money, 11, 14
   and simplicity, 16
   and social convention, 281–290
   definition, 12
   in clothes for occasion, 14–15
Terry, Walter, on Margot Fonteyn, 50
Texture, appreciation of, 118–121, 140–142
   art of combining, 136–140
   grain in fabric, 126–127
   hand, feel, touch of fabric, 122–123, 126
   light reflected by, 121–122
   meaning of, 117–119
   silhouette in relation to, 127–136
Textures, cotton and cotton-like fabrics, 300–302
   modern fabric, 298–300
   linen-like fabrics, 305
   silk and silk-like fabrics, 305–308
   wool and wool-like fabrics, 302–304

Unity or harmony, in costume, 68, 113–114
   in idea or theme, 16–17

Value, a dimension of color, 187–188
   dissonance, reversal of natural order, 188–189, 198–200
   home value of colors, 187–188
   natural order of colors, 188, 198

Value or tone quality (*see also* Dark-light), 145–149
    gradation of, 152
    neutral value scale, 159
    value contrasts, 155–161
    value keys, 148–149, 155–160
Van Dyke, John C., on texture, 118–119
Vener, Arthur M. and Hoffer, Charles, on clothing and adolescents, 4–5
Voice, asset to charm, 22–23

Wardrobe building, accessories, 281–282
    afternoon occasions, 285
    analysis, 277–279
    basic color path, 281
    clothing inventory, 279–282

Wardrobe building, formal evening attire, 286–289
    informal evening and dinner, 285–286
    leisure and active sports, 289–290
    social convention, 282–290
Weight, an index of health, 37–38

Yang-Yin, a concept of opposing traits, 49–50
    evidenced in personalities, 49–50, 52–58
    expressed in costume, 64–65
    in nature, 50–57
    physical aspects, 63
    symbol, 52
    temperamental aspects, 63
Young, Agnes Brooks, on silhouette, 84
Young-Helmholtz color theory, 182–183